Managing Seizure Disorders

A Handbook for Health Care Professionals

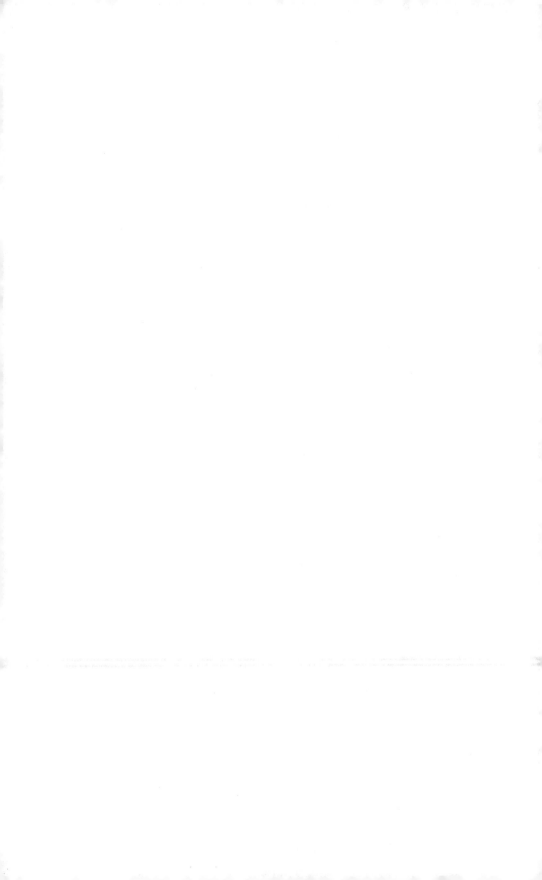

Managing Seizure Disorders
A Handbook for Health Care Professionals

Editor

Nancy Santilli, R.N., P.N.P., M.N., F.A.A.N.

Associate Professor of Neurology
Associate Director
Comprehensive Epilepsy Program
University of Virginia Health Science Center
Charlottesville, Virginia

Epilepsy Foundation of America®

Published by
Lippincott-Raven Publishers

Lippincott-Raven Publishers

Printed in the United States of America.

ISBN 0-397-51754-8

This book is intended to provide health care professionals with information on the management of epilepsy. Laypersons who read this material are warned against making any changes in their treatment without consulting a physician. Medical information about the diagnosis and treatment of epilepsy is improving constantly. Practitioners who want the most up-to-date information are invited to call the National Epilepsy Library's toll-free number (1-800-EFA-4050) for assistance.

Great care has been taken to maintain the accuracy of the information contained within this volume. However, neither the Epilepsy Foundation of America nor Lippincott-Raven Publishers can be held responsible for errors or for any consequences arising from the use of the information contained herein.

Epilepsy Foundation of America
4351 Garden City Drive
Landover, MD 20785-2267
1-301-459-3700
internet: postmaster@efa.org

EFA's Patient Information and
Referral
1-800-EFA-1000

EFA's National Epilepsy Library®
1-800-EFA-4050

9 8 7 6 5 4 3 2 1

Provided through an educational grant from
Ortho-McNeil Pharmaceutical

Preface

The Epilepsy Foundation of America has long recognized the important role of nurses and other health care professionals in the lives of people with epilepsy. The EFA's Professional Advisory Board members know that caring for people with epilepsy goes far beyond diagnosis and a prescription for medical or surgical management. Although a great deal of information has been published concerning the diagnosis and the medical and surgical management of people with epilepsy, the EFA noted 10 years ago that literature was lacking concerning the practical aspects of living with epilepsy from day to day. For nurses, social workers, occupational therapists, recreational therapists, physicians, advocates, and vocational counselors, the simple day-to-day exchanges that occur between health care professionals and individuals with epilepsy can make all the difference in supporting a positive quality of life.

The vast majority of people with epilepsy receive their care and treatment from primary care providers. Therefore, they do not have access to specialized centers dedicated to the treatment of epilepsy. It is critical for those individuals, especially in today's health care climate, to have as much knowledge as possible to help them self-manage their condition. Professionals working in primary care settings may encounter only two to five individuals living with a diagnosis of seizure disorders. It is the intent of the Epilepsy Foundation of America and the authors of this book to support health care professionals in providing an enhanced level of care for people with epilepsy and for their families.

The approach taken in developing this book has been collaborative. Monographs have been provided by nurse epileptologists, physicians, psychologists, therapists, and a number of other professionals working in the field of epilepsy. Each of us has also enjoyed the rewards of knowing that through this book we can assist the individual and the family to achieve the quality of life they desire. By sharing this information with others, we hope to provide the reader the same opportunities and experiences that we have all gained. We are all very grateful to our best teachers—people with seizures and their families. Moreover, it is important that we give credit to the collective wisdom and experience of our colleagues. Through collaborative efforts, we have come to this point in our own personal experiences and are therefore privileged to share our knowledge with others.

The leadership and staff of the Epilepsy Foundation of America warrant special acknowledgment for their insight and wisdom in developing this book and for their dedication and perseverance in carrying it out.

Nancy Santilli, R.N., P.N.P., M.N., F.A.A.N.
Chairman of the Board,
Epilepsy Foundation of America
August 1995

Foreword

This publication, designed primarily for use by health care professionals, is part of the Epilepsy Foundation of America's ongoing program to assist professionals in the management of epilepsy in all its forms. Through this book and with the support of other educational materials, the Foundation hopes to strengthen further the role of the health care professional as advocate and health educator concerned with the unique needs of individuals with seizure disorders.

We gratefully acknowledge the contributions of participants in EFA's Nursing Initiative, contributing authors and reviewers, and members of the Epilepsy Foundation's Professional Advisory Board. We particularly appreciate the work of Nancy Santilli, R.N., P.N.P., M.N., F.A.A.N., who has led EFA's nursing initiative since 1983. Ms. Santilli coordinated the development of EFA's "Count Me In!" project for school nurses and is the primary editor of *Managing Seizure Disorders: A Handbook for Health Care Professionals.* Special appreciation also is extended to Judith Beniak, R.N., M.P.H., and to Judy Ozuna, R.N., M.N., C.N.R.N., for serving on the Advisory Committee and coordinating the development of sections of the manuscript, and to Bonnie Kessler, Chris Merritt, and Ila Myers of EFA's staff who guided its development. We also gratefully acknowledge the guidance and assistance of Mark S. Yerby, M.D., M.P.H., Chairman of EFA's Continuing Education Committee, and Allan Krumholz, M.D., Chairman of EFA's Professional Advisory Board, in reviewing the manuscript and providing guidance in its development.

We are also very grateful to Abbott Laboratories for supporting the development of this collection of scholarly and practical monographs on epilepsy management, and to Ortho-McNeil Pharmaceutical for supporting its publication.

W. Edwin Dodson, M.D.
President
Epilepsy Foundation of America

Paulette V. Maehara
Chief Executive Officer
Epilepsy Foundation of America

Contents

Contributors

David R. Austin, Ph.D., *Professor, School of Health, Physical Education and Recreation, Indiana University, Indianapolis, Indiana*

Joan K. Austin, D.N.S., F.A.A.N., *Professor, Graduate Department of Psychiatric/Mental Health Nursing, Indiana University School of Nursing, Indianapolis, Indiana*

Mimi Callanan, R.N., M.S.N., *Clinical Nurse Specialist, Stanford Comprehensive Epilepsy Center, Stanford University Medical Center, Stanford, California*

David F. Chavkin, J.D., *Associate Professor of Law, Columbus School of Law, Catholic University of America, Washington, D.C.; and Former Director, Legal Advocacy, Epilepsy Foundation of America, Landover, Maryland*

Carol Maier Clerico, O.T.R., *Senior Occupational Therapist, Neuroscience Center, University of Virginia Health Science Center, Charlottesville, Virginia*

Joyce Cramer, B.S., *Project Director, Health Services Research, V.A. Medical Center, Yale University School of Medicine, West Haven, Connecticut*

Patricia Dean, R.N., M.S.N., *Clinical Nurse Specialist, Comprehensive Epilepsy Center, Miami Children's Hospital, Miami, Florida*

W. Edwin Dodson, M.D., *Professor of Pediatrics and Neurology, Associate Dean, Admissions, Washington University School of Medicine, St. Louis, Missouri*

Fritz E. Dreifuss, M.B., F.R.C.P., *Professor of Neurology, Director of Comprehensive Epilepsy Program, University of Virginia Health Sciences Center, Charlottesville, Virginia*

Chad R. Ellis, R.N., M.S., C.N.R.N., *Director, Zia Wellness Services, Columbia, Maryland*

Barbara Flock, R.N., M.Ed., S.N.P., *School Nurse Practitioner, North Allegheny School District, Pittsburgh, Pennsylvania*

Judith Harrigan, R.N., M.S.N., *School Nurse Practitioner, Monroe-Orleans Board of Cooperative Educational Services, Spencerport, New York*

W. Allen Hauser, M.D.,   *Professor of Neurology and Public Health, Associate Director, G. H. Sergievsky Center, Faculty of Medicine, College of Physicians and Surgeons, Columbia University, New York, New York*

Bruce P. Hermann, Ph.D.,   *Professor of Psychology, Department of Neurology, University of Wisconsin Medical Center, Madison, Wisconsin*

Dianne Chasen Lipsey, M.A.,   *Co-President, ADA Vantage, Inc., Washington, D.C.; and Former Director, Affiliate and Employment Services, Epilepsy Foundation of America, Landover, Maryland*

Marie Ormsby, M.S.W.,   *Former Director, Information and Referral Services, Epilepsy Foundation of America, Landover, Maryland*

Nancy Santilli, R.N., P.N.P., M.N., F.A.A.N.,   *Associate Professor of Neurology, Associate Director, Comprehensive Epilepsy Program, University of Virginia Health Science Center, Charlottesville, Virginia*

James R. Schimschock, M.D.,   *Child Neurologist, Emanuel Hospital and Health Center, Portland, Oregon*

Patricia A. Osborne Shafer, R.N., M.N.,   *Neuro-Epilepsy Nurse Specialist, Beth Israel Hospital, Boston, Massachusetts*

Jean Thatcher Shope, R.N., M.S.P.H., Ph.D.,   *Associate Research Scientist, University of Michigan School of Public Health and Transportation Research Institute, Ann Arbor, Michigan*

Tess L. Sierzant, R.N., M.S.N.,   *Nurse Clinician, Minnesota Comprehensive Epilepsy Program, Minneapolis, Minnesota*

Mariah Snyder, R.N., Ph.D., F.A.A.N.,   *Professor and Director of Graduate Studies, University of Minnesota School of Nursing, Minneapolis, Minnesota*

Nancy Stalland, M.A.,   *Licensed Psychologist, Stillwater, Minnesota*

Ann V. Walton, C.S.J.,   *Province Leadership, Sisters of St. Joseph, St. Paul, Minnesota*

Advisory Committee

Nancy Santilli, R.N., P.N.P., M.N., F.A.A.N., Chair, *Associate Professor of Neurology, Associate Director, Comprehensive Epilepsy Program, University of Virginia Health Science Center, Charlottesville, Virginia*

Judith A. Beniak, R.N., M.P.H., *Director of Student Services, University of Minnesota School of Nursing, Minneapolis, Minnesota*

Judy Ozuna, A.R.N.P., M.N., C.N.R.N., *Clinical Nurse Specialist, Neurology Section, V.A. Medical Center, Seattle, Washington*

EFA Project Staff

J. Joseph Giffels, *Director, Research and Professional Education*

Bonnie L. Kessler, *Former Director, Research and Professional Education*

Karen Lombardi, *Former Administrative Coordinator, Research and Professional Education*

W. Christopher Merritt, *Production Editor, Research and Professional Education*

Ila M. Myers, *Associate Director for Special Projects, Research and Professional Education*

Ann Scherer, *Director, Communications and Public Relations*

Managing Seizure Disorders
A Handbook for Health Care Professionals

Managing Seizure Disorders: A Handbook for Health Care Professionals, edited by N. Santilli, Lippincott-Raven Publishers, Philadelphia, 1996.
© 1996 Epilepsy Foundation of America.

1

Introduction and Overview

Nancy Santilli

The purpose of this book is to provide detailed information in support of the health professional's efforts to assist individuals with epilepsy to live the life they desire. A diagnosis of seizures may have little effect on a person's life or may be a profound disruption. A great deal has been written in the past concerning the classification of seizures and epileptic syndromes, with reviews of the diagnostic work-up and the medical and surgical treatments available. Although these topics are covered in this book, they are included to serve as a point of reference. More detailed information can be found in other publications available through the Epilepsy Foundation of America, or in many professional publications.

To provide the reader with an overview, some of this information is provided in a condensed format. "Epidemiology of Seizure Disorders and the Epilepsies," by Dr. Hauser, gives us new insights into the causes of seizures, the effects of the condition, and information on prognosis. "Classification of the Epilepsies: Influence on Management" provides the cornerstone on which all other efforts are based. Treatment issues include the diagnostic work-up, principles of acute and chronic medical management, surgical intervention, and information on currently available antiepileptic drugs. It was not possible to review all therapeutic approaches available to people with seizures, e.g., information regarding vagal nerve stimulation, cultural approaches, and religious supports. These can be found in other texts.

The authors' approach is a practical orientation to living daily with the condition. Although each section can stand on its own, many of the chapters build on themes and research that can be found in other areas. Because epilepsy affects individuals throughout the life cycle, there are critical issues for specific age groups that require special attention. Since new-onset epilepsy is most common in children and the elderly, Drs. Dodson and Dreifuss, respectively, review these issues for those age groups. Nancy Stalland and Mimi Callanan review reproductive health issues for women with epilepsy. The unique concerns and intervention strategies needed in working with individuals who have multiple disabilities are outlined in "Considerations for Individuals with Developmental Disabilities."

Dr. Shope outlines the knowledge, skills, and behaviors needed to accomplish successful management of epilepsy. Compliance is a major issue for both the person with seizures and the health care professional. This complex issue is reviewed and suggestions for intervention are provided. Nancy Stalland and Patty Shafer discuss the special issues faced when a person with epilepsy is considering parenthood and some of the adaptations that might be needed to safely fulfill the role of parent. Dr. Austin discusses the issue of parenting the child with a chronic illness such as epilepsy. Her longitudinal work in this area is extremely helpful to an understanding of the dynamics that families encounter in the process of learning to live with epilepsy. As children grow, they and their families face issues in the academic setting that present some unique challenges. These issues are reviewed in the chapter "The Student with Epilepsy in an Educational Framework." "Safety and Activities of Daily Living for People with Epilepsy" provides many tips on how to adapt both lifestyle and environment to reduce injury risks and seizures. Fear of injury continues to be a concern for employers, although, for the most part, their fears are unfounded. Dianne Lipsey discusses the "Impact of Epilepsy on Employability" and the possible accommodations available. Simply learning to live with epilepsy on a daily basis presents a large array of problems. Whereas some of these problems are common to all age groups, others are part of the normal growth and development process. Adjustment issues are discussed, with some suggestions on how to assess them, intervene, and minimize their impact on the individual's daily life. A detailed review of the legal issues that individuals with epilepsy face today is provided in the "Legal Advocacy" chapter. Finally, accessing community resources and supports can be critical to participating in community life. A review of resources commonly available is provided.

The appendices should help our readers to organize their efforts by identifying some of the issues in a concise manner, giving examples of intervention plans to deal with the various issues that people with epilepsy face, and listing resources available through the Epilepsy Foundation of America. This book is written to support health care professionals in the delivery of care to people with epilepsy.

THE SPECTRUM OF EPILEPSY[1]

Caring for patients and their families is the work of all health care professionals. Our efforts are directed toward restoring their health and supporting them in becoming well. Critical to this process in guiding the chronically ill is the assessment of something that has almost become a trite phrase: quality of life.

In the medical model, the focus is on defining and classifying seizure types and syndromes and on establishing appropriate therapeutic intervention. Equally important is identifying the psychosocial effects of seizures. Too often, success is measured only by a decrease in the number of seizures or a reduction in the

---

[1] Adapted with permission from Santilli N. The spectrum of epilepsy. *Clin Nurs Pract Epilepsy,* January, 1993.

amount of medication required. All too often, the patient's own experience of altered health is not addressed.

Physiologic and psychologic states are interdependent. Therefore, an individual's perception of symptoms, symptom labels, how distress symptoms are communicated, the inability to function normally, and the methods used to gain control over the seizure disorder are among the interdependent variables that determine quality of life.

HOW WIDE THE SPECTRUM

Every professional encounters individuals whose health status and support needs are so diverse that at times they may be overwhelming. This is especially true when attempts are made to effectively utilize institutional, community, and family resources. In addition, health care professionals recognize that their own skills vary when they attempt to provide direct personal care and long-term supportive care to individuals with epilepsy and their families. Because epilepsy cuts across all age groups, affecting people with a vast variety of abilities and needs, it is helpful to review the spectrum of epilepsy.

SEIZURE TYPES AND EPILEPTIC SYNDROMES

The spectrum of seizures and their effects ranges from people with no disability to people who are severely affected by their seizure disorder, by its treatment, and by lack of personal support. On the positive side, approximately 80% of people with seizures can now be completely controlled with proper diagnosis and treatment, enabling them to live normal, active lives. For the remaining 20%, however, their epilepsy may forever be an obstacle to a truly satisfying life.

Three Operational Categories

Although each individual's needs are unique, it is useful to use operational categories to describe the effect of epilepsy on the person's life. Use of these categories not only aids in individual assessments but helps to target high-risk patients. In addition, it supports the concept of functional assessment.

Marshall and Cupoli (1986) identified three categories of children with epilepsy, an approach applicable to all people with seizure disorders. These categories (Fig. 1), in increasing order of severity, are uncomplicated, compromised, and devastated. Because epilepsy is a chronic condition and life is a dynamic process, individuals may move in and out of these categories. Nor are these groupings mutually exclusive.

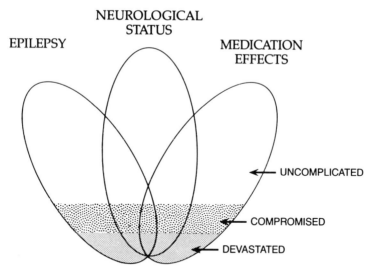

FIG. 1. Operational categories of students with epilepsy (courtesy of W. Edwin Dodson, M.D.).

Uncomplicated

The majority of people with epilepsy fall into the uncomplicated category. Their seizures are controlled and their medication causes minimal or no side effects. They have no concomitant problems, and family members and friends are supportive. Only rarely do they experience academic, vocational, or psychological problems secondary to their epilepsy. They are usually cared for by primary care providers. They may encounter a specialist only during the diagnostic work-up or when pathophysiologic or psychological changes threaten their functioning status and therefore affect their categorization.

For example, pregnant women with uncomplicated epilepsy are often considered "high risk." This is due in part to the pathophysiologic changes of pregnancy but can also be attributed to the lack of experience with epilepsy among other specialists. Prenatal care that fails to address the special needs of the patient with epilepsy can lead to adverse effects on emotional status, health perception, and role activities. Similar changes may occur when a school-aged child is transferred to a school that is less experienced with children with epilepsy, thus creating changes in the student's functional domains. However, these fluctuations are usually short-lived, and with appropriate support and intervention affected individuals usually return to their baseline functional state.

Compromised

People who are considered compromised have seizures that are usually controlled. Even though this group is free of serious mental and motor problems, they can experience difficulties that affect the domains of functional, social, and emotional status, cognition, health perceptions, and general quality of life. Professionals often overestimate how well these individuals are doing because, on the surface, everything may appear fine. These individuals are often cared for in primary care settings because they appear to have uncomplicated medical problems. Often, anything other than routine medical care is provided only when there is strong self-advocacy.

> Joseph, a 36-year-old man, developed epilepsy 16 years ago as the result of an AV malformation. He has recently become a new father, has been promoted, and has moved into a new house. During the past 3 months he has experienced two nocturnal seizures. He is suddenly having greater difficulty in concentrating, complains that his memory is worse, and feels tired all the time.
>
> Initially, his difficulties were attributed to the new baby and job stress. However, when these symptoms failed to resolve he insisted on a consultation with a specialist. A complete neurologic work-up revealed focal brain atrophy, EEG changes in the left occipital and temporal regions, and visual and fine gross motor changes. Therefore, a pathophysiologic basis for his difficulties was identified. The new baby and new job were not the underlying cause but simply made the problems more apparent.

Because Joseph appeared to be managing his life without too much difficulty, no one looked further. This case underscores the need for reevaluation when functional status changes. Through periodic reassessment of the individual's health, functional abilities, perceptions, and general life satisfaction, problem areas can be identified.

> Sally, a 65-year-old woman, was diagnosed with new-onset epilepsy 2 years ago. Her seizures are well controlled on monotherapy. Since her diagnosis, she finds it difficult to make the 2-h drive to the city that she used to do regularly. She is no longer comfortable about flying or traveling alone.

On the surface, everything may seem good for Sally, but it is clear that epilepsy has changed her life. Her hesitation may be related to fears, ineffective coping, or memory deficit. If the problem is unresolved, further problems may emerge, such as social isolation and role disturbance. These changes may have more far-reaching effects, especially when they involve cognitive, social, or role performance.

Devastated

Individuals whose condition is regarded as devastated by virtue of their multiple problems often have epilepsy as a result of brain disease that may also impair learning, motor, and emotional function. Often their seizures started early in life and may never have been truly controlled despite the use of aggressive therapy. Chronic overmedication is often the result of an effort to increase seizure control. Complicating conditions, such as mild to severe cognitive dysfunction, may be present because of underlying pathology, the frequency of seizures, overmedication, or a combination of the three. Family support may be strained or crumbling in response to the pressures.

By definition, individuals in this category require continuous intervention and reassessment. For selected patients, specific surgical resections for seizure control may result in improvement. Likewise, good comprehensive management can produce the same benefit.

> Kristin, an 11-year-old girl, was diagnosed with epilepsy 2 years ago. She has absence, generalized tonic–clonic, and myoclonic seizures. At present her seizures are uncontrolled. She was an A student, but now works very hard for Bs and Cs. She has lost many friends and now finds it difficult to participate in sports because of chronic fatigue and the extra time she needs to spend on school work. She loves to cook but is no longer allowed to because she burned her hand as a result of a seizure.
>
> Her mother has had to drop back to part-time employment because Kristin's father travels extensively. Although the family, in conjunction with the school, has been successful in developing an appropriate Individual Education Plan (IEP) for Kristin, they recognize that their two other children have received less attention. The family stays close to home, to be near the hospital where Kristin is treated. Epilepsy dominates this family's activities. They need support in almost every aspect of their lives.

The three cases illustrate the need for comprehensive management. After the correct diagnosis is made and appropriate therapy initiated, many of the issues individuals and their families face are secondary to the primary diagnosis but quite disruptive. Providing practical solutions to the day-to-day issues people face is paramount. Some solutions are identified in what follows. The most important thing for us to remember is to assist individuals with seizures to identify their passion for life and to do our best to support their efforts to live it.

REFERENCES

Marshall RM, Cupoli JM. Epilepsy and education: the pediatrician's expanding role. *Adv Pediatr* 1986;33:159–80.

Managing Seizure Disorders: A Handbook for Health Care Professionals, edited by N. Santilli, Lippincott-Raven Publishers, Philadelphia, 1996. © 1996 Epilepsy Foundation of America.

2

Epidemiology of Seizure Disorders and the Epilepsies

W. Allen Hauser

Instead of focusing on the individual patient, the epidemiologist is interested in patterns of disease occurrence within populations, with the ultimate goal of disease prevention. Descriptive epidemiologic studies provide information regarding the frequency of an illness as well as the disease course and prognosis. Analytic studies identify individuals at differential risk for the illness. Although epidemiologic information can only indirectly be extrapolated to the individual patient, these data do provide general information that may be useful in counseling individual patients. In addition, the data are useful for determination of disease burden in planning health care needs. This chapter reviews the epidemiologic data regarding the frequency of epilepsy in the population, the course of patients with seizures and epilepsy, and the risk factors for development of epilepsy.

For the following discussion, an epileptic seizure is defined as the clinical manifestation of an abnormal and excessive excitation of a group of cerebral neurons. The brain may respond to a variety of insults (i.e., head injury, stroke, metabolic disturbances such as uremia) with neuronal overactivity and seizures. There are many potential causes of a seizure. Seizures that occur at the time of an acute systemic disturbance or an insult to the central nervous system are termed *acute symptomatic seizures.* These seizures must be distinguished from *epilepsy.* Epilepsy is a unique condition characterized by a tendency toward recurrent seizures (two, three, or more) in the absence of an obvious insult (recurrent unprovoked seizures). Seizures that occur only with fever and those associated with acute systemic metabolic derangement or with acute central nervous system insult would be excluded from this definition.

HOW FREQUENTLY DO CONVULSIONS AND EPILEPSY OCCUR IN THE POPULATION?

Incidence

Incidence is a measure of the number of new cases of a disease occurring in a defined population. Incidence is important in the study of causes and in the determination of prognosis. For convulsions or for epilepsy, incidence is usually measured as new cases per 100,000 population per year.

Convulsions

Convulsions are among the most common neurologic conditions. Each year about 300,000 individuals in the United States come to medical attention because of a newly recognized seizure, an incidence of about 120/100,000. About 40% of these individuals are under the age of 18 at identification. The majority, 75,000 to 100,000, are young children younger than the age of 5 who have experienced only convulsions with a febrile illness.

Epilepsy

Each year 50/100,000 individuals in the United States will be diagnosed as having epilepsy (Fig. 1). This is equal to 125,000 new cases each year. Although epilepsy may start at any age, the incidence of epilepsy is highest in children under 2 years of age and in persons over 65 years of age.

Males are more likely to have a new diagnosis of epilepsy than females. The incidence is higher in black populations and in socially disadvantaged communities, although these two conditions may not be independent. Trends over

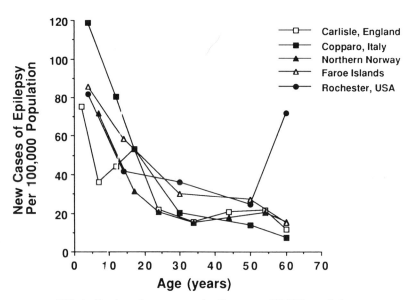

FIG. 1. Number of new cases of epilepsy per 100,000 population.

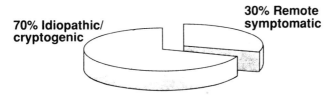

FIG. 2. Causes of newly diagnosed cases of epilepsy.

time suggest that the incidence of new cases of epilepsy in children has decreased in recent years, whereas the incidence has increased in the elderly.

In most cases of newly diagnosed epilepsy, no specific cause is identified (Fig. 2). Although a definite cause can be identified in a higher proportion of those with onset of epilepsy in adults and the elderly, even in these age groups more than half of newly identified cases have no clear antecedent. About half of all newly identified people with epilepsy will have generalized onset seizures (Fig. 3). Epilepsy manifest by generalized onset seizures is more common than partial (focal) seizures in young children, but after the age of 10 more than half of all new cases of epilepsy will have partial seizures.

Prevalence

Prevalence is defined as the number of cases of a disease in a population at a specific point in time. For epilepsy, prevalence is usually measured as the number of cases per 1,000 population and is primarily of value for determination of need for health care resources. The estimates for prevalence of epilepsy vary widely, from 3/1,000 to over 40/1,000 population, although most of this variation is related to differences in the definition of a prevalence case of epilepsy in the different studies (Fig. 4). Defining as an active prevalence case of epilepsy an individual with a history of epilepsy who has experienced a seizure or taken antiepileptic medication within the previous 5 years, the prevalence of epilepsy in the United States is 6–10/1,000 population. Therefore, more than 2 million people in the United States are presently affected by epilepsy.

In the United States, prevalence tends to increase with advancing age (Fig. 5).

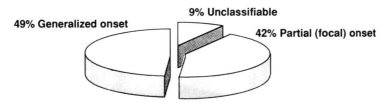

FIG. 3. Seizure type among newly diagnosed cases of epilepsy.

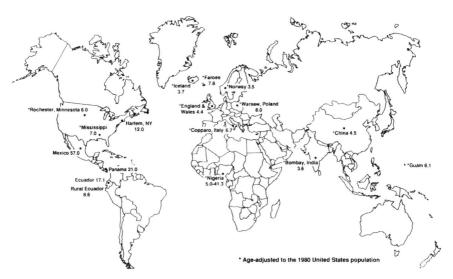

FIG. 4. Number of cases of active epilepsy per 1,000 population.

In preschool children, the prevalence of active epilepsy is about 1.5/1,000 (in the United States, about 27,000 cases). In schoolchildren through age 17, the prevalence is about 5/1,000 (about 300,000 cases). In persons over age 65, the prevalence is about 1% (about 300,000 cases). In the United States, the prevalence of epilepsy is higher among nonwhites compared with whites, although it is not clear whether these differences are related to race, socioeconomic factors, or both.

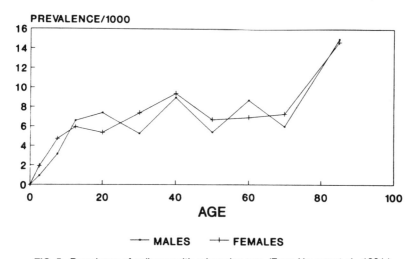

FIG. 5. Prevalence of epilepsy with advancing age. (From Hauser et al., 1991.)

Cumulative Incidence

The cumulative incidence is a measure of the risk for developing a condition by a particular age. By 20 years of age, 1% of the population can be expected to have developed epilepsy. More than 3% of the population can be expected to have had a diagnosis of epilepsy by age 75, and by this same age over 10% of the population can be expected to have experienced a seizure of some type.

WHAT FACTORS CAUSE EPILEPSY?

Many factors have been implicated in the etiology of epilepsy (Fig. 6). The most clearly established of these factors are severe head trauma, infections of

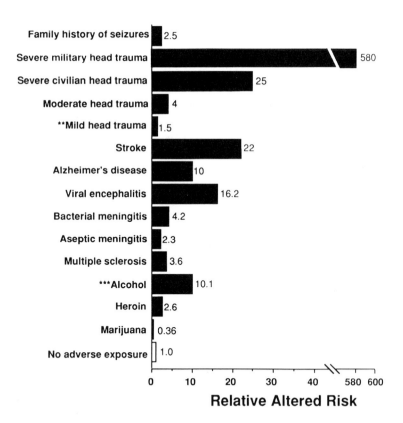

** Not statistically significant
*** One pint of 80 proof, 2 1/2 bottles of wine

FIG. 6. Factors associated with an altered risk of epilepsy (relative to people without these adverse exposures).

the central nervous system, and stroke, although many other factors are also important antecedents.

Severe head injury, as manifest by unconsciousness of more than 24 h or open head injuries, is associated with a substantial increase in risk for epilepsy. Unfortunately, most individuals with injury of this severity do not survive the initial insult, and the pool of such individuals is therefore small.

In general, adverse prenatal and perinatal events have not been shown to increase the risk for epilepsy, although some of these factors are associated with an increased risk for cerebral palsy (Fig. 7). Only children "small for gestational age" or with neonatal seizures have been shown to be at increased risk for epilepsy.

Children with motor handicaps present from birth, such as cerebral palsy (CP) and/or mental retardation (MR), have a substantially increased risk for epilepsy. Approximately 10% of children with moderate or severe MR alone, and about 10% of children with CP alone, can be expected to develop epilepsy during childhood, although the frequency may increase with increasing disability. When both conditions coexist, 50% or more can be expected to develop epilepsy by the age of 20 (Fig. 8).

Children who experience febrile seizures are at increased risk for developing epilepsy during their lives. As with mental retardation and cerebral palsy, febrile seizures do not cause epilepsy but are a marker for a common antecedent.

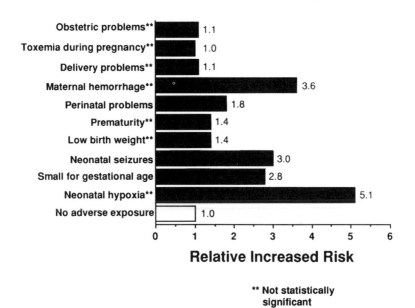

Relative Increased Risk

** Not statistically
significant

FIG. 7. Perinatal factors possibly associated with an increased risk of epilepsy (relative to people without these adverse exposures).

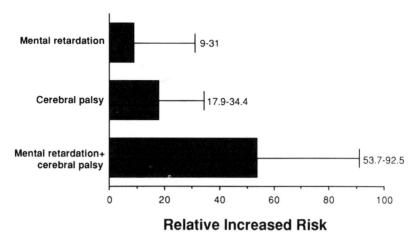

Relative Increased Risk

FIG. 8. Risk of epilepsy among people with mental retardation or cerebral palsy (relative to people without these conditions).

ARE FAMILY HISTORY AND GENETICS IMPORTANT IN THE DEVELOPMENT OF EPILEPSY?

If one considers the basic frequency of epilepsy, about 10% of the general adult population will have a first-degree relative with epilepsy, and almost one in three adults will have a first-degree relative with seizures.

Epilepsy frequently occurs in families. The parents, siblings, and offspring of a person with epilepsy are more likely than the general population to have epilepsy. This familial aggregation does not necessarily imply a genetic mechanism. In addition to genes, families share environmental exposures that may also increase the risk for epilepsy.

More than 200 syndromes inherited as Mendelian traits are associated with seizures or epilepsy. For these individuals, the risk for the syndrome (but not necessarily for seizures, because not all will manifest these symptoms) may be as high as 25% for recessively inherited diseases and 50% for dominantly inherited diseases. These syndromes account for less than 1% of all cases of epilepsy.

Thus far, a genetic locus has been identified for three specific epilepsy syndromes. A gene for benign familial neonatal convulsions is located on chromosome 20. A gene involved in juvenile myoclonic epilepsy and other generalized idiopathic juvenile-onset epilepsies is linked to a marker on chromosome 6. A gene for Baltic myoclonic epilepsy is located on chromosome 21.

The risk for epilepsy to siblings or offspring of individuals with epilepsy is increased above that of the general population by a factor of 2 to 3. This translates to a modest rate of 3–5% by the age of 20. Certain factors are associated with a higher risk for epilepsy among family members (Fig. 9 and 10). The risk is higher

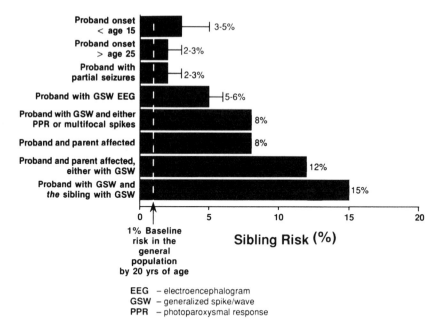

FIG. 9. Sibling risk for epilepsy.

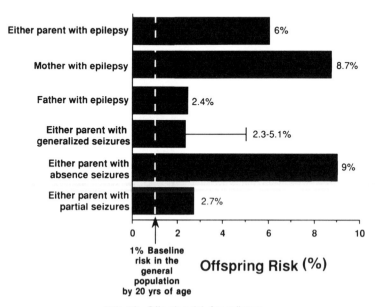

FIG. 10. Offspring risk for epilepsy.

for relatives of individuals with childhood-onset epilepsy, higher for the offspring of affected mothers than fathers, and higher when a parent also has a history of epilepsy. The electroencephalogram (EEG) may be a predictor of increased risk for other family members, but seizure type (other than absence seizures) and presumed etiology appear less important.

The increase in risk for children and siblings is substantially less than many assume, and laws regulating marriage and reproduction for people with epilepsy in many countries (including the United States into the 1970s) clearly were not justified.

WHAT IS THE LONG-TERM PROGNOSIS FOR PEOPLE WITH EPILEPSY?

This is a question with many aspects. The first and most important aspect relates to whether epilepsy is a lifelong illness. Other important questions relate to whether people with epilepsy are at increased risk for other medical conditions and for premature death.

Is the Epilepsy a Lifelong Condition?

For most individuals who experience seizures, the event occurs in the context of an acute illness (acute symptomatic seizures). In such circumstances, additional seizures tend to occur primarily with recurrence of the underlying condition. Most conditions that can cause acute symptomatic seizures also are risk factors for epilepsy, and individuals with these acute seizures are at increased risk for future epilepsy compared with those who have experienced the same insult but without a complicating seizure. Nevertheless, in most situations only a small percentage will experience further seizures.

For individuals who have experienced a single, unprovoked seizure, slightly more than one-third go on to have additional unprovoked seizures, although this risk varies from less than 20% to almost 100% depending on the presence or absence of specific clinical factors. The risk for seizure recurrence is increased for patients with a history of a neurologic insult and for patients with an abnormal EEG, and may be increased after a first partial seizure, in those with an abnormal neurologic examination, or in those with a sibling who also has epilepsy. Among individuals with none of the above factors, only one person in five experiences a second seizure. Once an individual has had recurrent seizure episodes, the likelihood of additional seizures approaches 100%.

For most individuals with epilepsy the seizures can be completely controlled, and approximately 70% can be expected to enter remission, defined as 5 or more years without seizures (Fig. 11). Remission of epilepsy is more common among patients with generalized onset seizures (especially generalized tonic–clonic seizures), in those with childhood-onset epilepsy, and those with a normal neurologic

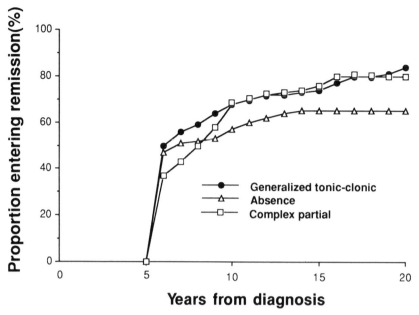

FIG. 11. Proportion entering remission following the diagnosis of epilepsy.

examination. Patients with epilepsy and associated MR and/or CP have a decreased likelihood of remission compared to other groups. Only about 35% of these patients can expect to achieve remission.

The favorable prognosis is not limited to control of seizures. Of individuals who remain seizure-free for 2 to 5 years, 75% can be successfully withdrawn from antiepileptic medication. Successful withdrawal of medication is more likely among patients whose EEG, neurologic examination, and intelligence are normal.

Approximately 10% of newly identified patients fail to achieve control of seizures despite optimal medical management. In some patients with intractable epilepsy, surgery represents a reasonable alternative. Seizure freedom or reduced seizure frequency can be expected in about 75% of appropriately selected patients (range 59.5–95%).

Are People with Epilepsy at Increased Risk for Death?

Most studies show a slight excess in mortality for people with epilepsy compared with the general population. For people with symptomatic epilepsy, the risk is substantial and is related to the underlying illness. For those with idiopathic epilepsy, the risk is modest and is increased only during the first few years after diagnosis. Males with epilepsy appear to have an increased mortality, whereas females do not. Individuals with absence seizures and with idiopathic (cryptogenic) partial seizures do not have an increased mortality. Compared with the causes of death in the general population, the causes of death in individuals with epilepsy are more frequently attributed to accidents, suicide, cerebrovascular and other circulatory system disease, respiratory disease, and central nervous system tumors. Contrary to the findings of clinical and autopsy studies, population-based studies fail to identify an increased risk for sudden death among people with idiopathic epilepsy.

Mortality associated with status epilepticus is high, but more than half of those who experience status epilepticus do not have a prior history of epilepsy, and death is usually due to the underlying cause (e.g., a brain tumor) rather than to adverse effects attributable to treatment or to the prolonged seizures.

Are People with Epilepsy at Risk for Problems During Pregnancy?

Apart from the concerns for epilepsy in offspring previously discussed, there is often concern about the course of pregnancy in women with epilepsy. In general, these women are considered high-risk patients. Seizure control may be altered, but not in a consistent manner. The frequency of seizures during pregnancy decreases in one-third of patients, stays the same in one-third, and increases in one-third. Intragestational bleeding is more than twice as common among pregnant women with epilepsy. This is related in part to the decrease in levels of vitamin K brought about by antiepileptic drugs.

Infants of women with epilepsy are more likely to be premature. These infants are also at risk for hemorrhagic disease of the newborn, a result of vitamin K depletion. The risk for major and minor malformations is also increased, although this increase is related to exposure to antiepileptic medication during the first trimester of pregnancy rather than to the epilepsy per se. This risk is substantially less than many assume. The risk for a major malformation is increased by two- to threefold over that of the general population. As the general risk for a major malformation is 2–3%, major malformations can be expected in 6–8% of infants exposed to antiepileptic medication in utero during the first trimester. In other words, more than 90% of women with epilepsy who are taking antiepileptic medications can be expected to have normal children.

The risk for malformations appears to be the same for all of the antiepileptic drugs presently marketed in the United States. No scientifically based evidence supports the existence of specific antiepileptic drug syndromes, although drug-specific major malformations may occur, such as the association between valproate and spina bifida. Malformations are more common among patients receiving polytherapy compared to those receiving monotherapy.

OTHER AREAS OF CONCERN REGARDING PEOPLE WITH EPILEPSY

There are many misconceptions about the psychosocial function of people with epilepsy. The intellectual function of children with epilepsy, as measured by standard psychological tests, has a distribution similar to that of the general population. Psychosocial function may be impaired among people with epilepsy, although studies have tended to evaluate only patients with poor seizure control. Psychosocial impairment may be greater in those with many seizures compared with those who experience only a few seizures. The occurrence of status epilepticus is an even more important predictor of psychosocial impairment than seizure frequency. There is no evidence for organized, directed ictal aggression in people with epilepsy, and no sound population studies support an association between psychosis and epilepsy.

SUMMARY

Seizures and epilepsy are common conditions that can affect individuals of all ages. In general, no specific cause can be identified for the majority of cases at all ages. The prognosis for seizure control is usually excellent. An increased risk for death is seen primarily in individuals with an identified cause for their epilepsy and is associated with the underlying cause rather than with the epilepsy itself. For those with epilepsy there is a risk for complications during pregnancy and for congenital malformations in children exposed to maternal use of anti-epileptic medications, but over 90% of pregnancies are uncomplicated and the children are normal.

ADDITIONAL READING

Hauser WA, Annegers JF, Kurland LT. Prevalence of epilepsy in Rochester, Minnesota: 1940–1980. *Epilepsia* 1991;32:429–45.
Hauser WA, Hesdorffer D. *Epilepsy: frequency, causes, and consequences.* New York: Demos Publications, 1990.
Hauser WA, Hesdorffer D. *Facts about epilepsy.* New York: Demos Publications, 1990.

Managing Seizure Disorders: A Handbook for Health Care Professionals, edited by N. Santilli, Lippincott-Raven Publishers, Philadelphia, 1996.
© 1996 Epilepsy Foundation of America.

3

Classification of the Epilepsies: Influence on Management

Fritz E. Dreifuss

Once a diagnosis of epilepsy has been arrived at, therapy should be designed as individually as possible. Consideration must be given to the seizure type, the medication most specifically useful, and the determination of the syndrome to which the seizures belong. This, in turn, allows formulation of a prognosis on which the choice of therapy, possibly including consideration of surgery, can be predicated.

CLASSIFICATION OF EPILEPTIC SEIZURES

In the International Classification (1981) (Table 1), the main categories of seizures are generalized seizures and partial seizures. Under generalized seizures are included absence, myoclonic, tonic, atonic, and tonic–clonic seizures. Under partial seizures there are two main subdivisions, including simple partial seizures, in which consciousness is preserved, and complex partial seizures, in which consciousness is impaired. Simple partial seizures are subclassified depending on the area of cortex predominantly involved, and it is recognized that they may progress to complex partial seizures or to secondarily generalized tonic–clonic seizures. Complex partial seizures are those involving limbic structures and in which consciousness is impaired. These may further progress to secondarily generalized tonic–clonic seizures. From the practical point of view, it is essential to distinguish seizures that are primarily generalized epilepsies from those that are secondarily generalized epilepsies, because of the differential treatment response and the different medications required for their treatment. It is also of the greatest importance to distinguish seizures such as absence seizures from seizures such as complex partial seizures, which may be phenotypically indistinguishable without intensive monitoring and which respond to quite different medications, each of which has its own particular side effects. Inappropriate medication should be avoided at all costs by accuracy in diagnosis. Similarly, absence seizures with automatisms must be distinguished from complex partial seizures with automatisms and, again, the same reasons apply.

TABLE 1. *The International Classification of Epileptic Seizures*

I. Partial (focal, local) seizures
    A. Simple partial seizures (consciousness not impaired)
        1. Motor (abnormal movement of an arm, leg, or both; Jacksonian march)
        2. Somatosensory or special sensory (gustatory, olfactory, auditory)
        3. Autonomic (tachycardia, respiration, flushing)
        4. Psychic (déjà vu, fearful feeling)
    B. Complex partial seizures (with impairment of consciousness)
        1. Beginning as simple partial seizure and progressing to impairment of consciousness
            a. No other symptoms
            b. Motor, somatosensory, special sensory, autonomic, or psychic symptoms
            c. Automatisms
        2. With impairment of consciousness at onset
            a. No other symptoms
            b. Motor, somatosensory, special sensory, autonomic or psychic symptoms
            c. Automatisms
    C. Partial seizures evolving to secondarily generalized seizures
        1. Simple partial leads to generalized seizures
        2. Complex partial leads to generalized seizures
        3. Simple partial leads to complex partial leads to generalized seizures
II. Generalized seizures (convulsive or nonconvulsive, all associated with loss of consciousness)
    A. Absence (petit mal)
        Onset in childhood; approximately 50% ending in adolescence and 50% supplanted by tonic–clonic
        Symptoms include altered awareness or attention and blank stare, may include eye blinking lasting 5–30 s
        Can be mistaken as learning disabilities or behavior problems if unrecognized
    B. Myoclonic
        Characterized by short, abrupt muscular contractions of arms, legs, and/or torso
        Symptoms include symmetrical or asymmetrical, synchronous or asynchronous single or multiple jerks; possible brief loss of consciousness
    C. Clonic
        Symptoms include muscle contraction and relaxation usually lasting several minutes
        Distinct phases may not be easily observable
    D. Tonic
        Symptoms include an abrupt increase in muscle tone (contraction), loss of consciousness and autonomic signs, lasting from 30 s to several minutes
    E. Tonic–clonic (grand mal)
        Tonic—may begin with a shrill cry caused by secondary expulsion of air due to abrupt closure of the epiglottis; rigidity, opisthotonos, extension of arms and legs; jaw may snap shut; temporary (up to 1 min); cessation of respiration; nonreactive, dilated pupils; decreased heart rate
        Clonic–begins suddenly and ends gradually, characterized by quick, bilateral, severe jerking movements; stertorous respirations; autonomic symptoms; lasts 2–5 min
        Postictal—muscle flaccidity; gradual return of consciousness; amnesia related to the seizure; patient may need 0.5–1 h of sleep
    F. Atonic
        Characterized by abrupt loss of muscle tone followed by postictal confusion; injury likely if seizure uncontrolled
III. Unclassified epileptic seizures—cannot be classified because of inadequate or incomplete data; include some neonatal seizures, e.g., rhythmic eye movements, chewing, and swimming movements

Adapted from Commission on Classification and Terminology of the International League Against Epilepsy, 1981.

Partial (Focal, Local) Seizures

Partial seizures are those in which the first clinical and electroencephalographic (EEG) changes indicate initial activation of a system of neurons limited to part of one cerebral hemisphere. A partial seizure is classified primarily on the basis of whether or not consciousness is impaired during the attack. (Impaired consciousness is defined as the inability to respond normally to exogenous stimuli by virtue of altered awareness and/or responsiveness.) When consciousness is not impaired, the seizure is classified as a simple partial seizure. In complex partial seizures, impairment of consciousness may be the first clinical sign, or simple partial seizures may evolve into complex partial seizures. In patients with impaired consciousness, aberrations of behavior (automatisms) may occur. A partial seizure may not terminate but instead may progress to a generalized tonic–clonic seizure.

There is considerable evidence that simple partial seizures are usually associated with unilateral hemispheric involvement and only rarely involve both hemispheres, whereas in complex partial seizures there is often bilateral hemispheric involvement.

Partial seizures can be classified into one of the following three fundamental groups:

1. Simple partial seizures (consciousness not impaired)
   With motor symptoms
   With somatosensory or special sensory symptoms
   With autonomic symptoms
   With psychic symptoms
2. Complex partial seizures (with impairment of consciousness)
   Beginning as simple partial seizure and progressing to impairment of consciousness
      With no other features
      With features as described under simple partial seizures (above)
      With automatisms
   With impairment of consciousness at onset
      With no other features
      With features as described under simple partial seizures (above)
      With automatisms
3. Partial seizures secondarily generalized
   Simple partial to generalized tonic–clonic
   Complex partial to generalized tonic–clonic
   Simple partial to complex partial to generalized tonic–clonic

Generalized Seizures (Convulsive or Nonconvulsive)

Generalized seizures are those in which the first clinical changes indicate initial involvement of both hemispheres. Consciousness may be impaired, and this impairment may be the initial manifestation. Motor manifestations are bilateral. The ictal electroencephalographic patterns initially are bilateral, and presumably reflect neuronal discharge which is widespread in both hemispheres.

1. Absence seizures
   Atypical absence seizures
2. Myoclonic seizures
3. Clonic seizures
4. Tonic–clonic seizures
5. Atonic seizures

Unclassified Epileptic Seizures

This category includes all seizures that cannot be classified because of inadequate or incomplete data and some that defy classification in hitherto described categories. This includes some neonatal seizures, e.g., rhythmic eye movements, chewing, and swimming movements.

CLASSIFICATION OF EPILEPTIC SYNDROMES

Syndromes are series of symptoms that include seizure type, etiology, precipitating factors, age of onset, severity, chronicity, diurnal and circadian cycling, family history, and prognosis (Table 2). Syndromes are also conditions about which clinicians communicate rather than seizure types, including such disorders as infantile spasm syndromes, Lennox–Gastaut syndromes, and benign juvenile myoclonus syndromes.

A review of the natural history of the epilepsies reveals that the concept of prognosis has been studied since the earliest days of effective antiepileptic drug (AED) therapy. Gowers (1884) asked, "What is the prospect of cure of the disease, or arrest of the fits by treatment? Of all the questions in the prognosis of disease it is the most difficult to answer, and no other is perhaps, put with the same anxiety and frequency." He also stated that the longer the interval between attacks, the more likely will be the arrest of seizures, and that the prognosis is most favorable for patients whose epilepsy has lasted less than a year. One problem in ascertaining prognosis is that the larger series emanate from epilepsy centers which deal with a particularly intractable population where terminal remission is relatively rare. On the other hand, Annegers et al. (1979), analyzing a prospective population group, and Elwes et al. (1984), prospectively looking at persons newly diagnosed with seizures, demonstrated remission rates of at least 70%.

It has recently become apparent that there exist among the epilepsies syndromes of such benign natural history that the risk/benefit ratio might well incline towards no treatment. Such syndromes include benign neonatal convulsions, benign in-

TABLE 2. *International Classification of Epilepsies and Epileptic Syndromes*

1. Localization-related (focal, local, partial) epilepsies and syndromes
   1.1 Idiopathic (with age-related onset)
       Benign childhood epilepsy with centrotemporal spike
       Childhood epilepsy with occipital paroxysms
       Primary reading epilepsy
   1.2 Symptomatic
       Chronic progressive epilepsia partialis continua of childhood (Kojewnikow's
         syndrome)
       Syndromes characterized by seizures with specific modes of precipitation
   1.3 Cryptogenic
       Cryptogenic epilepsies are presumed to be symptomatic and the etiology is
         unknown; this category thus differs from the previous one by the lack of etiologic
         evidence
2. Generalized epilepsies and syndromes
   2.1 Idiopathic (with age-related onset, listed in order of age)
       Benign neonatal familial convulsions
       Benign neonatal convulsions
       Benign myoclonic epilepsy in infancy
       Childhood absence epilepsy (pyknolepsy)
       Juvenile absence epilepsy
       Juvenile myoclonic epilepsy (impulsive petit mal)
       Epilepsy with grand mal seizures (GTCS) on awakening
       Other generalized idiopathic epilepsies not defined above
       Epilepsies with seizures precipitated by specific modes of activation
   2.2 Cryptogenic or symptomatic (in order of age)
       West syndrome (infantile spasms, Blitz–Nick–Salaam Krämpfe)
       Lennox–Gastaut syndrome
       Epilepsy with myoclonic–astatic seizures
       Epilepsy with myoclonic absences
   2.3 Symptomatic
       2.3.1 Nonspecific etiology
             Early myoclonic encephalopathy
             Early infantile epileptic encephalopathy with suppression burst
             Other symptomatic generalized epilepsies not defined above
       2.3.2 Specific syndromes
             Epileptic seizures may complicate many disease states
             Under this heading are included diseases in which seizures are a presenting or
               predominant feature
3. Epilepsies and syndromes undetermined whether focal or generalized
   3.1 With both generalized and focal seizures
       Neonatal seizures
       Severe myoclonic epilepsy in infancy
       Epilepsy with continuous spike-waves during slow-wave sleep
       Acquired epileptic aphasia (Landau–Kleffner syndrome)
       Other undetermined epilepsies not defined above
   3.2 Without unequivocal generalized or focal seizures; all cases with generalized tonic–
       clonic seizures in which clinical and EEG findings do not permit classification as clearly
       generalized or localization-related, such as in many cases of sleep-grand mal (GTCS),
       are considered not to have unequivocal generalized or focal features
4. Special syndromes
   4.1 Situation-related seizures (Gelegenheitsanfälle)
       Febrile convulsions
       Isolated seizures or isolated status epilepticus
       Seizures occurring only when there is an acute metabolic or toxic event due to
         factors such as alcohol, drugs, eclampsia, nonketotic hyperglycemia

Adapted from Commission on Classification and Terminology of the International League Against Epilepsy, 1989.

fantile myoclonus, febrile seizures, Rolandic seizures, and possibly some cases of pyknoleptic petit mal. Unfortunately, the proponents of the view that AEDs "cure" epilepsy make it difficult to study the natural history of the epilepsies, particularly now that they have been so well classified that confusion between the idiopathic and the symptomatic forms need no longer obscure the issue. Suspicion that vigorous AED therapy might in fact be counterproductive was early raised by Hunter (1959/1960), who observed historically that reports of status epilepticus appeared to become more common after the introduction of bromides into therapy, and the paradoxical ill effects of vigorous therapy have been attested to many times. The recognition of precipitating factors, such as is seen in some reflex epilepsies and other "Gelegenheitsanfälle," may lead to their elimination without the need for pharmacologic intervention.

Childhood Epilepsy Syndromes

Childhood epilepsy syndromes can be regarded as classifiable in an age-related manner. Thus, the earliest to appear are neonatal seizures, then infantile spasms, febrile seizures, astatic myoclonic seizures, absence seizures, benign childhood partial seizures, juvenile myoclonic epilepsy, reflex epilepsies, the syndromes of the generalized tonic–clonic seizures, and the syndromes of partial seizures, such as limbic and extralimbic complex partial epilepsies.

It is extremely important to realize that most of these categories consist of two main syndrome subgroups, i.e., the primary generalized epilepsies and the secondary, lesional, or symptomatic epilepsies.

The primary epilepsies are unassociated with underlying pathology, and there is often a positive family history of a similar seizure type. The child has usually made normal progress up to the time of seizures development, and very often the seizures are relatively self-limited and respond to appropriate medication.

The secondary (lesional or symptomatic) epilepsies often have an anatomico–pathologic substrate, there are neurologic abnormalities, and there may be abnormal neurologic development. The seizures are frequent and are more difficult to control. There may be a family history of seizures other than those under consideration.

These subdivisions can be applied to almost all of the childhood seizure syndromes, e.g., neonatal convulsions may be benign and familial and may require no treatment. On the other hand, they may be secondary or lesional, with a very severe prognosis.

The infantile spasms may be idiopathic primary epilepsy with normal development before the onset of the condition, with relatively good prognosis and relatively good response to therapy. On the other hand, they may be of early onset and associated with severe cerebral disease (e.g., anoxic encephalopathy, metabolic encephalopathy), with a poor outlook and poor response to therapy, yet with a seizure type identical to that of the more benign variant.

Febrile seizures come in two varieties, i.e., the idiopathic benign febrile seizures characterized by normal neurologic development, a strong family history of similar seizure type, and a seizure that is short, nonfocal, and although it may recur is usually not associated with the development of subsequent epilepsy. The converse is true for secondary or lesional febrile seizures. The importance of the distinction here is that simple febrile seizures of the benign variety require no treatment and the risk/benefit analysis may be in favor of withholding therapy because of the side effects of phenobarbital and the potential side effects of valproate, which are the drugs of choice in the prevention of febrile seizures. On the other hand, the risk/benefit analysis may be in favor of treatment for the secondary variety, in which the recurrence rate is great, the chance for severe seizures is increased, and the prognosis is less good for development of subsequent epilepsy.

Astatic myoclonic seizures consist of two varieties, including a relatively benign form described by Kruse and Doose and a severe form, the Lennox–Gastaut syndrome. The former variety responds relatively well to valproate therapy, whereas the latter is relatively intractable to most AEDs and the prognosis for normal intellectual development is not favorable.

The absence seizures can be classified into the same two categories. Primary generalized epilepsy (pyknoleptic petit mal) presenting as absence seizures responds well to treatment, whereas a very similar appearing secondary or lesional epilepsy is relatively intractable. The prognosis for spontaneous remission is much greater for the former than for the latter variety.

Some patients with benign partial epilepsy of childhood, such as Rolandic seizures, probably do better without therapy. They serve as examples of a primary epilepsy presenting as a partial seizure. The characteristics of primary epilepsy are the age of onset, strong family history, and the benign outlook.

The benign partial seizures of childhood must be distinguished from lesional or secondary partial seizures. There is no family history, the seizures carry a different connotation, and the outlook is based on the underlying process rather than on the benign syndrome itself.

These examples illustrate the practical rationale for classifying seizures and syndromes, not merely for purposes of communication but with the following goals in mind: utilization of the most appropriate treatment; judicious withholding of treatment; and determination of prognosis. The latter helps in the decision as to whether and when to attempt termination of treatment.

OVERVIEW OF MANAGEMENT

Recent advances in the management of persons with epilepsy have been achieved through the realization that this consists of more than the delivery of drugs. Overall management includes prevention. This concept includes prevention of epilepsy itself by adoption of appropriate measures to reduce epileptogenic processes, prevention of individual seizures achieved by the use of appropriate drug therapy, avoidance and elimination of precipitating factors, and prevention of the consequences of seizures, including neurologic consequences of repeated and prolonged epilepsy, psychosocial consequences, and deleterious consequences of AED therapy, particularly when this is inappropriately applied.

All AED therapy represents a compromise between therapeutic efficacy and unwanted side effects. Tempering of therapeutic enthusiasm with an acknowledgment of the risk for adverse side effects is a dilemma faced by everyone who manages seizure disorders. Adverse reactions (Dreifuss, 1983) can be divided into those that are the result of augmented pharmacologic effects and occur at the limit of the dose–response curve, and those that represent severe and unpredictable idiosyncratic reactions.

Pharmacologic effects are common and are largely dose-related. Examples of these include endocrinologic effects, such as changes in plasma cortisol caused by phenytoin, changes in antidiuretic hormone caused by carbamazepine, steroid metabolism alteration, and transient amenorrhea and changes in protein binding of thyroxine with valproate. Other metabolic effects include changes in calcium and folate metabolism by phenytoin. Immunoglobulin metabolism is altered by phenytoin, and this may have a bearing on gingival hypertrophy. Neurologic side effects include alterations in learning and cognitive function, effects on behavior ranging from inattentiveness to thought disorders and psychotic behavior, and the appearance of abnormal movements. These changes are particularly likely to occur with use of the sedative AEDs, such as phenobarbital, phenytoin, and primidone.

Idiosyncratic effects are less related to pharmacologic actions of medications than to unexpected toxic or immunologic reactions. These include dermatologic effects, such as skin rashes, Stevens–Johnson syndrome, necrotizing or hemorrhagic lesions, and exfoliative dermatitis, and systemic lupus erythematosus, which may occur with phenytoin, ethosuximide, and rarely, with other AEDs. Blood dyscrasias may accompany the use of most AEDs and should be particularly guarded against with phenytoin, primidone, carbamazepine, ethosuximide, valproate, and felbamate. Thrombocytopenia in isolation is not uncommon in valproate given in large doses. Effects of AEDs on lymphoid tissue, leading to a lymphadenopathy syndrome akin to infectious mononucleosis and a lymphoma-like reaction, may occur, particularly with phenytoin. Effects of AEDs on the liver and pancreas are particularly worrisome with treatment with valproate, for which fatal hepatic reactions and pancreatitis have been reported quite frequently. Similarly, fatal hepatic reactions have been reported for felbamate, carbamazepine, and occasionally phenytoin. In addition to these effects, drug interactions are common in patients receiving polytherapy.

For all the above reasons, AED therapy should not be entered into lightly and, once therapy is begun, from time to time during the treatment process consideration should be given to future discontinuation of medication. In other words, discontinuation of medication may be as important a decision as its commencement. In every case, discontinuation should be considered as soon as reasonably possible, although some patients will have to continue medications indefinitely.

For the same reasons, a diagnosis of epilepsy must be definitely arrived at, which means that the differential diagnosis must receive careful attention. Causes of episodes of loss of consciousness other than epilepsy must be rigorously excluded before a person is subjected to long-term therapy. A detailed discussion of management and drug therapy is found in Chap. 8.

DIFFERENTIAL DIAGNOSIS OF EPILEPTIC SEIZURES

Not all recurrent episodes of loss of consciousness represent epilepsy, and not all episodes of loss of consciousness in persons with epilepsy are epileptic. Syncope, either cardiac, vasovagal, or reflex, may present with loss of consciousness and episodes of loss of consciousness accompanied by pallor, with sensations of fainting or with evidence of severe vagal tone (pallor, sweating, bradycardia), and should be fully evaluated. Vertigo and periodic syndromes of children, including recurrent abdominal pain and/or headache (which may represent childhood migraine, hyperventilation, breath-holding, and various episodic attacks occurring during sleep) should be carefully evaluated for differential diagnostic consideration.

Pseudoseizures are common, both by themselves and in association with epilepsy. Many persons are treated with inappropriate amounts of AEDs because of persistence of seizures when, in fact, this decision is made on the basis of attacks other than epilepsy. The absence of ictal EEG abnormality, of incontinence with seizures, or of a postictal confusional state, and the presence of combativeness, resistance to medication, and attacks exacerbated by stress all suggest the possibility of pseudoseizures, which require specialized handling other than pharmacologic manipulation.

Transient ischemic attacks (TIAs) are not usually confused with epilepsy. Difficulty arises most often when the TIA is manifested by disturbed sensation over part or all of one side of the body or when muscle weakness results in a fall. In general, focal sensory symptoms associated with epilepsy show sequential spread from one body area to another, whereas ischemic paresthesias lack this segmental spread and instead develop simultaneously over affected areas. Lack of clonic motor activity and significant alteration in consciousness favor focal ischemia over epilepsy. The age group involved, the "negative" nature of the predominant symptoms, and the absence of a history of seizures are further arguments against an epileptic disorder, even when the history is unclear.

Hyperventilation attacks are often overlooked by clinicians who see patients with episodic complaints. The principal symptoms of dizziness, a sense of floating or levitation, feelings of anxiety, epigastric or substernal discomfort, paresthesias, and tetany may occasionally be mistaken for epileptic manifestations.

The cataplexic attacks of narcolepsy may sometimes be confused with atonic seizures, but preservation of awareness and the invariable presence of an emotional triggering factor, especially laughter, should resolve most uncertainty, even in the absence of other features of narcolepsy.

An automatic behavior syndrome has been defined in patients with excessive daytime sleepiness due to narcolepsy or sleep apnea. Affected individuals give a history of periods of altered mental function, usually lasting for more than a few minutes, for which they are amnesic except for an awareness of "lost time." When observed during an episode, patients appear distracted, detached, or blank, apparently out of touch with their surroundings. The eyelids may droop or even flutter, and a Bell's phenomenon may be observed. Attacks tend to occur in situations that predispose to drowsiness: performance of monotonous repetitive tasks, driving, or writing. The patient may vocalize a few words or simple sentences, and the episode may terminate with a hallucinatory experience. The automatic behavior occurs during repeated episodes of "microsleep" that intrude into wakefulness. Superficially, the automatic behavior syndrome resembles the automatisms seen with complex partial seizures.

Miscellaneous conditions that occasionally must be distinguished from epilepsy include the episodic mental symptoms of acute intermittent porphyria and the abnormal movements of paroxysmal choreoathetosis.[1]

Nonepileptic paroxysmal behaviors in infants and children are discussed in Chap. 8.

Treatment of epilepsy requires accurate diagnosis, proper classification of seizure types and, when possible, classification of the type of epilepsy. This allows appropriate selection and administration of AEDs on the basis of sound pharmacologic principles.

REFERENCES

Annegers JF, Hauser WA, Elveback LR. Remission of seizures and relapse in patients with epilepsy. *Epilepsia* 1979;20:729–37.

Commission on Classification and Terminology of the International League Against Epilepsy. Proposal for revised clinical and electroencephalographic classification of epileptic seizures. *Epilepsia* 1981;26: 268–78.

Commission on Classification and Terminology of the International League Against Epilepsy. Proposal for revised classification of epilepsies and epileptic syndromes. *Epilepsia* 1989;30:389–99.

Dreifuss FE. Adverse effects of antiepileptic drugs. In: Ward AA, Penry JK, Purpura DP, eds. *Epilepsy.* New York: Raven Press, 1983.

Elwes RDC, Johnson AL, Shorvon SD, Reynold EH. The prognosis for seizure control in newly diagnosed epilepsy. *N Engl J Med* 1984;311:944–7.

Gowers WR. *Epilepsy and other chronic convulsive diseases.* 2nd ed. London: J & A Churchill, 1901: 250.

Hunter RA. Status epilepticus: history, incidence and problems. *Epilepsia* 1959/1960;1:162–88.

---

[1] The previous four paragraphs are modified from Pedley TA, Hauser WA. Classification and differential diagnosis of seizures and epilepsy. In: Hauser WA, ed. *Current trends in epilepsy: a self-study course for physicians.* Unit I. Landover, MD: Epilepsy Foundation of America, 1988:8.

Managing Seizure Disorders: A Handbook for Health Care Professionals, edited by N. Santilli, Lippincott-Raven Publishers, Philadelphia, 1996. © 1996 Epilepsy Foundation of America.

4

Overview of Treatment Issues

Fritz E. Dreifuss, James R. Schimschock, and Tess L. Sierzant

DIAGNOSTIC WORKUP

No diagnosis of epilepsy can be arrived at without a careful history. This includes an exact description of the seizures as well as antecedent factors, including the mother's pregnancy, the process of birth, and the child's developmental history. This must include a history of previous illnesses, possible complications of vaccination, and a history of head injury, child abuse, or encephalopathic illnesses. The family history is of utmost importance.

The diagnosis of epilepsy is made on the basis of a variety of criteria and studies. First of all, a thorough physical and neurologic examination is completed. The clinical presentation of the individual is established not only to provide pertinent information regarding the current health status but to serve as a baseline from which future changes, if any, can be identified. Laboratory data are also obtained to establish a reference point and to determine any contribution of metabolic factors to the occurrence of seizures. For example, a person with undiagnosed diabetes could be experiencing swings in blood glucose that might account for seizures. Laboratory studies are also important for identifying the possible effects of antiepileptic drugs (AEDs) on liver or bone marrow function. Some elevation of liver function parameters is seen in many people receiving AEDs.

A detailed seizure history must be obtained. This should include birth history, developmental history, any possible precipitating factors (e.g., trauma or infectious processes), and a comprehensive description of the seizures themselves. The person with epilepsy may not always be able to give a good account of the seizures, and this must therefore be amplified by an observer who can detail such nuances as the presence of focal features, the nature of the beginning of the attack, and whether there is immediate return of awareness or a prolonged period of confusion. In most situations, it is therefore crucial to obtain a description from a person who has witnessed the seizure activity. Specific questions should be asked regarding each phase of the seizure activity (i.e., before, during, and after), because approaching the interview in an open-ended fashion usually yields incomplete information. The availability of video cameras allows individuals to produce visual examples of their seizures for professional review. At present, however, nothing can substitute for a detailed description of the event, as home videotapes may not be produced with sufficient technical detail.

Physical Assessment

The physical examination is the portion of the evaluation that may detect signs of localized brain abnormality. This can be evidenced by a functional deficit such as weakness, sensory disturbance, reflex alteration, and disorders of the thought processes or memory.

The electroencephalogram (EEG) is an integral part of the diagnosis and treatment of epilepsy. The EEG provides information regarding the electrophysiologic activity of the brain, and identification of the various patterns and waveforms can aid in diagnosis. Routine EEGs are usually obtained every 2–5 years. They are performed more often when the seizure pattern has changed, when epilepsy surgery is being considered or has been performed, and when the patient's clinical presentation has changed.

The α-rhythm is the primary background rhythm seen in the posterior portions of the brain. These are waves that occur within a specified frequency of 8–13 Hz. Variations from this frequency can indicate a pathologic condition, such as medication toxicity or an encephalopathic process. Interictal activity (an ictus is an event or a rhythmical stress, and here refers to the occurence of a seizure), or that which occurs between seizures, can also be diagnostic. Spikes, sharp waves, and slowing are abnormal variations that can be seen on an EEG. θ- and δ-waves are those that occur at frequencies less than α-activity, and except in the case of a sleeping individual are considered abnormal. The EEG of a person who is sleeping progresses through various stages, and variations in this progression can also be of help in the diagnosis.

A variety of techniques are available for use in EEG monitoring. The most reliable is the video EEG, in which the individual is viewed by a video camera and is simultaneously wired for EEG. This provides an opportunity to view the clinical event and the EEG at the same time. Activation procedures, such as photic stimulation with a strobe light at a variety of frequencies, hyperventilation, and sleep deprivation, may produce changes on the EEG, and in some individuals may actually stimulate seizure activity. The choice of technique is dependent on a variety of factors, including availability, patient age, and degree of clarification needed. Intensive monitoring for epilepsy is becoming more widely available. The term usually indicates an ability to perform prolonged video and EEG monitoring. In about 5–10% of patients, intensive video and EEG monitoring may be necessary to provide a definitive diagnosis and to exclude conditions other than epilepsy as etiologic in the episodes of loss of consciousness.

It is crucial to remember that a normal EEG does not exclude the diagnosis of epilepsy. It is not uncommon for a 2- or even a 4-h tracing to be completely normal. Therefore, the EEG cannot be relied on as the sole determinant of the diagnosis; the subjective report and the other objective findings are also important contributing factors.

Specialized diagnostic imaging techniques include computed tomography (CT), magnetic resonance imaging (MRI), and positron emission tomography (PET). Virtually all persons with epilepsy undergo CT or MRI. It is important to determine whether structural abnormalities, such as tumor or arteriovenous malformation, are contributing to the epilepsy. In some situations, surgery may become necessary if the lesion proves to be progressive. In the majority of situations, however, a structural cause for seizures cannot be determined.

MRI is a particularly useful technique for evaluating brain structure without subjecting the individual to dye injections or radiation. However, injection of gadolinium as a contrast agent may greatly enhance the usefulness of the MRI and may demonstrate lesions not visible by other means. A radiologic imaging study is essential in patients with focal epilepsy and is often useful in the generalized epilepsies. MRI has eclipsed CT scanning in the majority of cases, largely because of the MRI's ability to obtain coronal and sagittal images in addition to the axial images of a CT scan, the use of a magnetic field and radio waves to create the image rather than the ionizing radiation of the CT scan, making it safer in many respects, and the improved resolution of the images obtained. However, a contrast-enhanced CT scan can prove invaluable for diagnosis of a vascular tumor. Repetition of a structural study may be indicated when the clinical examination of the patient changes or when there is a significant change in seizure frequency, type, or duration. Evaluation of the medication regimen would, in these situations, take place concomitantly. Some physicians obtain routine structural studies every 5 years regardless of the patient's clinical status.

Selected individuals benefit from PET scanning, which records glucose metabolism by brain cells as a means of locating areas of abnormal activity. Localization of these areas is particularly important when surgical intervention is being considered.

Neuropsychological evaluation may also be a part of the diagnostic process. Information regarding higher cortical functions, such as memory, concentration, and cognitive flexibility, as well as personality assessment, may prove helpful. Standardized tests used in various batteries are administered, with the pattern of test results contributing information regarding any toxic effects of the AEDs, localization of dysfunction relative to other areas of the brain, and overall intellectual capacity. This information can be very important for academic and vocational planning.

DRUG THERAPY

The goal of management with medications is twofold: maximal control of seizures with minimal medications and side effects. Many patients with epilepsy must continue to take medications throughout their lifetimes. More than half of these patients are completely controlled with medications. An additional 20–30% experience improvement, and the remainder, unfortunately, are intractable. It is important to remember, however, that approximately 70% of people with epilepsy can be expected to enter remission, defined as 5 years without seizures. Further, once they remain seizure-free for 2–5 years, 75% of these patients can be successfully withdrawn from medication (Hauser and Hesdorffer, 1990).

Determination of the most appropriate medication is based on a variety of factors. First, the type of seizure plays a major role. Treatment for partial seizures is different from that for primary generalized seizures. However, there are no hard-and-fast "rules" to be followed in this regard. Medications believed to be effective only in the case of certain seizure types may, in certain instances, be effective for other types. One important principle, however, is that the medication trials should be performed in a systematic fashion; random changes in medications, inadequate trial periods, failure to reach maximally tolerated dosages, and simultaneous changes in medication dosages can affect the objective determination of a medication's effectiveness.

Second, lifestyle factors should be taken into account. Economic considerations play a role, because some AEDs are more expensive than others. Patients may "spread out" their doses at the end of a month or pay period because they are unable to afford more medication to meet the prescribed dosing schedule until the arrival of their next paycheck or support check. Generic preparations of the AEDs are becoming more widely available, and in some health plans are mandated. Although these may sometimes be more affordable, it is important that the same generic preparation be consistently used to monitor its efficacy accurately. Changes in generic brands purchased by pharmacies can contribute to fluctuations in blood levels of the medications, and thus may have an ultimate impact on seizure control. It is important for the health care provider with whom the patient is working, be it nurse, physician, or pharmacist, to be aware of the patient's use of generic medications.

In addition to economic considerations, the patient's understanding of the need to take medication, the acceptance of this need, and the ability to remember to take the medications at the prescribed times must be taken into consideration. Dosing three or four times a day may be more difficult for some patients than once- or twice-daily dosing. In some cases, a medication with a longer half-life would be more appropriate if the patient remembers twice daily dosing more consistently.

Monotherapy (i.e., treatment with a single medication) is usually adequate to achieve seizure control. In fact, a higher dose of a single medication may be better tolerated than when a lower dose of the same medication is used in combination with other drugs. More is not necessarily better in the management of seizures. A lesser number of medications at higher doses may produce fewer side effects and provide the same or even better seizure control than multiple medications. If additional medications are required, only one should be added at a time so that its efficacy, as well as any side effects, can be determined. The greater the number of medications being taken, the greater the chance for drug interactions, side effects, and toxicity. Fine tuning of doses may be a time-consuming and frustrating process.

Introduction of AEDs should be initiated with a single drug of choice, depending on the type of seizure under consideration. The drugs should be administered on an mg/kg basis and carefully monitored with drug level determinations. Monitoring weight changes for dosage determination is critical, especially in children. The drugs should be pushed to levels of toxicity if seizures are not controlled. If this is unsuccessful, an alternative drug should be started and the first drug gradually withdrawn. Throughout this process, re-evaluation of the patient may be necessary for confirmation of diagnosis both of epilepsy and of seizure type. Results of treatment are usually better in persons with primary epilepsy, i.e., those in whom there is no underlying structural neurologic disorder as evidenced by neurologic abnormalities, delay in neurologic development, mental retardation, or evidence of progressive neurologic deficit. Prognosis is more favorable when response to treatment is good.

An important principle of medication management is to treat the individual, not the blood level. Although therapeutic ranges have been designated for most AEDs and the majority of patients respond best when their levels are maintained within these ranges, some patients achieve good seizure control below the established therapeutic range. Conversely, there are patients whose doses must be pushed to a point above the therapeutic range before control is achieved but who do not experience side effects. A therapeutic range should be determined for each individual, and predetermined laboratory values should serve only as guidelines. Treat the individual, not the level.

Two definitions are helpful in understanding how dosing is determined and when an accurate blood level can be obtained. First, the half-life of a medication is the amount of time required for half of the drug to be metabolized by the body. The level of the medication in the blood therefore drops by one-half over the period of the half-life. For example, carbamazepine has a half-life of 9–19 h. Therefore, if the level in the blood is 10 μg/ml at 8 A.M., it would be expected to be 5 μg/ml 9 to 19 h later if no additional doses are taken. To maintain a steady level of the medication in the blood, it is important to base the dosage relative to the half-life. Phenobarbital has a long half-life and can usually be dosed once per day; valproate has a much shorter half-life and must be taken more frequently.

The second definition helpful to remember is steady state. This is the amount of time required for the medication to reach a relatively constant level in the blood, with only minor peak–trough variations when maintenance medications are taken properly. Steady state is usually reached in about five half-lives of the medication. It is therefore apparent that steady state is reached more rapidly with some medications than with others. A loading dose (i.e., an amount based on body weight that will increase the level more rapidly than if a daily maintenance dose only is taken) can be given when the drug is first introduced. The patient will be more prone to side effects if a loading dose is given, although most individuals tolerate them without difficulty. When side effects do occur they are usually short-lived. Medications with a longer half-life are usually the ones that would be initiated with a loading dose.

In addition to drug therapy, careful instruction of the person with epilepsy and significant others is essential to achieve compliance through understanding of the need for continuous therapy for prolonged periods of time. Lack of understanding of the effect of medications, including side effects, is a major cause of noncompliance (see Chap. 13 for further information on compliance). Choice of drug includes attention to the age and occupation of the patient. For example, a teenaged patient may respond better to a drug given once a day than one requiring repeated administration, which may be forgotten in the press of the day's activities. The choice of drug may also be influenced in a female patient by considerations of potential teratogenicity if she is sexually active. The effects of birth control medications, of anticoagulants, and of antibiotics may have to be carefully considered and discussed. Concurrent use of other pharmacologic agents should be carefully reviewed and discussed for possible interactions. This is especially true for birth control pills, anticoagulants, antibiotics, and antihistamines.

Factors that can precipitate seizures, such as sleep deprivation, light/dark pattern stimulation, and alcohol and recreational drugs must be discussed with patients. These factors and how they may affect the patient are a part of the overall therapeutic plan in which the person with epilepsy is an active and informed participant. Ultimately, these factors should also be considered when the time has come for a decision about discontinuation of medications.

BLOOD LEVEL MONITORING

Evaluation of the effect of AEDs takes into account, most importantly, the subjective report of the patient regarding response to the medication. In addition, monitoring of the level of drug in the blood and for potential hematologic, hepatic, or renal effects, must take place. Blood levels are obtained after a medication has reached steady state following a dosage adjustment, when a change in seizure frequency, duration, or type occurs, or when toxicity is suspected. Routine monitoring of levels and other parameters in individuals whose seizures are controlled is done every 6–12 months.

Once AED therapy has been commenced, drug level monitoring is important to optimize management. Each drug has a therapeutic range that has been statistically defined as the blood level range most likely to be associated with seizure control and least likely to be associated with side effects, although this range may vary from patient to patient. In addition to routine laboratory determinations by gas chromatography or high-pressure liquid chromatography (HPLC) assays, the AccuLevel assay can be used. Blood obtained from a finger-stick is used and the level is determined in approximately 20 min. A color bar is used to compare results to a reference scale. The use of such an efficient assay holds promise for the long-term monitoring of medication levels.

Because of potential effects on liver, renal, and bone marrow function, other laboratory studies should be obtained, including CBC, SMAC, liver enzymes, platelet count, and red cell folate. Acceptance of various degrees of abnormal laboratory results varies from physician to physician, and no "general rule" can be provided. There are, for example, those who tolerate virtually no decrease in white cell count below the normal lower limit, whereas others are comfortable if the white cell count drops no lower than $2,000,000/mm^2$. Likewise, for liver function studies, some physicians accept values of twice the top of the normal range, whereas others change medications with virtually any change in liver functions studies. It is therefore important to determine the acceptable limits of the individual's physician and to work within those parameters.

When more than one drug is used, drug interactions may change the blood levels. Therefore, more frequent monitoring may be necessary. Blood levels may be influenced by intercurrent illnesses, particularly those that affect the liver or kidney and those that may interfere with absorption of the AED from the gastrointestinal tract. Patients with intercurrent illnesses require more frequent blood level monitoring. Hormonal changes, particularly around the menses and during pregnancy, may lead to alterations in drug metabolism. Likewise, maturation of the person from childhood to adulthood can lead to metabolic changes, with alterations in blood levels that may mandate modification of the dose. Finally, blood level estimations are essential for information concerning compliance. There is evidence that compliance increases proportionately to the frequency of blood level monitoring (Porter, 1983).

When a patient does not respond to medication in the expected way, and when there is a question of drug compliance or drug interactions, intensive blood level monitoring under controlled conditions may be necessary. Rapid and accurate blood level monitoring technology is now available, making it easier to manage such situations.

For drugs that are highly bound to protein, entry of the drug into the nervous system is predicted on the portion of the drug that is free. Free blood levels may have to be obtained when the therapeutic efficacy is less than expected or when neurologic toxicity is greater than expected. Not all laboratories are equipped to run free AED blood levels. When a free level is needed, serum can be sent to a laborabory equipped to perform the analysis.

It is essential with all AEDs to know their pharmacologic characteristics, such as elimination half-life, for dosage frequency to be determined. It is important to realize the relationship of half-life to steady state so that the blood levels can be performed at the most appropriate times. Trough serum blood levels (before first morning dose, except when a drug is taken only at bedtime) are commonly performed. This is necessary because some of these drugs have large drug level fluctuations in relation to dosing times. A discussion of currently available agents and drugs under investigation can be found in Chap. 5.

SPECIALIZED CENTERS

Persons with uncomplicated epilepsy can be successfully managed by individual neurologists or primary care physicians without the assistance of other members of a comprehensive specialized team. Even in these cases, an initial and comprehensive evaluation or periodic consultation by a specialized team may be helpful or necessary. When people are compromised or devastated by their seizure disorders, referral to a specialized center is warranted.

A number of specialized centers exist around the country. A full range of services might include a thorough inpatient medical evaluation in a center with dedicated epilepsy beds for intensive EEG and video monitoring that can be done for extended periods of time and with presurgical evaluation as well as the surgery itself. These centers should include a nurse, psychologist, social worker, and/or vocational or educational counselor with expertise in the management of epilepsy. Smaller centers may not perform surgery or have long-term monitoring capabilities but might have a neurologist specializing in epilepsy and inpatient and outpatient facilities suitable for evaluation of some patients. The need for a specialized center will depend on the patient's unique set of circumstances. As a general rule, if the patient is still experiencing seizures and/or side effects from AED treatment after 18 months, then referral to a specialized epilepsy center is usually warranted.

EFA maintains a database of individual physicians and specialized centers around the country. For additional information, refer to Appendix D.

KETOGENIC DIET[1]

Although this diet itself is not a drug, the metabolic products of the diet act as pharmacological agents. The ketogenic diet is accepted for the treatment of intractable seizures in childhood. Although the idea may be helpful in other seizure types, it has been used primarily to treat severe childhood epilepsy with infantile spasms, atypical absence, myoclonic, tonic, and atonic seizures.

The diet consists of foods that are high in fat and low in carbohydrate and protein. Usually the ratio at the beginning of the diet is three to four parts fat to one part protein and carbohydrate. The beneficial component of the diet is not clear, although many investigators feel that the ketone bodies may have an antiepileptic effect.

Reference materials are available for diet planning and recipe selection. A hospital stay is indicated to get the child started. Usually the diet begins with

---

[1] Adapted from Holmes, 1987.

a period of fasting from 2 to 3 days until the urine becomes positive for ketone bodies, although in rare cases a longer fast is required. Transient hypoglycemia is not unusual during the fasting and requires no action unless the child becomes symptomatic. Once the diet is initiated, it is important for the child to remain ketotic. The parents can monitor this at home using urine specimens. A great deal of care must be exercised when other medications are being administered, as these may contain sugar to make them more palatable for children. In addition, vitamin supplements are recommended, including vitamin D at 500 IU per day to prevent osteomalacia.

A medium-chain triglyceride (MCT) regimen may be used instead of the conventional ketogenic regimen. This regimen has the advantage of providing more carbohydrate and protein; however, gastrointestinal side effects, including cramping and diarrhea, are more common and occasionally preclude its chronic use.

Drug interactions with the ketogenic diet have not been well studied. For example, in some individuals serum levels of phenytoin and phenobarbital may increase, and the use of valproate while on this diet can cause potential metabolic problems.

Children may be maintained on the ketogenic diet for months or years with no significant side effects. Hyperuricemia may accompany the ketogenic diet but only rarely leads to renal calculi. Like other antiepileptic drugs, the ketogenic diet should be tapered rather than stopped abruptly. This can be accomplished by gradually reducing the ratio of fat to carbohydrate until the child resumes a normal diet.

UNPROVEN APPROACHES

In recent years techniques such as chiropractic manipulation, megavitamin therapy, elimination diets, biofeedback, and relaxation therapy have gained increasing attention. However, their effectiveness has not been established. These approaches should not take the place of antiepileptic medication, nor should they be undertaken without the knowledge of the treating physician.

REFERENCES

Hauser WA, Hesdorffer DC. *Facts about epilepsy.* New York: Demos Publications, 1990.

Holmes GL. *Diagnosis and management of seizures in children.* Philadelphia: WB Saunders Company, 1987:101–103.

Porter RJ. Intractable seizures. In: Browne TR, Feldman RG, eds. *Epilepsy: diagnosis and management.* Boston: Little, Brown, 1983:355–61.

Managing Seizure Disorders: A Handbook for Health Care Professionals, edited by N. Santilli, Lippincott-Raven Publishers, Philadelphia, 1996. © 1996 Epilepsy Foundation of America.

5

Selection and Discontinuation of Antiepileptic Drugs[1]

Nancy Santilli

Two aspects of seizure management deserve special attention: the chance for recurrence of seizures and the need for a comprehensive approach to therapy.

The patient should be carefully evaluated to determine whether recurrent seizures are likely and the risks associated with recurrence. The findings vary and must be balanced against the risks and benefits of the proposed treatment. It is important to remember that the patient and family, not the physician, must incur the consequences and benefits of either treatment or nontreatment. Therefore, the decision to initiate therapy must be made by them, aided by the physician's advice.

The second important aspect is comprehensive management. Whether or not antiepileptic drug (AED) treatment is initiated, management should always be comprehensive. Such an approach should include a thorough understanding by the individual and family of (a) what seizures are and are not, (b) how to manage a recurrent seizure should one occur, (c) realistic adaptations that may need to be made to avoid secondary problems, and (d) the quality-of-life issues faced by every person with epilepsy.

THE DECISION TO INITIATE THERAPY

The likelihood of recurrence depends on the seizure type, the type of epilepsy, and perhaps on age. For a child who experiences a single generalized tonic–clonic seizure, the chance for recurrence may be as high as 30%. A study by Shinnar et al. (1990) suggests that for the child who is otherwise normal, with a relatively normal EEG, the chance for a second seizure may be as low as 15%. For the child who is neurologically abnormal or has an abnormal EEG, the chance for a second tonic–clonic seizure may be as high as 50–60%. Whether

---

[1]Adapted from *Students with seizures: a manual for school nurses.* This chapter includes material adapted with permission from the following sources: Dodson, 1987; Leppik, 1988; Santilli and Sierzant, 1987; Shinnar and Kang, 1988; and Vining and Freeman, 1988.

these numbers are considered high or low depends on the age of the child and the attitude of the family.

Children with absence seizures or partial complex seizures are rarely identified after a single first seizure. Most likely, brief episodes of staring have occurred before the condition was recognized as a seizure disorder. Therefore, the chance for recurrence or continuance of these seizure types is high.

The consequences of recurrence must be weighed in conjunction with all these chances for recurrence. Children differ from adults with seizures because the consequences of a recurrence depend on the person's age. The adult who experiences a single seizure may suffer severe consequences should a second generalized tonic–clonic seizure occur. Fear, embarrassment, or the possibility of losing a job or driving privileges may lead the adult to elect treatment to prevent a recurrence. In children, the consequences of a recurrence vary with age. For the school-aged child or the adolescent, embarrassment may also be a severe problem, and the fear of losing driving privileges may have a major effect. Such consequences would not affect young children. Although injury and death are more common in persons with seizures, the increment in risk for those who have had only one or two seizures is probably not substantial.

DRUG SELECTION

Medical management is aimed at control of seizures using the fewest number of AEDs possible, with minimal side effects. AEDs provide complete control for more than half of patients with epilepsy and partial control in another 20–30% (i.e., they have fewer seizures but are not seizure-free); the remaining 20% of cases are intractable.

With regard to the issue of control, consideration must be given to the seizure type and frequency. Achieving seizure control with minimal side effects relies on several principles. It is essential that the diagnosis be as accurate as possible because treatment for partial seizures differs from that for primarily generalized seizures. In addition, data collection is crucial, as the AEDs are specific for various seizure types. Periodic reassessment is indicated because the course of epilepsy is not predictable and the degree of seizure control is not static.

In most cases, seizures can be controlled with monotherapy. The AED should be started at a low average dosage that is gradually increased until seizures are prevented or until side effects become intolerable. Several AEDs should be tried alone before more than one drug is given simultaneously (polytherapy). When polytherapy is necessary, only one new medication should be added at a time so that the causes of side effects or toxicity can be properly assigned. The process can be frustrating, time-consuming, and tedious, as it requires fine adjustments in dosage and administration schedules.

Selection of an AED must be individualized and is based on several factors, the primary consideration being seizure type or type of epilepsy. Other factors include potential side effects, half-life, and cost of the prescribed medication, as

TABLE 1. *Antiepileptic medications*

Generic name	Trade name	Therapeutic dosage	Therapeutic AED level	Seizure type	Common side effects
Carbamazepine	Tegretol	10–15 mg/kg/day Half-life: 9–19 h	4–12 µg/ml	Secondary tonic–clonic Complex partial Simplex partial	Lethargy, dizziness, ataxia, behavioral changes, blurred or double vision, aplastic anemia
Clonazepam	Klonopin	0.05–0.20 mg/kg/day Half-life: 18–20 h	20–80 µg/ml	Absence Myoclonic	Drowsiness, slurred speech, double vision, behavior changes, increased salivation
Divalproex sodium, Valproate	Depakote Depakene	20–60 mg/kg/day Half-life: 6–18 h	50–150 µg/ml	Myoclonic Absence, tonic–clonic, mixed seizure types	Hair loss, tremor, elevated liver enzymes, irregular menses, increased appetite, nausea and vomiting (not as common with Depakote)
Ethosuximide	Zarontin	15–35 mg/kg/day Half-life: 24–72 h	40–100 µg/ml	Absence	GI upset, loss of appetite, headache, lethargy, behavior changes, dizziness
Phenobarbital	Luminal	4–6 mg/kg/day Half-life: 53–104 h	10–40 µg/ml	Tonic–clonic	Changes in sleep pattern, drowsiness, excitability, irritability, cognitive impairment
Phenytoin	Dilantin	5–10 mg/kg/day Half-life: 7–22 h	10–25 µg/ml	Tonic–clonic Complex partial Simple partial	Nystagmus, blurred or double vision, gingival hyperplasia, ataxia, skin rash, folate deficiency
Primidone	Mysoline	12–25 mg/kg/day Half-life: 3–12 h	5–12 µg/ml	Tonic–clonic Complex partial Simple partial	Drowsiness, hyperactivity in children, ataxia, behavior changes

Adapted with permission from Santilli and Sierzant, 1987.

well as the age of the patient, the acceptance of the treatment plan by the patient and family, and the use of other chronic medication, as in the case of the elderly. Table 1 contains a list of common AEDs.

RISKS AND BENEFITS

Although the obvious benefit of AED therapy is prevention of seizures, this is achieved in only about 70% of cases. If the drug causes no side effects and is efficacious, the individual will have the opportunity to pursue a seizure-free life. However, side effects occur in 30–40% of people and must be carefully monitored. These range from life-threatening problems, such as liver failure and other severe idiosyncratic reactions, to changes in appearance, behavior, and cognitive function. After weighing the unknown risks posed by a second seizure against the unclear benefits of initiating treatment after a single generalized tonic–clonic seizure, most physicians elect to counsel and educate parents rather than to administer medication to such children. However, the risks are greater for teenagers, adults, and the elderly.

The effectiveness of AEDs in preventing recurrence of a single generalized tonic–clonic seizure is open to question. In several studies the recurrence rate after treatment of a single generalized tonic–clonic seizure with carbamazepine or phenytoin appeared to be similar to the rate in untreated cases. Therefore, it is not clear that administering AEDs after a first seizure will prevent recurrence. However, for the individual who has had recurrent seizures (two, three, or many), AED therapy is clearly preferable to recurrence. The choice of the drug depends on the type of seizure or the type of epilepsy.

SPECIAL CONSIDERATIONS

Phenobarbital, which is the cheapest AED and the easiest to use, has substantial effects on learning and behavior. Hyperactivity occurs in 40% of children given this drug. Sleep disturbances and irritability are common, as are subtle effects on learning and behavior that are difficult to detect. Unlike the adult, who may complain of mild sedation, the child, who is less articulate, and the family, who are less aware of the child's true potential, may often not recognize these subtle disabling effects until after the AED has been discontinued and they note dramatic improvement in personality and performance. The same may be true for the elderly. Mild sedation, irritability, and forgetfulness may be confused with senility.

Phenytoin can cause hirsutism and gum hyperplasia. These cosmetic effects alone may preclude use of this medication as a first-line drug in some people.

Severe and even fatal liver damage can occur with *sodium valproate.* The incidence of fatal hepatic dysfunction among children 0–2 years old who are receiving polytherapy with valproate is approximately one in 500. Even monotherapy in this age group has a fatality rate of approximately 1 in 7,000. The

TABLE 2. *New antiepileptic drugs*

Drug	Therapeutic dosage (mg/day)	Status in USA
Felbamate	1,800–3,600	Approved July, 1993
Gabapentin	600–2,400	Approved December, 1993
Lamotrigine	300–700	Approved December, 1994

rate decreases considerably above the age of 2, with a rate of approximately one in 12,000 when the drug is given in combination, and is even lower in people over the age of 10. Valproate is effective and safe overall, but it should be used with extreme caution in children under 2 years of age, particularly in the severely disabled group who often receive polytherapy.

NEW MEDICATIONS

Much effort has gone into the clinical testing of a number of new antiepileptic compounds during the last decade. Most have been tested against complex partial seizures. One study has involved children with the Lennox–Gastaut syndrome. Table 2 includes a list of drugs approved for use by the FDA in the past few years. New AEDs under investigation that have demonstrated some promising results are listed in Table 3.

Felbamate (Felbatol) showed minimal toxicity in animal models and in controlled human studies. Since its release, however, fatal side effects of aplastic anemia and hepatic failure have been reported, severely limiting its use. It is effective in complex partial seizures (Leppik et al., 1991) and in the Lennox–Gastaut syndrome. Its half-life is approximately 20 h. Doses of 1,800–3,600 mg/day have been used in children and adults. It has interactions with phenytoin, carbamazepine, and valproate, and appears to be best used as monotherapy.

Gabapentin (Neurontin) is a GABA-related amino acid that penetrates the blood–brain barrier. Doses of 600–2,400 mg/day have been effective in studies of add-on therapy in adults with complex partial seizures (Schmidt, 1989). It is not metabolized in the liver and therefore does not have significant interactions with standard AEDs. Somnolence, fatigue, and dizziness were the most common side effects reported in one of the clinical drug trials (Andrews et al., 1990).

TABLE 3. *Antiepileptic drugs under investigation*

Drug	Therapeutic dosage (mg/day)	Status in USA
Oxcarbazepine	900–3,600	Testing planned
Tiagabine	N/A	Clinical testing in progress
Vigabatrin	1,500–3,000	Clinical testing in progress
Zonisamide	7–10 mg/kg/day	Efficacy studies completed, safety studies pending
Topiramate	200–600 mg/day	Initial efficacy studies completed

Because its half-life is 5–7 h, t.i.d. dosing is recommended. Gabapentin poses a potential risk to the developing fetus by causing delayed ossification of bone.

Lamotrigine (Lamictal) is a phenyltriazine unrelated to any established AED. It has an elimination half-life of approximately 24 h. Studies have established its efficacy in various types of epilepsy (Binnie et al., 1987; Gram, 1989; Ramsay et al., 1991). It is well tolerated. The most common adverse effects of diplopia, drowsiness, dizziness, ataxia, headache, and nausea and vomiting are dose-related. Drug adjustments can alleviate the symptoms (Binnie et al., 1989; Jawad et al., 1989; Loiseau et al., 1990; Risner et al., 1990; Sander et al., 1990; Richens and Yuen, 1991; Wolf, 1992).

Oxcarbazepine (Trileptal) is a relative of carbamazepine now being marketed in Europe. It does not have an epoxide metabolite (Dam et al., 1989). Therefore, it has a similar therapeutic profile but improved tolerability compared to carbamazepine (Jensen and Dam, 1990).

Vigabatrin (Sabril) is an inhibitor of GABA-transaminase. It induces increases in brain GABA concentrations in animals and elevations of CSF GABA in humans. Clinical studies using doses of up to 3 g/day have shown it to be effective for complex partial seizures (Browne et al., 1987). It is not yet approved by the FDA, but is currently being tested in adults and children.

Zonisamide has been shown to be effective in a number of animal models of epilepsy. (Wilensky et al., 1984). Early human studies in the United States were suspended because of a higher than expected incidence of nephrolithiasis. However, zonisanide is now marketed in Japan and is being restudied in the United States. It appears particularly effective in myoclonic seizures (Henry et al., 1988) and is now being tested for control of complex partial seizures.

Topiramate (Topamax) is a novel AED with four potential mechanisms of action. Although not yet approved by the FDA, clinical trials have shown it to be effective in the treatment of partial seizures (Reife, 1995).

All AEDs should be used for as short a time as possible. Most authorities recommend considering withdrawal of therapy after the person has been seizure-free for 2 years for the primary epilepsies. During administration, it is essential to monitor the drug's effects on academic or vocational performance as well as the psychosocial consequences of taking medication daily and of having epilepsy. Repeated assessment of blood AED levels, to be sure that they remain within the therapeutic range, is not enough. Generally speaking, the "right" drug and dose for any given person is the drug, or combination of drugs when necessary, that will control the person's seizures with the fewest side effects. Although monotherapy is preferable to polytherapy, it is sometimes necessary to treat with more than one drug.

INTERCURRENT ILLNESS

Intercurrent illness and its therapy are sometimes associated with changes in both seizure threshold and drug levels. Precariously balanced phenytoin levels are most likely to change. Phenobarbital is eliminated very slowly and is usually unaffected. The effect of illness on carbamazepine concentrations is probably intermediate, but carbamazepine is more often affected by drug interactions. When seizures occur with fever, AED therapy is needed only during times of illness. In these situations, intermittent treatment with benzodiazepines can be particularly helpful.

Phenytoin biotransformation is modified by intercurrent illness and other factors. Infectious mononucleosis, flu immunization, streptococcal pharyngitis, and nonspecific viral illness causing fever have been implicated. During a febrile illness, phenytoin levels can decrease by approximately 50%, leading to seizure recurrence. Because there are no changes in absorption or binding, it appears that the febrile illness per se leads to accelerated phenytoin biotransformation. In one recent study, phenytoin levels fell from 16 to 8 μg/ml but phenobarbital levels were unchanged.

Among children taking a variety of AEDs, 21% had significant changes in drug levels during febrile illnesses. Four of the 14 children studied had increased carbamazepine concentrations caused by co-medication with erythromycin. Macrolide antibiotics inhibit carbamazepine elimination. Carbamazepine toxicity appears 8–12 h after erythromycin is discontinued. Trimethoprim/sulfamethoxazole caused doubling of the unbound carbamazepine fraction. Three children with fever had lowered phenobarbital levels, and one developed phenytoin toxicity. Therefore, changes in seizure control must always be evaluated in relation to concurrent illness and treatment.

DISCONTINUING ANTIEPILEPTIC DRUGS

The major risk associated with discontinuing AED therapy is seizure recurrence. Although a seizure is a dramatic and frightening event, the main impact of a brief seizure in a child is predominantly psychosocial. There is no convincing evidence that a brief seizure causes brain damage. Reports of injury associated with brief seizures in children are primarily related to loss of consciousness and the resultant fall; serious injury from a brief isolated seizure is rare. No cases of injury were reported when medications were discontinued in controlled trials that involved more than 700 subjects. In general, the physical and emotional consequences of a seizure in a child, who is usually in a supervised environment and is not yet driving, are less serious than in a teenager or an adult, who faces loss of driving privileges and possible problems with after-school or full-time employment.

When risk for recurrence is being assessed, the possibility of status epilepticus must be considered. Clinical data suggest that the risk of injury from status epilepticus in the context of AED withdrawal is low. In recent studies of almost 200 children with status epilepticus, adverse outcomes were primarily related to an underlying neurologic insult, such as meningitis or anoxia. In the absence of an acute neurologic insult, the morbidity and mortality of status are very low.

The actual incidence of status epilepticus after controlled withdrawal of medications also appears to be very low. Although the reasons for this are not completely clear, it may be related to the characteristics of the population under study and to the protective effect of withdrawing the medication gradually. Many subjects experience recurrence shortly after the initiation of withdrawal while the AED is still being tapered, and the remaining drug may offer some protection against status epilepticus. Most clinicians gradually decrease the dosage over 1–3 months. Although longer tapering periods (over several years) have been advocated and may be associated with slightly lower rates of recurrence, this practice might needlessly prolong exposure to these drugs without significantly improving the long-term outcome.

RISKS OF CONTINUING DRUG TREATMENT

AEDs are potent medications, and their continued use is associated with a variety of side effects. Drug-related morbidity must be weighed against the risk for seizures if the medications are stopped. Of special concern are the long-term side effects of AEDs, including systemic effects such as cosmetic changes, altered bone metabolism, or possible hematologic or immunologic changes. More importantly, there is now ample evidence that AED treatment causes behavioral and cognitive impairment. Although the extent of these neuropsychological effects differs among medications, probably no AED is completely free of them, even when serum levels are in the therapeutic range. Therefore, it is important to discontinue unnecessary drug therapy.

A hidden side effect of continued AED treatment is the stigma attached to this condition. A person who had epilepsy as a child, has not had a seizure for many years, and is off medication is considered to have outgrown epilepsy. Such individuals can lead normal lives with few restrictions. In contrast, remaining on chronic medication implies ongoing illness to both the person and those around him. Continued use of AEDs requires ongoing medical care to prescribe and monitor drug levels. In addition, it implies certain driver's license restrictions and may adversely affect employment and the ability to obtain health insurance. The problems associated with having epilepsy are compounded by the perception that any chronic illness will adversely affect the normal psychosocial maturation process, particularly in adolescents.

DURATION OF THERAPY

The decision about how long to treat with AEDs must be individualized and must take into account (a) the probability of the person remaining seizure-free without medications, (b) the possible adverse consequences of a seizure, and (c) the side effects of long-term AED therapy. Given the consequences of long-term treatment, it appears reasonable to attempt withdrawal of AEDs at least once in the vast majority of children and adolescents with epilepsy, regardless of risk factors, before committing them to lifelong therapy. Whatever the decision, it must be arrived at jointly between the physician and the family after careful discussion. This discussion should include not only an assessment of the risks and benefits of withdrawing medication but also a review of measures to be taken in the event of recurrence. Even children with idiopathic epilepsy who have had only a few seizures and have a normal EEG will experience recurrence in at least 10% of cases. Similarly, children at risk for recurrence may remain in remission without medications. It is far easier to take such risks while the child is still in the supervised environment of the home and school. For many families, even if the chances of success are remote, withdrawal of medications is worth pursuing.

REFERENCES

Andrews J, Chadwick D, Bates D, et al. Gabapentin. *Lancet* 1990;1:1114–17.

Binnie CD, Beintema CJ, Debets RMC, et al., Seven day administration of lamotrigine (Lamictal) for refractory partial seizures. *Epilepsy Res* 1987;1:202–8.

Binnie CD, Debets RM, Engelsman M. Double-blind crossover trial of lamotrigine (Lamictal) as add-on therapy in intractable epilepsy. *Epilepsy Res* 1989;4:222–9.

Browne TR, Mattson RH, Penry JK. Vigabatrin for refractory complex partial seizures: Multicenter single-blind study with long-term follow-up. *Neurology* 1987;37:184–9.

Dam M, Ekberg R, Loyning Y, et al. A double-blind study comparing oxcarbazepine and carbamazepine in patients with newly diagnosed, previously untreated epilepsy. *Epilepsy Res* 1989;3: 70–6.

Dodson WE. Special pharmacokinetic considerations in children. *Epilepsia* 1987;28(suppl 1):S56–70.

Gram L. Potential antiepileptic drugs: lamotrigine. In: Levy R, Mattson R, Meldrum B, et al., eds. *Antiepileptic drugs,* 3rd edition. New York: Raven Press, 1989:947–53.

Henry TR, Leppik IE, Gumnit RJ, et al. Progressive myoclonic epilepsy treated with zonisamide. *Neurology* 1988;38:928–931.

Jawad S, Richens A, Goodwin G, et al. Controlled trial of lamotrigine (Lamictal) for refractory partial seizures. *Epilepsia* 1989;30;356–63.

Jensen PK, Dam M. Oxcarbazepine. In: Dam M, Gram L, eds. *Comprehensive epileptology.* New York: Raven Press, 1990:621–9.

Leppik IE. Drug treatment of epilepsy. In: Hauser WA, ed. *Current trends in epilepsy: a self-study course for physicians.* Unit II. Landover, MD: Epilepsy Foundation of America, 1988:12–22.

Leppik IE, Dreifuss FE, Pledger GW. Felbamate for partial seizures: Results of a controlled clinical trial. *Neurology* 1991;41:1785–9.

Leppik IE, Fisher J, Kreil R, Sawchuck RJ. Altered phenytoin clearance with febrile illness. *Neurology* 1986;36:1367–70.

Loiseau P, Yuen W, Duche B, et al. A randomized, double-blind, placebo-controlled, crossover add-on trial of lamotrigine in patients with treatment-resistant partial seizures. *Epilepsy Res* 1990;7: 136–45.

Ramsay RD, Pellock JM, Garnett WR. Pharmacokinetics and safety of lamotrigine (Lamictal) in patients with epilepsy. *Epilepsy Res* 1991;10:191–200.

Reife RA. Topiramate: a novel antiepileptic agent. In: Shorvon SD, ed. *Treatment of epilepsy.* London: Blackwell Science, 1995.

Richens A, Yuen W. Overview of the clinical efficacy of lamotrigine. *Epilepsia* 1991;31(suppl 2): S13–16.

Risner M, et al. Multicenter double-blind, placebo-controlled, add-on crossover study of lamotrigine (Lamictal) in epileptic outpatients with partial seizures. *Epilepsia* 1990;31:619–20.

Santilli N, Sierzant TL. Advances in the treatment of epilepsy. *J Neurosci Nurs* 1987;19:141–58.

Sander J, Patsalos P, Oxley J, et al. A randomized, double-blind, placebo-controlled, add-on trial of lamotrigine in patients with severe epilepsy. *Epilepsy Res* 1990;6:221–6.

Schmidt D. Potential antiepileptic drugs: Gabapentin. In: Levy R, Mattson R, Meldrum B, et al., eds. *Antiepileptic drugs,* 3rd edition New York: Raven Press, 1989:925–35.

Shinnar S, Kong H. Discontinuing antiepileptic drug therapy in children with epilepsy. In: Hauser WA, ed. *Current trends in epilepsy: a self-study course for physicians.* Unit III. Landover, MD: Epilepsy Foundation of America, 1988:43–50.

Shinnar S, Berg AT, Moshe SL. Risk of seizure recurrence following a first unprovoked seizure in childhood: a prospective study. *Pediatrics* 1990;85:1076–85.

Vining EPG, Freeman JM. Epilepsy and children. In: Hauser WA, ed. *Current trends in epilepsy: a self-study course for physicians.* Unit III. Landover, MD: Epilepsy Foundation of America, 1988: 34–42.

Wilensky AJ, Friel PN, Ojemann LM. Pharmacokinetics of CI-912 in epileptic patients. In: Levy RH, Pitlick WH, Eichelbaum M, Meijer J, eds. *Metabolism of antiepileptic drugs.* New York: Raven Press, 1984:209–15.

Wolf P. Lamotrigine: Preliminary clinical observations on pharmacokinetics and interactions with traditional antiepileptic drugs. *J Epilepsy* 1992;5:73–9.

Managing Seizure Disorders: A Handbook for Health Care Professionals, edited by N. Santilli, Lippincott-Raven Publishers, Philadelphia, 1996
© 1996 Epilepsy Foundation of America.

6

Surgical Management of Seizures[1]

Nancy Santilli and Tess L. Sierzant

Although most persons with epilepsy are able to lead normal lives, approximately 20% continue to experience seizures or serious side effects from medication. In the United States, between 250,000 and 1.25 million people have disabling seizures. Refinements in diagnostic and treatment techniques have made surgery an increasingly available option for certain individuals with epilepsy. This option should be pursued after medical management has proven ineffective for certain individuals with epilepsy.

Increasingly, health care professionals play an important role in educating the patient and the family about surgery and potential outcomes. First, the health care professional must be familiar with the types of procedures available and the complex process involved in determining candidacy. All of those concerned must understand that, even after a considerable investment of time and money, surgery may be eliminated as an option because diagnostic testing may show unusual risk for postoperative complications or because the outcome would cause damage to memory and other higher cerebral functions. Second, epilepsy surgery must be presented to the patient and family as an option that offers no guarantee of success. It may be necessary to clarify information regarding surgery so that each step in the process is understood. Professionals play a key role in this regard and also in supporting the patient and family throughout the decision-making process. Third, because the decision to perform surgery and the type of surgery selected are influenced by the correlation between clinical events and EEG data, the patient's family may be asked to assist in precisely documenting the seizure type and frequency.

Finally, the health care professional may be asked to provide assessments of the patient's behavior and abilities. The ability of the patient and family to tolerate a long period of confinement, particularly with indwelling monitoring devices, is crucial to a successful outcome. Everyone involved should communicate with the treating physician about any changes observed in the patient's seizures, behavior, and academic performance, because 6–18 months may elapse between the time of the initial workup and the surgery.

---

[1] Adapted with permission from Santilli N, Sierzant T. Advances in the treatment of epilepsy. *J Neurosci Nurs* 1987;19:141–158.

Surgery offers the greatest benefit to people whose seizures originate from clearly delineated, unilateral, anterior temporal lobe foci. Generally accepted criteria for selecting candidates for surgery were summarized by McNaughton and Rasmussen (1975). These criteria limit surgery to persons whose EEG and clinical evaluations indicate that seizures are clearly focal in origin and arise in an area of the brain that can be excised with a reasonable expectation that serious neurologic deficits will not be produced or that existing ones will not be increased.

Other surgical procedures are used as well. Localized cortical excisions are indicated in cases of simple partial epilepsy, which usually result from malformation, trauma, or infection. Surface or depth ictal EEG recording may be necessary; recordings from subdural electrodes are often helpful, and the role of a subdural grid (a map of the focal area) is widely recognized. Advances in neuroimaging techniques are decreasing the need for invasive monitoring by assisting in identifying the site and spread of epileptic foci. Other surgical procedures are corpus callosotomy and hemispherectomy. These resections are recommended in specific cases where other treatment options have been unsuccessful.

PRESURGICAL EVALUATION

Presurgical evaluation of a patient begins with a complete physical and neurologic examination and a thorough seizure history (Surgery for Epilepsy, 1994). EEG recordings and video recordings are obtained to allow the epileptologist to correlate more closely the electrical findings with clinical presentation of seizure activity. If epileptiform discharges are emanating from the temporal lobe and stereotypic activity is observed clinically, some clinical centers utilize nasopharyngeal or sphenoidal electrodes (Table 1). EEG information gathered by these means is evaluated in conjunction with surface electrode recordings. Both ictal and interictal EEGs are evaluated. Interictal recordings (made between seizures) can provide information regarding brain tissue that is more excitable. However, it is crucial to the surgical workup that ictal events be captured on EEG to localize the epileptic focus as precisely as possible. The number of events needed to clarify the diagnosis of seizure type varies from person to person. Clarification is achieved with the aid of supplemental information obtained from neuroimaging studies, neurologic and neuropsychological examinations, and clinical presentation.

If a question remains as to the epileptic focus, subdural or epidural electrode placement is used to evaluate candidates for surgery. The area of seizure focus can be mapped before, rather than during, the operation. The resection is performed after a sufficient amount of information has been gathered from the subdural or epidural electrode placement.

Depth electrode placement may be employed to obtain additional EEG data. Mapping the areas of depth electrode placement is completed using CT or MRI techniques. A highly specific computer program is employed, with coordinates determined by CT or MRI. The electrodes must be inserted carefully in the precise location to monitor structures deep in the brain. There is a waiting period after removal of the electrodes before the resection can be performed.

Determining hemispheral dominance is essential in presurgical evaluation for temporal lobectomy, because the dominant hemisphere usually contains the speech center. This parameter is assessed by the *Wada* or *amobarbital test.*

Complete neuropsychological evaluation using standardized tests is also a crucial part of the presurgical workup. These tests provide information regarding higher cortical function and are of significance in localizing dysfunction. The positive correlation of EEG data with neuropsychological data provides additional support in identifying appropriate candidates for surgery.

Electrocorticographic surface brain recordings (electrodes placed directly onto the brain to identify functional areas), which can be used at the time of surgery, may help to determine the extent of a temporal resection and to identify functional areas of the cerebral cortex.

Presurgical evaluation is time-consuming, costly, and can be frustrating. To alleviate these problems, the professional can help the patient and family to understand:

The many steps in the workup

That findings from depth, subdural, or epidural electrodes may rule out surgery

That the patient is not obligated to undergo the procedure even if it is recommended

That the patient with a space-occupying lesion may be urged to have surgery

That even after spending considerable time, energy, and money there may be little or no improvement in long-term seizure control

That there are no guarantees with temporal lobectomy, corpus callosotomy, or extratemporal resections, although the chances are good that temporal resection will be successful.

TEMPORAL LOBECTOMY

Resection of the temporal lobe to treat epilepsy has been performed for many years. With recent refinements in diagnostic methods the procedure is now available to more people. It is estimated that approximately 30% of persons with partial epilepsy are not well controlled with medications and could benefit from temporal lobectomy.

Immediately after the operation most patients are monitored in an intensive care unit for 24–48 h. In addition to reviewing the components essential to the assessment of any craniotomy patient, the nursing staff should be alert for any changes in speech if the lobectomy was performed in the dominant hemisphere. Difficulty in finding words may be temporary. Frequently, vision will be lost in the upper quadrant of each eye (superior homonymous quadrantanopsia) owing to interruption of the visual pathways that pass through the temporal lobe. Although these visual deficits are permanent, they usually do not cause problems.

TABLE 1. *Neurodiagnostic approaches to epilepsy*

Type of test	Definition	Length of test	Care considerations
Routine hard-wire	Individual remains in a stationary position connected to an EEG machine	$1\frac{1}{2}$ h to unlimited length	Patient's hair must be clean. Must be prepared to stay in stationary position.
Nasopharyngeal leads	EEG lead inserted through the nares into the nasopharynx to record discharges originating from deeper mesiotemporal structures	Same length as routine EEG	Patient preparation important. Insertion of lead can be painful. Discomfort may be present throughout procedure. Leads produce artifact to respiration. Patient cannot blow nose while leads are present. Maximal toleration of electrodes usually 2 days for prolonged studies.
Sphenoidal electrodes	Inserted using sterile technique and local anesthesia, inferior to the zygomatic process and directed into the pterygopalatine fossa to obtain EEG information from the anterior mesial temporal region. The electrode is threaded through a 22-gauge $3\frac{1}{4}$ in. spinal needle. The needle is withdrawn and the electrode remains.		Risks include infection, facial paralysis, paresthesias, and bleeding. Does not require operating room. Initial discomfort when opening mouth, yawning. Eating not usually impaired, except for 1–2 days when trying to bite foods such as apples.
Sleep deprivation	EEG performed after the individual has been deprived of sleep for 24 h so that natural sleep will occur during recording. This physiologic state is an activation procedure.	2 h once patient goes to sleep	Scheduling usually requires individual to stay up all night. Can be difficult for pediatric population and/or concurrent disabilities.

Depth electrode placement	Used to help localize seizure focus. Can identify multifocal seizure onset undetectable by scalp and sphenoidal electrodes. Placed under local anesthesia using stereotactic techniques in the mesial temporal lobe, occipital lobe, hippocampus, or other area suggested by clinical and EEG data.	Several hours (includes time in radiology for CT/MRI scan and in operating room)	Operating room; checking and rechecking coordinates is time consuming. Head is shaved completely before electrode placement. Risks include intercerebral hematoma, subdural hematoma, and infection.
Subdural–epidural electrodes	Inserted via burr holes or craniectomy to monitor the EEG. Electrodes may be in strips or grid form and may substantially reduce artifact. Subdural electrodes may be stimulated to map areas of speech, motor, and sensory function.		Similar to persons undergoing neurosurgical interventions, including extensive pre- and postoperative patient instruction.
Closed circuit television (CCTV/EEG)	Video picture is obtained simultaneously with EEG recording. Can be done with any method of EEG technique, but limits mobility according to the number and position of video camera(s).	Unlimited	Individual may initially be uncomfortable with being recorded. Can serve as a visual teaching tool for the individual and family. However, can be emotionally stressful for individual to see himself having a seizure and suffering loss of privacy.
Ambulatory cassette	Ambulatory EEG monitoring allows unlimited mobility. Recording can occur while hospitalized, in school, at work, or at home	Unlimited	Outside hospital setting, patient and/or family must be responsible for regluing electrodes every 24 hours. Equipment can be concealed by wearing a hat, high collar, and jacket or bulky top. Individual may need a break in recording to wash hair. Useful to record seizure activity occurring in specific situations and/or infrequently. Assists in the differential diagnosis of seizure episodes.

continued

53

TABLE 1. *Continued.*

Type of test	Definition	Length of test	Care considerations
Telemetry	An ambulatory EEG that allows some mobility Must occur within range of an antenna; therefore, the patient's environment is limited to a given unit.	Unlimited	Requires wearing headgear to hold the recorder in place. This restricts mobility somewhat and can be uncomfortable during sleep.
Special procedures using EEG monitoring (Neonatal)	EEG recording for neonatal seizures attempt to measure state changes	2 h minimum	Explain testing to parents. Electrode placement and removal to maintain skin integrity.
Wada	Used to measure hemispheral dominance, as part of an epilepsy surgical evaluation. Usually there is simultaneous video and audio recording. Each hemisphere is anesthetized by injecting amobarbital into the carotid artery. Dysphasia or speech arrest indicates hemispheral dominance	1 to 4 h per hemisphere	The anesthetic arrests speech and produces a temporary hemiparesis lasting 20 min to 1 h after the testing session. During memory testing, speech and motor functions are assessed by immediate identification of objects and ability to read, identify shapes, and speak. Prepare for cerebral angiography and inform patient of temporary nature of paralysis. Catheter insertion and position may be uncomfortable.

From Santilli et al., 1991.

Sixty to 90% of individuals who undergo temporal lobectomy have an excellent outcome, defined as a decrease in seizure frequency of 95% or more 1 year after surgery. Therapeutic serum levels of antiepileptic drugs (AEDs) should be maintained postoperatively for 1 year, at which time tapering may be attempted.

CORPUS CALLOSOTOMY

Sectioning, or separating, the corpus callosum was first reported in the medical literature in 1940. By separating the cerebral hemispheres, the spread of an epileptic discharge can be confined to one cortex, reducing generalized seizures. Since the initial conceptualization, various combinations of interhemispheric tracts have been sectioned, although outcomes have varied greatly. This surgical technique will probably be further refined.

Indications for corpus callosotomy vary from institution to institution. The procedure may be performed when it is not possible to localize an epileptic focus or when resection of a localized focus would cause a pronounced neurologic deficit. Indications have also been defined on the basis of tonic or atonic seizures occurring several times weekly and resulting in falls and injuries, combined with EEG data indicating a secondarily generalized seizure disorder and active interictal abnormalities.

Hemispherectomy may be recommended for children with hemiparesis when the seizures are having a devastating effect on the patient. As our understanding of brain dysfunction is enhanced, surgical interventions will be recommended for a greater variety of patients with uncontrolled seizures.

Preoperative evaluation includes a complete physical and neurologic examination. A thorough seizure history is essential, including detailed descriptions from both the patient and those who have observed the seizure(s). Past and present seizure types should be noted, including age of onset, possible causative factors (e.g., trauma, infection), duration of the seizure type over the patient's lifetime, any increase or decrease in severity or frequency of seizures, duration of a single event, frequency, precipitating factors, and any pattern of occurrence. Multiple EEG recordings, CT scans, cerebral angiography, MRI, complete neuropsychological assessment, and Wada testing are also performed. The health care professional should be prepared to answer questions the patient may have about each of these procedures, either preoperatively or postoperatively.

REFERENCES

McNaughton FL, Rasmussen T. Criteria for selection of patients for neurosurgical treatment. *Adv Neurol* 1975;8:37–48.
Santilli N, Dodson WE, Walton AV, eds. *Students with seizures: a manual for school nurses.* Landover, MD: Epilepsy Foundation of America, 1991.
Surgery for epilepsy (brochure). Landover, MD: Epilepsy Foundation of America, 1994.

Managing Seizure Disorders: A Handbook for Health Care Professionals, edited by N. Santilli, Lippincott-Raven Publishers, Philadelphia, 1996.
© 1996 Epilepsy Foundation of America.

7

Prolonged Seizures (Status Epilepticus) or Serial Seizures

Tess L. Sierzant

According to the International League Against Epilepsy, "the term 'status epilepticus' is used whenever a seizure persists for a sufficient length of time or is repeated frequently enough to produce a fixed and enduring epileptic condition" (Gastaut, 1970). Difficulty in applying this definition in the clinical setting arises when one tries to clarify such terms as "sufficient length of time" or "frequently enough." More recently, the Epilepsy Foundation of America's Working Group on Status Epilepticus (1993) has defined the condition as more than 30 min of continuous seizure activity or two or more sequential seizures without full recovery of consciousness between seizures.

Any type of epileptic seizure can progress to status epilepticus. Consistent with the International Classification of Seizures presented in Chap. 3, this condition is divided into generalized and partial status epilepticus. It can also be divided into convulsive and nonconvulsive types.

The evolution of convulsive tonic–clonic seizure activity into status epilepticus is the most commonly discussed and certainly the most dangerous. Because convulsive status epilepticus (CSE) is a life-threatening condition, it is crucial for health care professionals to learn to recognize it and to be aware of the various treatment modalities. Administration of an antiepileptic drug (AED) should be initiated if a convulsive seizure has lasted for 10 min or if two or more generalized tonic–clonic seizures occur without full recovery of consciousness between them. Brain damage and death can usually be avoided with prompt and appropriate intervention.

CSE is a medical emergency. In addition to the potential for irreversible damage to the central nervous system, this condition poses a threat to life. Medications used to manage status epilepticus may have adverse effects, and knowing a patient's medication allergies is of the utmost importance. Nursing preparedness cannot be overemphasized in the management of generalized CSE.

Nonconvulsive status epilepticus includes continuous absence seizures or continuous complex partial seizures. Partial status epilepticus may present in various ways, including speech arrest, automatisms, and alteration of consciousness.

Consciousness is preserved in status with simple partial seizures, a condition sometimes called epilepsia partialis continua.

Even though nonconvulsive status epilepticus is not life-threatening, as CSE is, treatment is still important. In children, absence status epilepticus is perhaps the most commonly observed type, in which the child may exhibit a change in level of consciousness, behavior, and academic performance. The child may appear uncoordinated, clumsy, or postictal. If untreated, these problems may last for days. Diagnosis relies on demonstrating continuous generalized spike-and-wave activity on the EEG. Drug therapy varies.

Complex partial status epilepticus may also have various expressions, including altered consciousness, cessation of speech or activity, or both, and oral and motor automatisms. Diazepam and phenytoin may be used, as may intramuscular lorazepam. Prolonged periods of nonconvulsive status (absence and complex partial) interfere with academic performance, nutritional intake, and a multitude of activities of daily living.

Status epilepticus has many causes, and most people who develop it have not been previously diagnosed with epilepsy. Hauser (1990) reports that status epilepticus will occur in 50,000–60,000 individuals annually in the United States. DeLorenzo et al. (1992) estimated 250,000 cases per year, or about one per thousand. Status epilepticus will be the presenting symptom in patients with a first unprovoked seizure or with epilepsy in about one-third of these cases. In another one-third, the condition is due to an acute cerebral insult in individuals with no history of epilepsy (Hauser, 1990).

A number of these causes have been identified, including brain tumor, infections, craniocerebral trauma, cerebrovascular disease, and toxic or metabolic disorders. Among people with epilepsy who develop status epilepticus, about one-third of cases (Hauser, 1990), the most common cause is medication withdrawal or noncompliance with their prescribed medication regimen. This group can usually be identified by measuring AED levels, although in some cases these levels will be within the usual range for the individual, and no cause can be pinpointed (Cranford et al., 1979).

According to Leppik (1990), three factors contribute to morbidity and mortality secondary to status epilepticus: (a) direct damage to the brain caused by an acute insult that precipitates the condition; (b) systemic stress from repeated generalized tonic–clonic (GTC) seizures; and (c) injury from repetitive electrical discharges within the brain.

Death may occur as a result of CSE but is more frequently due to the acute precipitating illness (Cranford et al., 1979; Hauser, 1983). Although mortality was previously estimated to be 5–50%, more recent figures place the expected death rate at 10–12% for adults (Delgado-Escueta et al., 1983) and less than 5% for children. Mortality caused by status epilepticus itself has been reported to be 1–2%, but Hauser (1990) suggests that this may be an overestimate in light of the more effective methods of treatment now available.

MANAGEMENT OF CONVULSIVE (GENERALIZED TONIC–CLONIC) STATUS EPILEPTICUS

Convulsive (generalized tonic–clonic) status epilepticus (CSE) is a medical emergency requiring aggressive treatment. The subsequent quality of life for the affected individual depends on stopping the seizures as quickly as possible. If seizures last longer than 30 min, damage to the central nervous system may begin. Nurses must be able to identify the point at which a generalized convulsive seizure becomes status epilepticus and to initiate emergency interventions. To establish a time limit after which a generalized tonic–clonic seizure becomes status, one must allow for individual assessment and consider a multitude of other factors. This assessment includes, but is not limited to, the following:

Does the person have a history of epilepsy or of generalized tonic–clonic seizures that routinely last around 4 min or occur in clusters?

If the individual's seizures have been previously observed and documented, do similarities or differences exist between the present occurrence and past seizures?

Is this the first episode of seizure activity the person has ever experienced?

What medications is the person taking?

Is manipulation of medications taking place?

Is there a history or potential of street drug use?

Is there a postictal phase and adequate recovery of respiratory function and consciousness, or do the seizures continue to occur one after another?

Obtaining a complete seizure history is essential to determine whether a patient is in a dangerous seizure state.

Maintaining vital signs and oxygenation during a seizure is essential in treating status epilepticus. The affected individual should be transported promptly to an emergency facility equipped to handle this problem. Various medications are effective in treating status epilepticus, although debate continues as to which drugs are most effective and appropriate. Many comparative studies have been performed (Delgado-Escueta and Enrile-Bascal, 1983; Greenblatt and Divoll, 1983; Leppik et al., 1983; Sorel et al., 1981; Treiman et al., 1985), but no protocol has been universally agreed on. One of the most important aspects of treating this condition is identifying the cause and providing specific therapy when possible. In managing the initial phase of CSE, it is imperative that nurses know the variety of medication options available in order to anticipate specific needs and precautions in administration and to monitor correctly patient response to these medications. Ready command of the knowledge of the treatment protocol existing in one's area of professional practice is crucial to efficient management of the patient during status epilepticus. The medications most commonly administered during generalized tonic–clonic status epilepticus include diazepam, lorazepam, phenytoin, and phenobarbital.

Assessment and management of patient responses to the effects of the status epilepticus and to the medications must take place. Management of the airway is of primary importance to achieve the goal of maintenance of adequate ventilation, proper oxygenation, and minimization of potential for aspiration. Cerebral hypoxia may be a cause and a result of status epilepticus. It is desirable to administer oxygen via face mask, because nasal prongs may not provide an adequate supply. This should be verified by oximetry or arterial blood gas determinations. Use of oral, nasopharyngeal, and tracheal suction must be instituted to remove excessive secretions. Although use of an oral airway is helpful in gaining more effective access to the secretions and in providing adequate oxygenation, it may be difficult or impossible to insert and endotracheal intubation may become necessary. Seizures must be stopped to avoid injury during intubation. Short-acting barbiturates or neuromuscular blockers can be administered to temporarily stop the seizures during intubation. With a secure airway established, attention can be given to other aspects of patient management.

Vital signs must be monitored closely. Maintenance of adequate cerebral perfusion is another top priority. Initially, hypertension occurs with status epilepticus, and may persist for 30–45 min. Blood pressure may then return to baseline or below. It is important that systolic blood pressure be maintained at normal or high normal level during episodes of status, using vasopressors as necessary (Working Group on Status Epilepticus, 1993). Blood pressure checks should be done at intervals not to exceed 5 min; more frequent checks are usually necessary. During tonic–clonic activity or with a decrease in blood pressure, auscultation may prove increasingly difficult and an external monitoring device may be useful.

Tachycardia, bradycardia, and cardiac arrhythmias may occur during CSE. Use of a cardiac monitor is imperative. Attaching adhesive electrode patches may be difficult because of the excessive diaphoresis patients often experience, and additional adhesive tape may have to be applied. Tincture of benzoin applied to the skin before application of the electrodes may also be helpful.

Axillary temperature assessment may be the most accessible in this situation, but rectal determination is more accurate and desirable. One can expect an increase in temperature with episodes of CSE, primarily as a result of increased motor activity (Simon, 1985). A pronounced increase in body temperature may contribute significantly to epileptic brain damage and should be treated aggressively. The degree of elevation may be important in the determination of the underlying cause of the episode.

Intravenous access must be established during an episode of status epilepticus. Avoidance of solutions containing glucose is an accepted rule of thumb because of the precipitation that occurs when glucose is combined with some of the medications used in management. Monitoring the amount of fluid administered and avoiding overhydration (which has complications of its own) are also important. Placement of an indwelling bladder catheter is usually necessary to more accurately assess fluid status.

Various laboratory studies may be performed, including serum electrolytes, complete blood count, AED serum concentrations, glucose, calcium, and urea nitrogen. Urine and blood toxicology screens may be ordered. Arterial blood gas determinations may be made at various points during the episode. Correction of acidosis with sodium bicarbonate is not usually necessary except when the patient is severely acidotic.

Once the patient is stabilized, other diagnostic studies may follow. These include electroencephalography, lumbar puncture (although this may be done earlier in patients with fever), and brain imaging with CT or MRI. Several factors contribute to the decision as to which studies will be done, including pre-existing knowledge of the patient, the patient's clinical condition, the institutional setting, response to therapy, and suspected causes (Working Group on Status Epilepticus, 1993).

MEDICATIONS

A discussion of the various medications administered during CSE follows. Not all of the medications are routinely administered, nor is the order in which they are presented intended to convey a priority in administration. Once again, it must be emphasized that there is no universally accepted treatment protocol. Knowledge of the institution-specific protocol is a key nursing responsibility. Knowing a patient's medication allergies is also of utmost importance. An allergy to phenytoin, for example, obviously would preclude administration of this mainstay of management.

Many drugs are effective in the treatment of CSE. They must be administered promptly and in adequate doses. Nurses play an essential role in the successful treatment of CSE. A key principle is that both short-acting and long-acting medications are usually needed for effective management. The short-acting benzodiazepines are administered initially in patients who are actively having seizures. Because of their short-acting nature, the benzodiazepines are followed with administration of a long-acting agent, most usually phenytoin. The benzodiazepines will in most cases stop the seizures long enough to allow administration of the longer-acting agent.

Glucose

Glucose was once routinely administered to patients with generalized CSE. Most of the time, hyperglycemia occurs initially, followed by hypoglycemia caused by the early increase in insulin secretion. It is important to determine blood glucose when possible and then to administer 50 ml of 50% glucose (in adults) i.v. if hypoglycemia is present. The Working Group on Status Epilepticus (1993) recommends administration of 100 mg of thiamine before glucose administration (see also Slovis and Wrenn, 1994).

Diazepam

Diazepam, a potent benzodiazepine, is in many instances the first medication administered to a patient in CSE. A main advantage of use is its rapid onset of action, with the majority of GTC seizures being stopped within 5 min (Delgado-Escueta et al., 1983). However, it has a short central nervous system half-life, and therefore seizures may recur in 15–20 min. Diazepam is usually used to "buy time" until longer-acting medications can be infused. Other disadvantages include its potential for depression of respiration, hypotension, and cardiac arrhythmias. Recommended rate of infusion is no greater than 2 mg/min, with an initial dose of 5–10 mg. A total dose of 20 mg is not unusual, with some patients requiring more. Continuous diazepam infusion can be used in patients who do not respond to more conventional treatment. Intramuscular administration is not recommended because of its erratic absorption from the tissues. Rectal diazepam is being used more often to terminate prolonged or frequently repeated serial seizures in patients with severe epilepsy, particularly children. A school nurse or family member may be asked to administer it under the guidance of a physician as emergency treatment.

Lorazepam

Lorazepam, another potent benzodiazepine, has been studied extensively (Greenblatt and Divoll, 1983; Leppik et al., 1983; Levy and Krall, 1984; Treiman et al., 1985) for use in treatment of CSE. Some advantages of lorazepam include its longer central nervous system half-life, the rapidity with which it can be administered, and its safety compared to other medications used in management of CSE. For these reasons it is becoming the benzodiazepine of choice. As with diazepam, administration of a long-acting medication usually follows. The primary side effect is sedation; others that may be observed include respiratory depression, confusion, and hallucinations. To administer i.v. lorazepam correctly, it must be diluted with an equal volume of compatible diluent. Doses that have been utilized range from 2 to 10 mg (Levy and Krall, 1984). One study (Leppik et al., 1983) recommended administration of an initial dose of 4 mg followed by another 4 mg if seizures have not stopped in 10 min. Administration over 2 min is recommended (Coniglio and Garnett, 1989).

Phenytoin

Phenytoin is often used in the management of status epilepticus. One of its hallmark advantages is its long half-life compared to the benzodiazepines. Another is its relative lack of central nervous system depression. However, there are disadvantages, including potential for cardiac arrhythmias because of the prophylene glycol vehicle in which phenytoin is contained and the time required for administration of a full loading dose, 18–20 mg/kg with rate of administration recommended at no greater than 50 mg/min. Even this rate may have to be slowed because of patient intolerance of the burning at the i.v. site or development of hypotension or cardiac arrhythmias. Continuous i.v. infusion is the safest method of administration. Direct i.v. push of this medication must be done with caution; some institutions require a physician to be present during an i.v. push loading dose. Cardiac and blood pressure must be closely monitored throughout the administration. Intramuscular administration is discouraged because phenytoin may precipitate at the injection site and is quite painful when given in this manner. In addition, as with diazepam, absorption when administered intramuscularly is erratic at best. A new form of phenytoin, a prodrug, is being developed and may be available for both intramuscular and intravenous use in the future.

Phenobarbital

Phenobarbital has proven to be effective with both partial and generalized seizures. It has the advantage of a very long half-life and can be given fairly rapidly. It is, in fact, the drug of choice in some institutions for management of CSE. Its primary disadvantage is its depressive effect on the respiratory status and the level of consciousness. The loading dose is 20 mg/kg and the rate of administration should not exceed 100 mg/min. Care should be taken if phenobarbital is given after a dose of diazepam, because the depressive effects may be more pronounced.

Paraldehyde

Paraldehyde can be given orally, intravenously, or rectally. It is rarely the first medication administered for status. Intravenous administration is recommended as a 4% solution of the medication in normal saline. Because the medication is sensitive to light and air, care must be taken to store it properly. Unused portions should be discarded 24 h after opening (Browne, 1983). Glass utensils and equipment should be used for administration, as the drug tends to decompose plastic. This has implications for all routes of administration. Availability of this agent is scarce, and it therefore has limited usage.

Last Resorts

These include pentobarbital coma (Yaffe and Lowenstein, 1993) and general anesthesia. When pentobarbital coma is utilized for management of status epilepticus, the EEG should be monitored continuously for burst-suppression activity. Labar et al. (1994) report on the use of high-dose lorazepam as an alternative to pentobarbital coma. Use of midazolam (Kumar and Bleck, 1992; Parent and Lowenstein, 1994), lidocaine (Aggarwal and Wali, 1993), and propofol (Borgeat et al., 1994) has also been reported in select cases for which standard treatment of CSE was unsuccessful. General anesthesia may be called for when all other medication options have been exhausted and it becomes therapeutically necessary to prevent major metabolic and neurologic complications.

NONCONVULSIVE STATUS EPILEPTICUS

Although nonconvulsive status epilepticus is not life-threatening in the sense that CSE is, treatment is nevertheless important (Cascino, 1993). It is estimated that 25% of people who experience status epilepticus have absence or complex partial status epilepticus (Celesia, 1976). Absence status epilepticus is the most commonly observed type. The individual may exhibit a change in level of consciousness and behavior may be altered. Diagnosis is via EEG, with demonstration of spike-and-wave activity. Treatment is with intravenous or oral AEDs, including benzodiazepines, ethosuximide, valproate, or clonazepam.

Complex partial status epilepticus may be seen with various expressions. These can include alteration of consciousness, cessation of speech and/or activity, and oral and motor automatisms. Because of this variability, recognition may be difficult. EEG is an essential part of diagnosis, and brain imaging may be needed if a structural lesion is suspected. Pharmacologic management is similar to that for CSE, and includes use of short- and long-acting medications.

SUMMARY

Determination of the cause and identification of precipitating factors play an important role in the successful management of nonconvulsive status epilepticus and CSE. CSE produces an array of effects in the patients. In addition to the threat to life, the potential exists for irreversible damage to the central nervous system. Medications used in the management of CSE introduce additional possibilities for adverse effects. The importance of nursing preparedness in the management of CSE cannot be overemphasized. Knowledge of institution-specific treatment protocols, the medications that are routinely utilized or potentially prescribed, as well as anticipation of equipment needed and parameters to monitor are crucial nursing responsibilities. Intimate knowledge of a patient's seizure history, skilled assessment of the patient and of the seizure activity, and recognition of a deterioration in the patient's condition lie in the treatment team's hands. Gathering the treatment team and confidently delegating tasks, in addition to providing support to family members, must follow. These are indeed major responsibilities contributing to the overall effectiveness of management.

ACKNOWLEDGMENT

Special thanks to Margaret Jacobs and Ilo Leppik, M.D., for their thoughtful critiques of this manuscript and their many helpful suggestions.

REFERENCES

Aggarwal P, Wali JP. Lidocaine in refractory status epilepticus: a forgotten drug in the emergency department. *Am J Emerg Med* 1993;11:243–4.

Borgeat A, Wilder-Smith OHG, Jallon P, Suter PM. Propofol in the management of refractory status epilepticus: a case report. *Intensive Care Med* 1994;20:148–9.

Browne TR. Paraldehyde, chlormethiazole, and lidocaine for treatment of status epilepticus. In: Delgado-Escueta AV, Wasterlain CG, Treiman DM, Porter RJ, eds. *Status epilepticus: mechanisms of brain damage and treatment.* New York: Raven Press, 1983:509–17.

Cascino GD. Nonconvulsive status epilepticus in adults and children. *Epilepsia* 1993;34(suppl 1): S21–8.

Celesia GG. Modern concepts of status epilepticus. *JAMA* 1976;235:1571–4.

Conigilio AA, Garnett WR. Status epilepticus. In: DiPiro JT, Talbert RL, Hayes PE, Yee GC, Posey LM, eds. *Pharmacotherapy: a pathophysiologic approach.* New York: Elsevier, 1989:599–610.

Cranford RE, Leppik IE, Patrick B, Anderson CB, Kostic B. Intravenous phenytoin in acute treatment of seizures. *Neurology* 1979;29:1476–9.

Delgado-Escueta AV, Enrile-Bascal F. Combination therapy for status epilepticus: intravenous diazepam and phenytoin. In: Delgado-Escueta AV, Wasterlain CG, Treiman DM, Porter RJ, eds. *Status epilepticus: mechanisms of brain damage and treatment.* New York: Raven Press, 1983: 477–85.

Delgado-Escueta AV, Wasterlain CG, Treiman DM, Porter RJ, eds. Status epilepticus: summary. In: *Status epilepticus: mechanisms of brain damage and treatment.* New York: Raven Press, 1983: 537–41.

DeLorenzo RL, Towne AR, Pellock JM, et al. Status epilepticus in children, adults and the elderly. *Epilepsia* 1992;23(suppl 4):515–25.

Gastaut H. Clinical and electroencephalographic classification of epileptic seizures. *Epilepsia* 1970;11: 102–13.

Greenblatt DJ, Divoll M. Diazepam versus lorazepam: relationship of drug distribution to duration of clinical action. In: Delgado-Escueta AV, Wasterlain CG, Treiman DM, Porter RJ, eds. *Status epilepticus: mechanisms of brain damage and treatment.* New York: Raven Press, 1983:487–91.

Hauser WA. Status epilepticus: frequency, etiology, and neurological sequelae. In: Delgado-Escueta AV, Wasterlain CG, Treiman DM, Porter RJ, Eds. *Advances in Neurology.* Vol. 34. *Status epilepticus: mechanisms of brain damage and treatment.* New York: Raven Press, 1983:3–14.

Hauser WA. Status epilepticus: epidemiologic considerations. *Neurology* 1990;40(suppl 2):9–13.

Kumar A, Bleck TP. Intravenous midazolam for the treatment of refractory status epilepticus. *Crit Care Med* 1992;20:483–8.

Labar DR, Ali A, Root J. High-dose intravenous lorazepam for treatment of refractory status epilepticus. *Neurology* 1994;44:1400–3.

Leppik IE. Status epilepticus: the next decade. *Neurology* 1990;40(suppl 2):4–9.

Leppik IE, Derivan AT, Homan RW, Walker J, Ramsay RE, Patrick B. Double-blind study of lorazepam and diazepam in status epilepticus. *JAMA* 1983;249:1452–4.

Levy RJ, Krall RL. Treatment of status epilepticus with lorazepam. *Arch Neurol* 1984;41:606–11.

Parent JM, Lowenstein DH. Treatment of refractory generalized status epilepticus with continuous infusion of midazolam. *Neurology* 1994;44:1837–40.

Simon RP. Physiologic consequences of status epilepticus. *Epilepsia* 1985;26(suppl 1):S58–66.

Slovis CM, Wrenn KD. Treatment of status epilepticus [Letter, comment]. *JAMA* 1994;271:980–1.

Sorel L, Mechler L, Harmant J. Comparative trial of intravenous lorazepam and clonazepam in status epilepticus. *Clin Ther* 1981;4:326–36.

Treiman DM, DeGiorgio CM, Ben-Menachem E. Lorazepam versus phenytoin in the treatment of generalized convulsive status epilepticus: report of an ongoing study. *Neurology* 1985;35:S284.

Working Group on Status Epilepticus: Epilepsy Foundation of America. Treatment of convulsive status epilepticus. *JAMA* 1993;270:854–9.

Yaffe K, Lowenstein DH. Prognostic factors of pentobarbital therapy for refractory generalized status epilepticus. *Neurology* 1993;43:895–900.

Managing Seizure Disorders: A Handbook for Health Care Professionals, edited by N. Santilli, Lippincott-Raven Publishers, Philadelphia, 1996.
© 1996 Epilepsy Foundation of America.

8

Issues in the Comprehensive Management of Epilepsy in Children and Young Adults[1]

W. Edwin Dodson

This section deals with methods of identification of seizures and referral resources in newborns, children, and young adults who are having seizures. Factors that increase the risk of seizures are also considered. Although neurologic or systemic disease predisposes people to seizures and in some cases to developing epilepsy, most people who develop epilepsy do not have risk factors and are otherwise normal.

Many behaviors in addition to generalized convulsions are manifestations of seizures. In newborns this is an especially important issue because they do not have generalized tonic–clonic seizures like older children. Because the behaviors that indicate seizures in newborns differ from those in older children and adults, neonatal seizures have a separate classification system. In these children, as in adults, it is better to carefully document the behavior rather than to say only that the person had a seizure.

RISK FACTORS IN NEWBORNS ASSOCIATED WITH NEUROLOGIC ABNORMALITIES AND NEONATAL SEIZURES

Many factors are associated with an increased risk for seizures in both sick and otherwise abnormal newborns (Table 1). Some of these factors increase the risk for later epilepsy. Risk factors for later epilepsy include the occurrence of neonatal seizures, the type of neonatal seizures, and the cause of the brain abnormalities. The most common cause of seizures in newborns is perinatal asphyxia or a lack of adequate brain oxygenation. Other causes include CNS infection, metabolic abnormalities, including abnormal blood glucose, electrolytes, calcium and magnesium, inborn errors of metabolism, plus brain malformations, cerebral infarction, and idiopathic cases. Among newborns who have seizures, the risk of later epilepsy is more closely linked to the cause of the neonatal seizures than to other factors such as seizure type.

---

[1] Portions of this chapter were adapted from Santilli N, Dodson WE, Walton AV, eds. *Students with seizures: a manual for school nurses.* Landover, MD: Epilepsy Foundation of America, 1991.

TABLE 1. *Factors associated with an increased risk for seizures in newborns*

Perinatal asphyxia
Metabolic disturbances
  Hypoglycemia
  Hyponatremia
  Hypocalcemia
  Hypomagnesemia
Infections
  Meningitis
    Group B streptococcus
    Gram-negative organisms
    E. coli
    L. monocytogenes
  Encephalitis
    Herpes simplex
  Septicemia
Congenital malformations
  Chromosomal disorders
  Malformation syndromes
  Isolated brain malformations
  Drugs and environmental teratogens
  Maternal substance abuse
Toxins and drugs (exogenous substances)
  Congenital addiction
    Alcohol
    Narcotics
  Neonatal drug therapy
    Local anesthetics
    Theophylline
Inborn errors of metabolism
  Phenylketonuria (PKU)
  Maple syrup urine disease
  Argininosuccinic aciduria
Disease of visceral organs
  Cardiac disease
  Pulmonary disease
  Renal disease

ASSESSMENT OF NEUROLOGIC FUNCTION IN NEWBORNS

Seizures are one of the most dramatic neurologic abnormalities that affect newborns. However, seizures often occur in the setting of other neurologic problems. The ability to recognize these associated background abnormalities is an important aspect of recognizing and characterizing seizures in newborns. Furthermore, knowing the clinical context in which a seizure occurs is an important diagnostic feature among patients of any age.

Although a complete description of the neonatal neurologic examination is beyond the scope of this chapter, certain features require emphasis. Observation and documentation of abnormalities of mental status, tone, and movement are essential for early diagnosis and early intervention. In some cases, when metabolic abnormalities such as hypoglycemia affect the nervous system, careful observation can lead to diagnosis and treatment before serious brain injury occurs.

The principal features of the neurologic examination of newborns include assessment of (a) the level of alertness, (b) the cranial nerves, (c) the motor system, (d) neonatal reflexes, and (e) the sensory system. Among these categories, assessment of the level of alertness and the motor system will be emphasized here. Readers who want a complete discussion of the neonatal neurologic examination are referred to the book by Dr. Joseph J. Volpe (Volpe, 1994).

As with older patients, the mental status is a sensitive indicator of neurologic disease in newborns. When disease of the nervous system is present the mental status is often abnormal. In newborns, the mental status is assessed by evaluating the level of alertness and responsiveness. The level of alertness is the most vulnerable neurologic function when there is a widespread insult to the nervous system such as hypoglycemia or hypoxia.

In normal full-term newborns, there are normal fluctuations between wakefulness and sleep and the newborn can be awakened with gentle stimulation. Fluctuations in level of alertness are also associated with hunger. Hungry babies wake up and cry until they are fed. Conversely, feeding difficulties, particularly easy fatigability and poorly sustained sucking, often occur when alertness and arousal are reduced. When there is diffuse brain abnormality, periods of wakefulness are abbreviated or absent. As the brain abnormality worsens the infant becomes progressively more difficult to arouse. In the most severe cases the newborn cannot be aroused even by painful stimulation. Therefore, a cornerstone of assessing newborn behavior is to be aware of the level of alertness or arousal, including whether the expected fluctuations occur.

Normal newborns respond to visual images and to sound. They should visually fixate on and follow large bright objects. The most readily available test object is the evaluator's face. Normal full-term newborns should directly look at a face and they should track it laterally with their eyes. Similarly, they should respond to sound by alterations in activity. A normal newborn startles to a loud noise, such as a clap, and slowly turns the head toward a milder persistent stimulus, such as a tinkling bell. Although the responsiveness of a newborn to do these tasks varies with the level of arousal, persistent inability to arouse to alertness, failure to visually fixate and track a target with the eyes, or inability to respond to sound indicate that a brain abnormality might be present. When an abnormality is suspected, a more detailed neurologic assessment by a physician should be obtained.

The muscle tone of newborns also varies with their level of arousal or alertness and in the presence of neurologic disease. Tone is defined as the resistance of a limb to passive movement. Newborns with brain abnormalities often have abnormal tone. The pattern of the abnormality is determined by the location of the brain dysfunction and its duration, but reduced tone or hypotonia is most common. With diffuse brain abnormalities, the hypotonic newborn is floppy or limp, making the infant difficult to lift and handle. The examiner has the sensation that the child might slip out of the examiner's hands. In assessing newborns who are at risk for seizures, it is important to evaluate the newborn's tone and the pattern of the tone. Is the tone symmetrical or equal on the right and left?

When abnormalities of tone are present, there is often a reduction of spontaneous movement. It is important to note whether spontaneous movements are occurring on both sides of the body with equal frequency. Reduced movement on one side of the body may indicate CNS disease, such as brain infarction or stroke, an abnormality that predisposes to neonatal seizures. Similarly, after partial or focal seizures there are often lateralized abnormalities of movement and tone.

NEONATAL SEIZURES

Neonatal seizures take a variety of forms that differ from seizures in older patients. In fact, neonatal seizures cannot be adequately categorized by the International Classification of Epileptic Seizures. Whereas older patients usually have a well-organized and often stereotyped ictal sequence, newborns have disorganized or fragmentary ictal patterns. In adults, for example, partial complex seizures that secondarily generalize begin with an abnormal mental experience that is followed by loss of responsiveness with automatic behaviors, which in turn may be followed by generalized tonic–clonic movements. The time and extent of progression through these stages vary, but each stage is stereotypic when it occurs. Newborns do not have generalized tonic–clonic seizures. Their seizure patterns tend to be more fragmentary and disorganized. Therefore, special classifications for neonatal seizures have been developed.

Newborns make many movements that look like seizures but are not. Jitteriness with tremor is the most important nonepileptic but paroxysmal behavior to distinguish from seizures. Furthermore, during sleep, newborns have a variety of paroxysmal twitches, rapid eye movements, episodic sucking, and limb movements, all of which are normal.

Jitteriness is paroxysmal and can be confused with seizures in newborns. The characteristic movement during jitteriness is tremor, whereas clonus is characteristic of seizures. Tremor is characterized by rapid to and fro movements. In clonus the movements are phasic, having a rapid phase followed by a slow phase in the opposite direction. The to-and-fro movements of tremor have the same velocity in both directions. Tremor varies with position or limb posture, such that repositioning the affected limb(s) quiets the movements. Jitteriness is usually associated with a mental state of extreme arousal and may be stimulus-dependent, being triggered by sound, movement, or other types of stimulation. Although tremor in jittery newborns is often triggered by stimulation, it can also occur spontaneously.

Over time, several classification schemes for classifying neonatal seizures have been developed. In considering contemporary classifications of neonatal seizures, it is important to be aware of the changes that have occurred in classifications of neonatal seizures during the 1980s.

Before the mid-1980s, classifications of neonatal seizures were based on clinical observation alone. However, as video–EEG recordings became available, it became possible to evaluate the newborns' behavior along with simultaneous EEG patterns. This has shown that not all paroxysmal behaviors in newborns are associated with epileptic discharges on the EEG. Accordingly, our thinking about neonatal behaviors that indicate seizures has been refined.

The clinical classification of neonatal seizures developed by Volpe (1994) is the most widely used. This classification was based on clinical observations of newborns' behaviors. Those behaviors that had a paroxysmal temporal profile and that did not attenuate with repositioning the newborn were judged to be seizures. The paroxysmal behaviors defined in this classification are summarized in Table 2.

The clinical classifications of neonatal seizures were devised before video–EEG recordings in newborns were possible. Subsequent video–EEG recordings in newborns who were believed to be having seizures have indicated that many of them do not have epileptiform EEG changes during their clinical spells. Furthermore, those behaviors that are not associated with epileptiform EEG discharges, not surprisingly, are not prevented by AEDs. Because the classifications of neonatal seizures continue to be refined, it is better for all health professionals to describe paroxysmal behaviors and movements in newborns rather than to simply label or call a paroxysmal behavior a seizure.

The most common paroxysmal behaviors in sick newborns are subtle. Subtle paroxysmal behaviors include sucking, rowing, pedaling, swimming, and apnea. These are caused by seizures in less than 5% of cases. When subtle movements indicate seizures, they are accompanied by abnormal eye movements and by other seizure types. Abnormal eye movements that indicate seizures include tonic or sustained eye deviation or combinations of tonic eye deviation and

TABLE 2. *Clinical neonatal seizure types[a]*

Paroxysmal behavior	Frequency of epileptiform EEG
Subtle	Rare
Ocular	Rare
Oral buccal	Very rare
Progressive movements	Very rare
Pedaling	Very rare
Rowing	Very rare
Swimming	Very rare
Apnea	Rare
Generalized tonic	Rare
Mutlifocal clonic	Common
Focal clonic	Usually
Myoclonic	Sometimes

[a] See Volpe, 1994; Mizrahi and Kellaway, 1987.

TABLE 3. *Neonatal paroxysmal behaviors likely to be associated with epileptiform EEG changes*

Focal clonic jerking
Focal tonic movements
Multifocal clonic jerking
Myoclonic jerking

jerking eye movements. However, paroxysmal subtle movements in newborns are rarely accompanied by epileptiform EEG patterns and most of them are probably not seizures. The frequency of epileptic EEG abnormalities in paroxysmal neonatal behaviors is shown in Table 2. Most of the time subtle, paroxysmal neonatal behaviors do not indicate seizures. The only sure way to substantiate whether subtle movements are seizures is to document simultaneous epileptiform discharges with the EEG.

In contrast to paroxysmal subtle movements, which rarely indicate seizure activity, other paroxysmal movements have a high probability of being caused by seizures (Table 3). The paroxysmal movements that usually indicate seizures include focal movements that affect a single limb on one side of the body. Focal movements may be either tonic (slow and sustained) or clonic (phasic to-and-fro movements having fast and slow phases in opposite directions). Generalized tonic stiffening in newborns rarely indicates seizures but is important to recognize because it indicates serious abnormalities of lower brain structures. Most of the time multifocal clonic jerking is associated with epileptic EEG discharges. Apnea in newborns is rarely due to seizures, with seizures accounting for less than 10% of apneic spells in newborns. When apnea is due to seizure activity, there are abnormal paroxysmal eye movements at the same time.

RISK FOR LATER EPILEPSY AFTER NEONATAL PROBLEMS

The risk for later epilepsy is increased by CNS disease during the perinatal period. However, the extent to which the risk for later epilepsy is increased depends on several factors, including the state of brain maturation at birth (premature vs. full term), the types of neurologic symptoms that are produced and, most important, the cause of the neonatal neurologic abnormalities. It is clear that newborns can have severe neurologic symptoms, including neonatal seizures, and still recover completely and develop normally if the cause of the abnormal brain functioning does not severely damage nerve cells. In this regard, neonatal hypoglycemia and hypoxia are most dangerous, whereas late neonatal hypocalcemia and certain drug intoxications or neonatal withdrawal from congenital addiction to narcotics are usually associated with a good outcome.

When perinatal abnormalities cause epilepsy later in childhood, they also cause abnormalities of the motor system, so-called cerebral palsy. In the absence of cerebral palsy there is no evidence that problems in the newborn period increase the risk for epilepsy later in life.

Whereas both full-term and premature newborns can be affected by similar diseases (Table 1), the patterns of brain injury and abnormal neurologic behavior differ according to the different states of brain maturation. The risk for epilepsy after perinatal problems is lower in premature newborns than in full-term newborns. The reason for this difference relates to the different degrees of brain maturation when the insult to the brain occurs. The extent of brain maturation determines the changing patterns of brain vulnerability to lack of oxygen and other insults. Because of this, full-term newborns are more likely to manifest neonatal seizures than prematures. The premature newborn's nervous system is not sufficiently developed to support the propagation of seizures. Whereas asphyxiated full-term newborns are highly prone to development of diffuse cortical injury and neonatal seizures, premature newborns are more vulnerable to injury of deeper brain structures that leads to intraventricular hemorrhage.

Long-term sequelae of perinatal asphyxia also differ in these groups. Full-term newborns who were severely asphyxiated at birth are more likely to have epilepsy in association with cerebral palsy and mental retardation than premature newborns. Prematures are more likely to have motor deficits, but epilepsy is less common. When motor sequelae are present, premature newborns usually manifest spastic diplegia, a distinctive pattern of cerebral palsy associated with spasticity, weakness, and poor control of the legs, with lesser or no involvement of the arms and face. On the other hand, full-term newborns more often have abnormalities of both upper and lower extremities in a pattern of quadriplegia.

Newborns who are otherwise normal may also have neonatal seizures. The seizures that occur in these babies are variably associated with an increased risk for epilepsy. However, in this situation the risk for epilepsy that persists into childhood is low, 10% or less.

FACTORS THAT INCREASE THE RISK FOR SEIZURES IN CHILDREN

Among infants and children, many factors increase the risk of seizures. Broad categories of risk factors include genetic disorders, a history of perinatal problems, such as asphyxia or CNS infection, and postnatally acquired CNS disease. Tuberous sclerosis is a prominent example of a genetic condition that carries a high risk for seizures. Nonspecific signs of brain abnormality increase the risk for seizures in children. One-third of children who have cerebral palsy develop epilepsy. The risk is greater when the child has quadriplegia than when the child has diplegia. Similarly, the risk for seizures is increased among children who have moderate to severe mental retardation (IQ less than 50).

Acquired CNS disease in childhood can also increase the risk for seizures.

After meningitis the risk of epilepsy is approximately 10%. The occurrence of seizures early during the meningitis heightens the risk for epilepsy. Most of the patients who develop epilepsy after meningitis do so within the first 5 years. Encephalitis also is associated with an increased risk of epilepsy. However, after encephalitis the increased risk for epilepsy continues for more than a decade.

Severe closed head trauma also increases the risk for both transient seizures and later epilepsy in children. Children are more likely than adults to have seizures within the first hour after head trauma. Seizures that occur during this time period usually are not associated with an increased risk for later epilepsy. However, seizures that appear thereafter are associated with an increased risk for epilepsy.

A family history of seizures also increases the risk for epilepsy in a child (Hauser and Hesdorffer, 1990). The extent to which this risk is increased depends on the cause of the seizures in the other family members.

Although more than 150 specific diseases with Mendelian inheritance have been identified that increase the risk for epilepsy, only a tiny fraction of patients with epilepsy have a diagnosable inherited disease that causes seizures. In the rare cases in which precise diagnosis is feasible, diagnosis is especially important because the risk for epilepsy as a symptom of the disease can be defined and a prognosis can be given. However, a majority of patients with epilepsy do not have identifiable causes.

The risk of epilepsy is increased when other family members have epilepsy. The extent of the increased risk varies with several factors. These include the type of seizure or epilepsy in other family members and the degree of relatedness to the specific child who is being considered. Depending on the diagnosis, the risk ranges from about 4 to 10%. When a parent has epilepsy the risk of the child having epilepsy sometime during the child's lifetime is approximately 4%. When a parent had febrile seizures as a child, the risk that the child will have febrile seizures ranges from 10% to more than 30% in various studies. If both a parent and a sibling have epilepsy, the risk that the child will develop epilepsy is approximately 20%.

SPECIAL TYPES OF SEIZURES THAT OCCUR ONLY IN INFANTS AND YOUNG CHILDREN

Febrile seizures occur in children who are younger than 5 years old who have fever and no other cause for the seizures. There are several important issues. Foremost is the principle that this is a diagnosis of exclusion. To make this diagnosis, the child must be evaluated to exclude other serious disorders. Approximately 2% of young children who are evaluated for seizures with fever have meningitis. Conversely, seizures can be a presenting symptom in children with meningitis and other serious disorders. The failure to diagnose meningitis and other severe brain disorders can be catastrophic for the child. These children must be referred to a physician for evaluation as soon as possible. This is a medical emergency.

Most young children who have fever and seizures do not have life-threatening problems. Most of them have febrile seizures, a transient disorder that affects 4% of children. The problems associated with febrile seizures include, first, a 33% chance of having more febrile seizures and, second, an increased risk for persistent epilepsy. The risk for later epilepsy (recurrent seizures not associated with fever) is increased when the seizure has a focal onset (partial seizure), when there are multiple seizures in a 24-h period, when the child has several bouts of febrile seizures, when the child is abnormal developmentally or neurologically, and when there is a family history of epilepsy. In the worst case the risk for later epilepsy is less than 20% and for most children the risk of epilepsy is only mildly increased. Therefore, most of the children with febrile seizures have only a temporary problem. When febrile seizures are diagnosed, reassuring the family is indicated.

Infantile spasms may be a particular problem to recognize because this seizure type is not associated with tonic–clonic convulsive movements. The seizures are typically brief and usually occur in clusters. Infantile spasms may be flexor, extensor, or a mixture of these forms. Flexion movements consist of a bending forward of the neck and trunk with the arms being outstretched forward, as if the infant were reaching out to be held. Extensor spells are characterized by brief tonic stiffening with the neck and trunk extending backwards and with the arms variably moving outward, much like the extension of the arms in the Moro reflex. The individual seizures are brief, lasting at most 2–3 s. However, they tend to occur in clusters of few to many seizures at one time. The clusters are most common when the infant is awakening from sleep either in the early morning or after a nap. Often the infant cries between the individual seizures, a feature that contributes to an erroneous diagnosis of colic.

The combination of infantile spasms with the EEG pattern of hypsarrhythmia and with developmental arrest or regression is West's syndrome. The EEG pattern of hypsarrhythmia is one of the most severely epileptiform patterns, with multifocal spikes and a disorganized abnormally slow background. Both the seizure-type infantile spasms and the EEG pattern hypsarrhythmia occur only in infants and young children. As the child grows older, the seizure type and the EEG pattern change.

There are many causes of infantile spasms (see Table 4). Virtually any disease that damages the brain can cause spasms. However, one-third of infants who begin to have spasms are normal at the time the spasms begin, and no etiology can be identified. This group is called *cryptogenic,* because it has no known cause. Diagnosis is especially important in this group because they have the best prognosis if therapy is started promptly.

Infantile spasms can also occur in infants who have had other types of seizures. Usually the other seizure types are partial, partial secondarily generalized, or generalized tonic–clonic. Similarly, infants whose epilepsy begins with spasms

TABLE 4. *Symptomatic causes*
of infantile spasms

Neurocutaneous disorders
   Tuberous sclerosis
   Hypomelanosis of Ito
Perinatal asphyxia
Postnatal metabolic disorders
   Hypoxia
   Hypoglycemia
Trauma
Cerebrovascular disease
   Stroke
   Venous thrombosis
Brain malformations
   Hydrocephalus
   Aicardi's syndrome
   Lissencephaly
Chromosomal disorders
   Down's syndrome
Infections
   Pre- and postnatal
      Toxoplasmosis
      Herpes simplex
      Syphilis
      Rubella
      Cytomegalovirus
   Meningitis
   Encephalitis
Inborn errors of metabolism
   Phenylketonuria (PKU)
   Maple syrup urine disease
   Pyridoxine dependency

may also develop other seizure types after the spasms appear. Therefore, one should be sensitive to the possible occurrence of other types of seizures when a child is having infantile spasms.

It is important to recognize that infants who have sudden movements that occur in clusters may be having seizures. The prognosis is improved in cases of infantile spasms when therapy is started within the first month after seizures appear. If infantile spasms are suspected, the child should be evaluated by a physician who has experience with epilepsy in infants.

The Lennox–Gastaut syndrome is a rare epileptic disorder of childhood. This syndrome is like infantile spasms in that many severe brain diseases can produce it. However, no cause is found in approximately 40% of children with this disorder. Children with Lennox–Gastaut syndrome have multiple types of seizures, but they usually begin by having partial or generalized tonic–clonic convulsions. Later they develop other features that lead to the diagnosis of Lennox–Gastaut syndrome. The other features include multiple types of seizures—especially atonic seizures (drop attacks) and absence or atypical absence seizures—developmental arrest or regression with subnormal intellect, and a characteristic EEG pattern of slow spike-and-wave. It is important to recognize the possibility that a child who has recent-onset epilepsy may develop other seizure types that indicate a more specific diagnosis and that require additional evaluation and possibly a change in AED therapy.

SPECIFIC CHILDHOOD DISEASES ASSOCIATED WITH INCREASED RISK FOR EPILEPSY

The presence of certain diseases increases the risk for epilepsy in children. Examples of diseases that are associated with an increased risk include tuberous sclerosis and Down's syndrome, for which the risks are approximately 80% and 6%, respectively. These conditions cause abnormalities in the general physical examination, but the manifestations of the former condition may be particularly subtle in infants and young children.

Tuberous sclerosis is an example of a neurocutaneous disorder (Table 5). It is characterized by the triad of epilepsy, subnormal mentality, and adenoma sebaceum. However, most children who have tuberous sclerosis do not have all three of these features, and some of the features do not develop until the mid-childhood years. At present, tuberous sclerosis is the most common cause of infantile spasms.

Skin abnormalities may be the first sign that tuberous sclerosis is present. Dermatologic signs include hypomelanotic (depigmented) patches that occasionally have the shape of an ash leaf. In pale children these may be difficult to see, but examination with a Wood's lamp helps. Among suntanned children the pale spots are easy to recognize. After the age of 4 years, patients with tuberous sclerosis develop adenoma sebaceum on the face in the area beside and over the bridge of the nose. During childhood it is bright red. Later during adolescence and adulthood the redness abates and the rash assumes a flesh-colored, warty appearance. Shagreen patches are another skin abnormality that occurs in patients with tuberous sclerosis. These are areas of skin that appear to be thickened, with the appearance of orange peel.

Tuberous sclerosis is transmitted genetically in an autosomal dominant fashion.

TABLE 5. *Neurocutaneous disorders associated with increased risk for epilepsy[a]*

Tuberous sclerosis
Sturge–Weber syndrome
Hypomelanosis of Ito
Linear sebaceous nevus
Incontinenti pigmenti
Neurofibromatosis type 1

[a] See Gomez, 1987.

Half of affected children have an affected parent. More than 80% of patients with tuberous sclerosis develop epilepsy.

Neurofibromatosis type 1 is another disorder that usually causes abnormalities of skin and also affects the nervous system in some cases. The risk for epilepsy is much lower in neurofibromatosis than in tuberous sclerosis. The abnormalities of skin in neurofibromatosis include multiple café-au-lait or coffee-colored spots, and lumps under the surface of the skin caused by either neurofibromas or lipomas. Neurologic involvement and seizures are less common among patients with neurofibromatosis than in tuberous sclerosis. Neurofibromatosis can cause many other medical problems in addition to neurologic dysfunction. Readers who want more information are referred to the book edited by Gomez (Gomez, 1987).

Chromosomal abnormalities such as Down's syndrome are associated with an increased risk for mental retardation, epilepsy, and other problems. Down's syndrome is easily recognized because it is associated with a characteristically abnormal physical appearance and with variable degrees of mental retardation. Other chromosomal problems associated with an increased risk for epilepsy include X-linked mental retardation, with or without fragile X chromosome, and extra chromosomes (trisomies) or deletions of parts of a chromosome, such as the rare condition called Angelman's happy puppet syndrome. As a general principle, children who have abnormalities of three or more systems should have a karyotype (the full chromosome set of the nucleus of a cell) evaluated. For example, a child who has mental retardation with seizures, abnormal skin creases on the palm of the hand, and foot deformities should be referred for genetic evaluation in addition to being evaluated and treated for the seizures.

NONEPILEPTIC PAROXYSMAL BEHAVIORS IN INFANTS AND YOUNG CHILDREN

Infants and toddlers have other paroxysmal behaviors that can be confused with seizures (Table 6). Among these, breath-holding spells are most common. Breath-holding spells are characterized by stimulus-induced loss of consciousness. When the loss of consciousness occurs only after the child has been injured or is crying for some other reason, breath-holding spells are the most likely diagnosis. Breath-holding occurs in older infants and toddlers. The nurse has an important role in gathering the history and in supporting the parent in this situation.

Breath-holding spells have been categorized into two types, blue (cyanotic) or pale (pallid). The blue spells are most common. Typically the child, usually a toddler, is frustrated and begins to cry. The crying begins with the child's making a prolonged exhalation and turning blue, which is invariably associated with loss of consciousness. Occasionally there are brief convulsive movements during the period of unconsciousness. It should be emphasized that in this setting the occurrence of a few convulsive movements does not indicate that the diagnosis is

TABLE 6. *Nonepileptic causes of paroxysmal behavior in children*

Breath-holding spells
  Blue
  Pallid
Migraine equivalents
  Benign paroxysmal torticollis
  Benign paroxysmal vertigo
Rage attacks
Cardiac arrhythmias
Movement disorders
  Tics
  Choreoathetosis
  Myoclonic jerks
Sleep disturbances
  Bedwetting
  Night terrors
  Sleepwalking
Staring spells/daydreaming

epilepsy. The key to the proper diagnosis is documenting that the spell always begins with the child's being frustrated or angry and crying.

Parents and other caretakers who witness breath-holding spells are usually frightened by the spells and fear that the child might die. This fear emotionally reinforces the breath-holding behavior in the child. The secret to treating breath-holding spells is to recognize and deal with the caretakers' fears and to modify their behavior so that they do not reinforce the child's behavior. In some cases this is difficult to accomplish. Simple reassurance is not enough. Considerable emotional support and developing a specific behavioral plan for the caretaker helps the caretaker begin to feel comfortable enough to ignore the spell and to not reinforce it by paying attention to it.

So-called pallid breath-holding spells are vasovagal syncope. These usually occur in susceptible people following a painful injury or a frightening stimulus, such as the sight of blood. Patients with epilepsy can also have vasovagal syncope. Again, the key to diagnosis is a carefully obtained history. When vasovagal syncope is suspected, having a good description of the events and a promptly obtained set of vital signs can make the diagnosis. Characteristically, the pulse is feeble and slow and the blood pressure is low. However, the vasovagal spells are usually brief, and pulse and blood pressure return to normal quickly. The patient is pale, ashen, and cold and clammy to the touch. Patients with vasovagal syncope should be evaluated by a physician to rule out an underlying cardiac abnormality.

Episodic dyscontrol syndrome is characterized by recurrent attacks of uncontrollable rage (rage attacks), usually with minimal provocation and often completely out of character for the person. The syndrome is usually seen in teenagers and young adults but can also affect younger children. In many individuals impairment is evident on neurologic examination. Attacks occur suddenly and can be explosive and characterized by uncontrollable behavior that consists of primitive physical violence such as kicking, gouging, scratching, spitting, hitting, and biting. In girls and young women the violence is often verbal and consists of obscene, profane language. Those affected often display remarkable strength and speed in their attacks.

During the attacks the individual often appears temporarily psychotic. Afterward, amnesia, fatigue, and occasionally remorse may prevail. Although such people are often referred to a neurologist to rule out the diagnosis of complex partial seizures, it is not difficult to differentiate the latter from rage attacks. Some individuals may become agitated and combative when restrained during a complex partial seizure, but directed violence is extremely unusual.

Migraine poses a special problem, especially in children, because its manifestations are so diverse (Table 7). When a characteristic headache is part of the attack, diagnosis is usually not difficult. However, in children, headache may frequently be inconspicuous or even absent. Cyclic vomiting with or without nausea, diarrhea, signs of vasomotor instability such as flushing or pallor, mydriasis, and photophobia can be the most prominent manifestations. In the past, these symptoms were often labeled "epileptic equivalents," although evidence for an epileptogenic basis is weak. Paroxysmal focal and generalized EEG abnormalities are common in migraines, even between attacks. However, in the absence of specific epileptiform patterns, these abnormalities should be interpreted with caution.

Two forms of migraine deserve special attention because of the frequency with which they are misdiagnosed as epilepsy in some children. In *confusional migraine,* attacks are characterized by a state of confusion with mood changes, lethargy, agitation, impaired memory, and disorientation. In most instances a careful history reveals past symptoms of visual or sensory phenomena, recurrent

TABLE 7. *Differentiation of migraines from seizures*

Clinical data	Migraines	Seizures
Family history	Often positive for migraine	Often positive for seizures
Headaches	Frequent during or after period of neurological symptoms	Frequent postictally
Impaired consciousness	Rare	Always seen in complex partial and absence
Automatisms	Rare	Frequent in complex partial and absence seizures
Clonic or myoclonic movements	Never	Common in absence; occasionally in complex partial
EEG		
Interictal	Occasionally abnormal	Frequently abnormal
During attacks	Often abnormal; diffuse or focal slowing	Abnormal; epileptiform activity

Adapted with permission from Holmes GL. *Diagnosis and management of seizures in children.* Philadelphia: WB Saunders, 1987:52.

TABLE 8. *Differentiation of parasomnias from seizures*

Clinical data	Night terrors	Sleepwalking	Seizures
Age	4–12 years	All ages, but more common in children than in adults	All ages
Timing	First third of night	First third of night	Shortly after going to sleep; early morning hours
Interictal EEG	No	No	Yes
Postictal EEG	Usually normal	Usually normal	Frequently abnormal

From Holmes GL. Diagnosis and management of seizures in children. Philadelphia: WB Saunders, 1987.

headaches, and a family history of migraine. In the acute phase, however, a nonconvulsive ictal state, such as absence status epilepticus, must be considered among the diagnostic possibilities; this can be excluded promptly by means of an EEG recording. *Basilar artery migraine* is a syndrome characterized by non-lateralized headache, vertigo, ataxia, bilateral visual disturbances, and cranial nerve (including oculomotor) disturbances. A prominent family history of migraine is typical. Although most common in adolescents and young adults, especially women, the syndrome may occur in preschool children.

Parasomnias, or disorders of sleep in children, may also be confused with seizures (Table 8). These include night terrors and somnambulism, nightmares, bruxism, and head banging. The attacks of muscle weakness (cataplexy) that occur in narcolepsy may sometimes be confused with atonic seizures, but preservation of awareness and the invariable presence of an emotional triggering factor, especially laughter, should resolve most uncertainty, even in the absence of other features of narcolepsy.

Involuntary movement disorders appear abruptly and can be confused with seizures. The most important issue is whether or not there is an alteration of consciousness. Tics are the most common movement disorder in children. They are very brief and abrupt. In some cases they are vocal, causing the child to grunt or make other utterances. Other movement disorders, such as paroxysmal choreoathetosis, are rare but can be dramatic and may last for several minutes. To assess whether consciousness is altered, one should be able to answer two types of questions. Can the child respond to simple commands during the episode? After the episode is over, does the child remember a simple phrase or instruction that was presented during the episode? Having this type of information is vital to making the proper diagnosis.

APPROACH TO THE CHILD WITH SUDDEN ALTERATIONS OF BEHAVIOR

Several aspects of observation and documentation are important to making a proper diagnosis when children have sudden or paroxysmal alterations of behavior. When there has been careful observation and documentation of an episode, the diagnosis is usually easy. When these are lacking the diagnosis of the episode is less certain, and therapy can be misguided.

There are several steps to diagnosing the cause of paroxysmal behaviors in children (Table 9). It is important to define the setting in which the episode occurs. Most seizures occur in a variety of settings whereas breath-holding occurs only when the child is angry or frustrated.

To help to determine the cause of paroxysmal behaviors in children, some questions to ask are:

> What is the relationship to previous meals or sleep? If the episode occurs only when the child has not eaten for a long period of time, check blood glucose during or soon after the episode to evaluate the possibility of hypoglycemia
> Is there a characteristic emotional context?
> During the episode, what is the sequence of events?
> What happens first? Second? Third?
> Where are the movements located? Do they migrate? Is only one or are both sides of the body affected?
> What is the duration of the episode? Time it.
> During the episode, is there impairment of consciousness?
> After the episode, is recovery immediate or delayed?
> If recovery is delayed, when can the patient speak or otherwise function normally?
> Is the speech pattern normal or abnormal?
> What is the sequence of recovery?

The importance of these steps is illustrated by considering the child who has episodic staring. Are the spells seizures or only daydreaming episodes? Occasional daydreaming is normal. However, absence or partial complex seizures can also cause episodic staring. This differential diagnosis is one of the most difficult but also one of the most important, because different medications are required for absence vs. partial complex seizures. Of course, children who are only daydreaming should not be treated with AEDs at all.

For the practitioner, the differential diagnosis of staring spells is easy when the child has atypical features and a characteristically abnormal EEG. However,

TABLE 9. *Steps in the diagnosis of paroxysmal behaviors*

Identify the setting
Describe the event
   Sequence of movements or behaviors
   Vital signs
   Blood tests
Describe the recovery period
   Duration
   Sequence of recovery
Document and communicate your observations

this is often not the case, and the practitioner must depend on an eyewitness description of the episodes. This is where careful observation and documentation of the episode are invaluable. A diagnosis of seizures is supported by documenting that the child's mental functioning is impaired during the episode. Does the child respond to and remember instructions that are issued while he is staring? How long does the episode last?

Typically, absence seizures are brief, lasting only a few seconds. Partial complex seizures usually last more than a minute, especially when the child is not taking AEDs. Does the child have any movements during the staring episode? Stereotyped repetitive movements, such as fumbling with clothing, lip smacking, or swallowing, are important features that suggest that the seizure was partial complex. Does the child experience a warning that the episode is beginning? The occurrence of an aura indicates that the seizure was partial complex.

Soon after the episode it is important to record the observations that were made. These should be communicated directly to the treating practitioner whenever possible, and a copy should be given to the child's parent or other caretaker. No matter how well-intentioned or how fastidiously collected, good information does not help if it does not get to the right place. In this case the "right place" is the person who will further evaluate the child and who will prescribe the child's treatment. It is also helpful to include your phone number in case the evaluator has other questions.

OUTPATIENT EVALUATION

When seizures occur in the office or clinic, careful observation and documentation of the episode are critical. The approach to identifying seizures in clinics and offices is similar to the methods that are used for inpatients. It is unusual for patients to have a seizure at the physician's office, but if this occurs the opportunity for observation and documentation should be capitalized on. The principles of observing and documenting seizures are summarized in Table 8.

Most patients with epilepsy do not oblige the practitioner by having an observable spell, and the diagnosis of epilepsy is therefore heavily dependent on the history. When the patient arrives at the office, the source of the history should be identified. Because an eyewitness account is so important in identifying the type of spell, it is important to locate the witness and to contact that person if a written description of the spell was not sent with the patient. In a referral situation, this information should be obtained in advance and forwarded to the physician. The widespread availability of video cameras may make it possible for the family to provide a videotape of the behavior.

COMPLIANCE WITH GLOBAL MANAGEMENT IN INFANTS AND CHILDREN

Compliance with an overall plan of management is necessary if the therapy of epilepsy is to succeed. Successful management occurs when the child is able to develop to his or her full potential unfettered by the effects of epilepsy or its treatment, insofar as possible. Note that this goal does not state that seizures must be prevented at any cost.

Achieving the best outcomes for children with epilepsy is a group endeavor. The group always includes the patient, parents, and health care providers, and it variably includes other caretakers, social service workers, psychologists and teachers, depending on what the patient needs. When the child is very young, the parent is largely responsible for care. As the child matures, he should become increasingly responsible for his own care.

Global care for a child with epilepsy includes adhering to medical regimens and providing the child with an environment and opportunity that encourages development into an independent adult. This means that children with epilepsy, like all other children, must develop emotional, intellectual, and occupational adult life skills. This developmental process always involves taking chances, something that is difficult for parents to accept even when there is no epilepsy. Helping parents of young children to avoid overprotection and to allow their children opportunities for growth is an important aspect of global care. When epilepsy affects older children and adolescents, the patient should progressively be assigned responsibility for his own care. The parents' role remains very important, but it is more difficult because of the ambiguity introduced by the evolving reassignment of responsibilities.

Studies of compliance among pediatric patients who depend on their caretakers for administration of medication indicate that compliance in children is subject to all of the problems that occur when the caretakers should be taking medication themselves. Stated another way, the same factors that affect compliance with their own medical care influence caretakers' compliance with the child's medical care.

Several factors affect compliance with medical care. These include, first, having a trusting relationship with the caregivers. Second, understanding and accepting the diagnosis are essential for building compliance. Third, the patient or the parent must feel able to control or at least influence the outcome. Fourth, dealing with illness-related and with coexistent although unrelated concerns is prerequisite for compliance. For example, a family's ability to comply with the treatment plan may be harder during difficult financial times. Fifth, the medical management should be woven into the family's daily routine to facilitate carrying out the treatment plan and to minimize illness-related disruptions of everyday family life. Having an objective means of documenting compliance reinforces the cooperation of parents and patients. Finally, all of the above factors must be considered and addressed within the cultural context of the patient and family.

TRUST AND COMMUNICATION

When a parent trusts the care providers, communication and compliance with the treatment process are abetted. Several factors help to build a trusting relationship with the parents. Effective communication skills and honesty are fundamental. The therapeutic relationship is built first with the parents, and in so doing their feelings and concerns must be considered. Emotional issues are paramount. If these are not dealt with, delivering the technical aspects of the child's care can be severely inhibited. This means that health care providers must first relate to the parents as individual people. In doing this, one must question how parents are coping with the feelings that have been generated by their child's illness. The manifestations of excessive anxiety and unresolved emotional issues are misunderstood medication changes, omitted doses, unkept appointments, and endless calls and questions about minor problems. These issues occasionally arise with any patient, but when they recur or persist it usually indicates a more basic problem. The way to begin to explore the area is to ask the parent, "How are you doing?" Then listen carefully.

Open communication builds trust. Families should be encouraged to address any of their questions to any of the care providers who participate in their child's care. They should also be encouraged to seek information from other sources. Parents should know as much as possible about their child's condition.

An open approach has several benefits. The facts are reinforced when the parents or patients hear them from several sources. Although having multiple sources of information introduces the risk of the parents being confused or receiving contradictory answers, resolving confusion and contradictions actually helps in the long run. In the process of resolving contradictions, the parents acquire deeper insight into the nuances of their child's situation and of epilepsy in general. There are few issues in the treatment of epilepsy that justify a dogmatic approach, because there are many unanswered questions about seizures and epilepsy. When the answer to a parent's question is unknown, it is important to say so. "I don't know" or "No one knows the answer to that question" is often the correct answer. In addition to trusting the care providers, the parents and patients need to trust the therapy that is prescribed. They need to believe in the therapy, feeling that there is a good chance that the therapy will work. Otherwise, why bother?

UNDERSTANDING THE DIAGNOSIS

Parents want reliable facts presented frankly but gently. The facts must be presented in straightforward language that they can understand; jargon is deadly. However, even clearly presented information must almost always be repeated. In explaining a child's epilepsy to the parent, it is best to begin by asking the parent to clarify their understanding of the problem. The information you want to convey should begin at the parent's point of understanding and build. Similarly, when parents have a specific question it is best to determine how much they know about the issue before offering an answer.

FACTS TO BE COMMUNICATED

It is very important to emphasize what is known about the patient's problem even when the information is negative. The answer "I don't know" is easier for the parent or patient to accept when it is followed by an affirmative statement of what is known. For example, "We don't know what is causing your child's seizures, but we do know that your child does not have a brain tumor or some other horrible brain problem." Even the most intelligent parent fears that the child might have a brain tumor or some other indiscernible, potentially lethal problem. Every family should be told that there is no brain tumor after the appropriate studies are negative.

There are many positive facts that parents need to know about epilepsy. They need to know that for more than 50% of children who develop epilepsy the problem is temporary and will not require lifelong therapy. Parents need to know that anyone can have a seizure when brain cells are stressed by certain illness or metabolic problems, and need to be told that seizures almost never harm the brain. They need to know that most patients who have seizures have no other brain problem. They need to know that AEDs control seizures in a majority of patients without troublesome side effects. Most of all, they need to know that there are many different types of epilepsy and that any given statement may not apply to their child.

Negative aspects of epilepsy should also be discussed. Parents should be told that the social stigma of epilepsy is unfounded and has no basis in fact. The stigma of epilepsy originated in ignorance, misunderstanding, and fear. It is important for patients' families to join and support organizations that advocate for persons with epilepsy, such as the Epilepsy Foundation of America and its state and local affiliates. (For more information call 1-800-EFA-1000. Internet: postmaster@efa.org.) The presence of epilepsy does slightly increase the risk for death in all age groups. Overall, however, the risk for death during a seizure is negligible. In very rare cases seizures cause brain damage, but this occurs only when the child has one of the rare epileptic syndromes or experiences status epilepticus. Any AED can interfere with behavior and learning skills, but this occurs when the dose is too high. This is why physicians who treat children with epilepsy try to use the lowest dose possible. When children with epilepsy have learning problems, these are usually related to antecedent underlying brain and developmental problems rather than to the epilepsy or its therapy. Finally, parents need to know that there is much to be learned about epilepsy. The causes of seizures, the brain mechanisms of seizures, the effects of seizures on other brain functions, and better ways to treat seizures are all ongoing areas of research.

For most parents and patients, the uncertainty about the cause of seizures is more difficult to deal with than a definite diagnosis, even when the diagnosis is inimical. The problem of uncertainty is a central issue in treating epilepsy because in a majority of patients the cause of the epilepsy is unknown. This problem must be addressed head on. It helps families to know that the caregivers have experience with idiopathic or cryptogenic cases similar to theirs. It helps parents and older children to know that they are like most other people who have seizures and epilepsy.

ACCEPTING THE DIAGNOSIS

Compliance is enhanced when the parents take the diagnosis seriously but it is hindered when their anxiety about the condition is excessively high and paralyzing. When a condition is too frightening or too anxiety provoking, the tendency is to deny the illness, to be noncompliant, or to seek a nonconventional, quack treatment that promises a cure. This is a formidable problem with epilepsy, because at some point virtually every parent of a child who has had convulsions fears that the child might die during a convulsion. Even when the child has nonconvulsive seizures, parents fear that the seizures might be causing brain damage. Later, they worry that the antiepileptic medications might be interfering with learning and school performance. These fears must be addressed realistically and frankly.

Many parents have difficulty accepting the diagnosis of their child's epilepsy. It is rare for young parents to imagine that their child might have problems or be imperfect in any way. When they are confronted with the fact that their child has a chronic problem, such as epilepsy, they usually feel responsible and guilty. Although this belief and feeling are irrational, they interfere with the parents' ability to comply with the child's overall management. A parent burdened with guilt finds it almost impossible not to overprotect the child, and no amount of attention and therapeutic manipulation satisfies this lingering concern. Parents who have children with epilepsy must be reassured that the child's problems are not their fault. At the same time they must be reminded that they could not have prevented the problems.

For most parents, simply expressing and discussing their concerns helps to reduce their anxiety so that they can carry out the technical details of their child's treatment. For most families of children with epilepsy, the anxiety about the diagnosis attenuates gradually. During the process, it helps the parents to know that the caregivers understand their concerns and have dealt with these issues before. Parents are reassured to know that their concerns are appropriate to the situation of having a child with epilepsy.

Parents who have persistent difficulty coping with the uncertainty of an idiopathic ("I don't know") diagnosis in the face of a chronic, difficult problem may be helped by talking to other parents who have come to grips with this issue. Support networks can be very helpful. If a parent is having other problems or cannot come to grips with the child's diagnosis, individual counseling may be needed.

TREATING THE WHOLE CHILD

Epilepsy tends to be blamed for all of the child's problems. This is usually a mistake. Seizures are a symptom, a manifestation of abnormal brain functioning, and therefore are no different from other neurologic symptoms. Because both seizures and other neurologic functions are caused by abnormal brain functioning, it is not surprising that, as a group, children with seizures have a greater chance of abnormalities in other aspects of brain functioning. Children with epilepsy are at higher risk for learning problems, behavior problems, and academic underachievement than children without epilepsy. Even though these problems are more common among children with epilepsy, it should be emphasized that the problems are usually independent of the epilepsy. Nevertheless, school problems ranging from learning disabilities to frank mental retardation are sometimes erroneously blamed on the epilepsy. For more information on seizures and developmental disabilities, see Chap. 2.

Some children who have seizures also have handicaps in other areas. An overall approach to these problems is an essential part of global care and treatment. The problems of seizures and epilepsy should be considered in the context of the child's global development and adjustment. For most children with epilepsy and learning problems, the seizures themselves are a minor and often overemphasized component of the child's overall situation.

Children who have school problems along with epilepsy need psychological testing and individualized educational programs, just like other nonepileptic but learning-impaired children. In these situations it is important for care providers to communicate with school nurses, counselors, psychologists, and educators to provide a coordinated program. It is also important to educate school personnel about the relationship of epilepsy to learning problems, clarifying the misconceptions that are commonly held by educators. The school nurse can play an important role in minimizing misconceptions among other school personnel by helping them to understand the child's condition. The communication link between the clinic nurse and the school nurse or the classroom teacher is essential. For a broader discussion of this topic, see Chap. 15. Also refer to the book *Students with seizures: a manual for school nurses,* available from the Epilepsy Foundation of America.

GIVING CONTROL

Because epilepsy is so unpredictable, parents feel better when they know that help is available if they need it. Knowing when to seek help and where alternative sources for help are located gives them a means of controlling the effects of their child's epilepsy. Because this cultivates compliance, care providers should discuss the facilities that are available if the family has a problem or question at odd hours. If there is a phone number to an on-call expert, they will usually test it. Family members also should know what they can reasonably expect of themselves when their child has a frightening seizure. What are their limitations? It helps if the care providers tell them that we expect them to be their child's parent, not their child's doctor or nurse (even when the parents are health professionals). The parents need to have a plan, knowing what they are going to do if their child has another a seizure. The plan should be simple. Parents need clear guidelines about when to call for help, even though they are unlikely to need it. For example, if the child is prone to prolonged seizures, the parents should know when and where to call for emergency help. They also must know what care providers mean by a "prolonged" seizure. Parents feel that all convulsions last too long.

Letting parents participate in therapeutic decisions, such as when to stop medication, when to switch medication, and when to obtain psychological testing also provides them with a measure of control in their child's care. The more they know about epilepsy, the better they can participate.

HELPING PARENTS ALLOW THEIR CHILDREN TO TAKE RISKS

In the process of growing up, children learn from successes and failures, and this process must allow them to take chances. In some cases the consequence of failure is negligible. In other situations the consequence of failure may be substantial physical harm. For example, if a child falls off his bicycle, a broken arm is a possible consequence.

All parents worry that something bad will happen to their child. It begins when the new baby first comes home. The parent looks in on the baby in the middle of the night to make sure that she is still breathing. After a while the parent goes in less often. The parent is learning to accept a risk and not watch the child's every breath.

As the child grows older, parents worry about different consequences for their children. Allowing the child to take chances for learning by success or failure is essential for a child's overall development. Parents must gradually allow their child to take more risks if that child is to develop normally. This general principle should be pointed out to parents of children with epilepsy.

Parents of children who have problems of any type are prone to overprotect the child. The problem is perhaps worse for parents of children with epilepsy because of the unpredictable nature of seizures. The parent never knows when the seizure will occur. If the seizure occurs while the child is involved with physical activity, there is risk for physical harm. What if the seizure occurs while the child is riding a bicycle, or climbing a tree, or swimming?

On the other hand, overprotecting the child has a serious impact on emotional and social development. If the child has no opportunity for participating in age-appropriate activities with peers, critical opportunities for social learning are lost. When interpersonal social skills are not acquired in childhood, the consequences in adulthood are severe. At a fundamental level, the child who is afraid to take a chance has no opportunity for success.

Overprotection of children with epilepsy should be avoided. Children with epilepsy need to do all of the things that other children do. They need to acquire the same social and personal abilities that other children need. In fact, if the epilepsy endures into adulthood, they need extra skills to adjust to their condition as independent adults. This means that, in some cases, parents of children with epilepsy must allow their children to take more chances than normal children take.

It is not easy for the parents of children with epilepsy to allow their children to take the extra chances. Fortunately, the risk of taking extra chances is over-exaggerated. Children who have convulsions rarely experience them while they are engaged in physical activity. Seizures are very uncommon when children with epilepsy are riding a bicycle, running, or swimming.

In most cases, children with epilepsy should participate fully in age-appropriate activities. As with other children, common sense and good judgment should prevail. For example, children who swim should always swim where there is a lifeguard on duty and should swim with a buddy. The same is true for children with epilepsy. On the other hand, children who have convulsions should take showers rather than tub baths because of the tendency of all parents to leave children playing in the tub unattended. The child's actual situation needs to be considered when guidelines are being formulated. Children who are experiencing many seizures daily should probably postpone riding their bicycles and should avoid climbing until the seizures are controlled. On the other hand, children who experience seizures only during sleep should not be restricted. The situation for most children lies somewhere between these extremes, and guidelines should therefore be discussed on an individual basis. For most children with epilepsy the aphorism applies: "Better a broken arm than a broken heart." In the balance, it is better to take a chance unless there is a clear justification for curtailing a child's participation in physical and social activities. A more detailed discussion of safety issues is found in Chap. 16.

MAKING THERAPY CONVENIENT AND ROUTINE

Taking medication and medication-related issues should be made as conve-nient as possible. Administration of medication should be woven into a patient's daily routine of living and linked to habitual daily activities. For most patients, minor variations in the timing of medication administration are insignificant. What is more important is that doses are not forgotten altogether. This means that it is better to link medication administration to meals or to arising or retiring than to set scheduled times. Specifically scheduled times for taking medication are rarely needed.

Avoid administering medication at school when possible. Not administering medication at school has several advantages. It affords a measure of privacy for the child, it avoids making the child different from other pupils because of the need to take medication, and it minimizes the number of people who are ad-ministering the medication, reducing the opportunity for miscommunication about dosage changes.

Visual reminder systems greatly help to avoid missing doses of medication.

Although these can take several forms, the pill reminder box is most widely used. Most pill reminder boxes have a separate compartment for each day of the week. Once a week it is necessary to load each day's compartment with that day's medications. Pill reminder boxes are helpful in all situations and are critical when multiple caretakers are involved with administering medication. Pill reminder boxes also make it much easier for youngsters to become responsible for taking their own medication. The parents can simply look in the box and tell whether the medication is gone. Verbal discussion and the potential for argument are avoided most of the time. Of course, the medicine's being absent from the pill reminders compartment does not guarantee that the child took it, but until proven otherwise it is reasonable to assume that if the medication is gone from the box, the child probably acted responsibly.

The major problem with pill reminder boxes is that they are not childproof safety containers. In households with toddlers or others who might accidentally ingest the patient's medication, it is safer to use childproof bottles, with a separate bottle labeled for each day of the week. For some older children and teens, a multialarm watch can provide the needed reminder necessary to ensure compliance.

OBJECTIVE MEASURES OF COMPLIANCE

Despite highly motivated parents' good intentions to comply, and despite attempts to make drug administration part of a daily household routine, doses of medications are occasionally forgotten. Pill reminder boxes or other visual reminders help to avoid potentially missed doses in many cases. However, when missed doses are discovered, the parent needs to know how and to what extent missed doses should be made up. This varies with the particular medication and with the frequency of drug administration. The procedure for making up doses should be discussed with the prescribing physician.

Patients should be advised to bring their medication with them when they come for checkups. Reviewing the names and doses of the medications with parent or patient helps them learn about the medication and reduces the chances of mistakes in dosing. It also provides a recurring check that the medication was dispensed and labeled as intended. When elixirs are prescribed, it may be necessary to check the volume of the measuring spoon used for administration to ensure proper dosing, since size can vary tremendously.

Measuring AED levels helps to reinforce compliance. If AED levels vary widely and unexpectedly, noncompliance is a leading possibility. When this happens, it is important to discuss the variation in drug levels with the caretaker or the patient. Usually the noncompliant individual confesses when the facts are presented. In fact, in advance of measuring levels it helps to indicate to the patient that you intend to measure AED levels but that if the medications have not been taken regularly the test will not be reliable. This gives patients an opportunity to acknowledge that they have missed doses, and the AED level measurement can then be postponed until the medication has been taken consistently. If AED levels are highly variable and omitted doses are denied, the clinician must look for other causes of varying drug levels. Several factors other than noncompliance can cause drug levels to vary. These include intercurrent febrile illness, drug interactions, and disorders of the gastrointestinal tract, liver, and kidneys.

Most laboratories report drug levels on computer-generated printouts. These printouts often include an asterisk or other indicator when the value is outside of the therapeutic or normal range. It is important for all care providers to understand that certain patients are best treated when their drug levels are lower or higher than these recommended ranges. When abnormal values are encountered, check with the practitioner for interpretation.

HELPING OLDER CHILDREN TO BECOME RESPONSIBLE FOR THEIR CARE

As children grow older they should become responsible for more and more of their own care. This means that they should know the names of medications they are taking, the doses, and the times of administration. They should load their own pill reminder boxes and keep track of their own seizure frequency if they have recurrent seizures despite treatment. When parents have a healthy and comfortable attitude about the disorder, it is easier for the them to support the the patient's assumption of responsibility.

Sooner or later, most adolescents who must take AEDs on a regular basis have a period of time when they avoid or refuse to take their medications regularly. This should be expected and dealt with matter-of-factly, emphasizing to the adolescent that it is they who are at risk for seizures if the medication is not taken regularly. Emotional overreaction by parents, physicians, or nurses only tends to polarize the situation, inhibiting the possibility that the youth will become more compliant. It is important for young people with epilepsy to know that health care providers and their parents can try to help them but that ultimately they are responsible for what happens to themselves. Virtually all teenagers want to drive an automobile. It sometimes helps to remind them that driving will not be possible until their seizures are controlled.

SPECIAL PROBLEMS IN ADOLESCENCE

Health care providers can help teenagers to assume an adult level of responsibility for taking care of their epilepsy. The process begins by treating the teen like an adult. Teenaged patients should be fully informed about their epilepsy and should be allowed to make their own decisions, within the limits of reason and experience. Allowing a teenager to make choices means that the teenager has the right to refuse therapeutic recommendations. What to do when this occurs depends on the teen's situation and the perceived consequences of failure to follow medical recommendations. In most cases in which teenagers rebel and refuse therapy, they eventually resume compliance if the lines of communication are kept open. When teenagers are oppositional and rebellious, they need regular appointments to enable them to work out the transition and to become responsible for their own care in a mature fashion. Health care providers, like parents, must avoid being caught up in emotional debates with teenagers. Peer support groups can also help when teenagers are having problems.

For many young people with well-controlled epilepsy, it is possible to discontinue AED therapy during adolescence. Teenagers who are candidates for withdrawal of therapy should be informed and should participate in the decision of whether to discontinue AED therapy. However, sometimes the decision is not clear-cut, and the teenager may have views that are different from those of the parent. At best, the withdrawal will be successful and the youth is freed of the inconvenience of medication. At worst, if the attempted withdrawal of therapy fails because seizures recur, the young person learns first-hand the importance and justification of AED therapy.

Teenagers with epilepsy must have education about their condition, just like the parents of young children who have epilepsy. They should be advised about the implications of epilepsy and its therapy on adult concerns, such as birth control and family planning. Teenaged girls in particular, must be informed about the teratogenic potential of AED therapy. Both boys and girls need to understand the potentially adverse effects of alcohol and substance abuse on epilepsy and its therapy.

The possibility of pregnancy in adolescence has important implications for teenagers with epilepsy. In particular, young women with epilepsy must be informed about the interactions between AEDs and contraceptive pills. Most AEDs induce metabolism of birth control pills such that women who take AEDs must take higher doses or stronger birth control pills. Breakthrough bleeding in the middle of the menstrual cycle is one sign that young women who take contraceptive pills along with AEDs may require a higher dose of the contraceptive pills. Unfortunately, an unwanted pregnancy is another sign.

Young women with epilepsy must also be informed about the potentially adverse effects of epilepsy and AED therapy on the developing fetus. Decisions about changing or reducing antiepileptic medication must be done *before* conception occurs. After the pregnancy is established, it is usually too late to change therapy because prolonged maternal convulsions are also hazardous for the fetus.

If a teenaged woman's seizures have been well controlled, an attempt to withdraw AEDs is usually indicated. Even when AED therapy cannot be discontinued, young women with epilepsy need to know that epilepsy and AEDs only slightly increase the risk of birth defects in their offspring. Even if they did not have epilepsy or did not take AEDs, they, like every other woman, would still face a 2.5% chance that their baby might have a major problem. There is increased risk associated with maternal epilepsy and AED therapy, but in most cases women with epilepsy have healthy, normal babies. See Chap. 10 for a more detailed discussion.

REFERENCES

Gomez MR. *Neurocutaneous diseases: a practical approach.* Boston: Butterworth-Heinemann, 1987.

Hauser WA, Hesdorffer DC. *Epilepsy: frequency, causes and consequences.* New York: Demos Publications, 1990.

Mizrahi EM, Kellaway P. Characterization and classification of neonatal seizures. *Neurology* 1987;37: 1837–44.

Volpe JJ. *Neonatal neurology.* Philadelphia: WB Saunders, 1994.

Managing Seizure Disorders: A Handbook for Health Care Professionals, edited by N. Santilli, Lippincott-Raven Publishers, Philadelphia, 1996.

9

Considerations for Individuals with Developmental Disabilities

Chad Ellis

Successful management of epilepsy often requires a complex coordination of services and efforts from individuals, health care professionals, and community resources. Treatment modalities may improve conditions in one aspect of a person's life yet create new problems in another arena (for example, medications causing sedation when the person is at work). When developmental disabilities (DDs) are present, new and complex variables are added, often making effective epilepsy management more difficult.

Although the actual treatment of seizures in people with DDs does not differ from that for seizures in those without DDs, special considerations must be taken into account in assisting the person to achieve optimal epilepsy management. This chapter discusses the unique needs of the developmentally disabled community.

DEFINITIONS, PREVALENCE, AND ETIOLOGY

The term "developmental disability" is a broad, catch-all term used to describe any number of conditions that significantly and indefinitely impair a person's cognitive, physical, or psychosocial functioning and that have an onset before the age of 22 years. There is considerable variation in ability in DD individuals, just as there is in the epilepsy community as a whole.

To clarify the definition for public financial assistance and entitlement purposes, the Rehabilitation, Comprehensive Services, and Developmental Disabilities Amendments of 1978 (PL95-602) further elaborated that the individual classified as DD must require a combination of extended services and must have substantial and chronic limitations in at least three of the following areas: language, learning, mobility, self-care, independent living skills, and economic self-sufficiency (United States House of Representatives, 1978). However, some of these functional areas are not readily applicable to children, so additional amendments allowed the recognition of early intervention and the provision of services to children (Morse, 1994).

Many conditions can be considered DDs, such as cerebral palsy, epilepsy, tuberous sclerosis, congenital birth defects, childhood trauma, and mental retardation.

Mental retardation is one of the most common developmental disabilities. Estimates of the prevalence of mental retardation in the United States range from 0.8 to 3% of the general population (Morse, 1994). Discrepancies in these estimates stem from the historic differences in defining mental retardation and the limitations of the tests used to diagnose mental retardation.

Mental retardation is diagnosed using a number of tests to evaluate cognitive functioning and adaptive skills. The familiar intelligence quotient (IQ) test ranks individuals who score below 70 as mentally retarded. However, clinicians and caregivers should remember that IQ scores must be interpreted in a proper context and in conjunction with other tests. To clarify and standardize evaluation processes, the American Association on Mental Retardation stresses the following points:

1. Valid assessments must consider cultural and linguistic diversity.
2. Limitations in adaptive skills occur within the context of the individual's community environment.
3. Limitations in adaptive skills often coexist with strengths in other adaptive skills.
4. With appropriate support, life functioning of the individual with mental retardation will improve.

Because mental retardation is frequently found in the DD community, many use the phrase *developmental disability/mental retardation* (DD/MR) to describe the community as a whole. This chapter addresses the community as being DD and discusses their needs specific to epilepsy, whether or not mental retardation is present.

The etiology of DDs is similar to that of epilepsy as a whole (Table 1). However, it is important to note that there is not a causal relationship between epilepsy and a DD condition such as mental retardation. Rather, the underlying etiologic mechanisms for the DD condition are probably involved in the etiologic mechanisms for epilepsy.

Estimates vary regarding the prevalence of epilepsy in the DD community. However, epilepsy appears to be more closely associated with mental retardation and cerebral palsy than with other DD conditions. Hauser and Hesdorffer (1990) estimate that 21% of people with mental retardation also have epilepsy and that 50% of people with both cerebral palsy and mental retardation have epilepsy. However, Freeman et al. (1990) reassure parents that otherwise normal children who develop epilepsy will not develop mental retardation.

One must suspect the accuracy of epilepsy prevalence statistics in the DD community, because the diagnosis of epilepsy is often difficult to obtain. Many individuals with DD are unable to provide the physical, behavioral, or communicative cooperation needed to complete an appropriate diagnostic work-up.

TABLE 1. *Common etiologies of developmental disabilities*

Prenatal
  Infections (e.g., AIDS, toxoplasmosis, rubella, syphilis)
  Maternal–fetal blood incompatibilities
  Substance abuse (e.g., alcohol, drugs)
  Uncontrolled maternal health problems (e.g., hypertension, diabetes)
  Chromosomal disorders (Down's syndrome)
  Congenital malformations (e.g., spina bifida)
Perinatal
  Premature birth
  Anoxia during labor or birth
  Cerebral trauma
Postnatal
  Trauma
  Infections (e.g., meningitis, encephalitis)
  Neoplasms
  Metabolic disorders (e.g, phenylketonuria)
  Toxins (e.g., lead, mercury, elevated bilirubin)
  Nutritional deficiencies

Diagnosis is sometimes left to clinical observation, and some of the observational data provided to clinicians come from unskilled personnel. Nevertheless, the prevalence of epilepsy in the DD community is significantly greater than in the general population. In addition, it is generally agreed that the more severe the DD condition(s), the more likely that epilepsy will be present, and the more likely that the epileptic condition will be difficult to manage.

HISTORICAL PERSPECTIVE OF THE DD COMMUNITY

As with the general epilepsy community, the DD community has had a long and dark history of routine denial of basic human rights and appropriate medical treatment. Many institutions during the eighteenth and nineteenth centuries housed residents with a variety of disorders. Distinctions were not made between mental illness, epilepsy, and DD/MR (of course, there were individuals with a combination of these disorders). Individuals were lumped together as being "insane" or "feeble-minded." As knowledge about these disorders increased during the twentieth century, institutions began to cater to specific types of conditions.

Not until the 1960s, with the Kennedy administration's focus on mental retardation, did services for the DD community begin to expand. It was at this time that the concepts of normalization (social role valorization), developmental model, least restrictive environment, and mainstreaming began to drive the approach used by service providers and health care professionals. Services and therapies became more available to the DD community in both institutionalized and noninstitutionalized settings. Nevertheless, most of the DD community with moderate to profound conditions resided in institutions, and many of these were slow to adopt new strategies in providing service. In 1972, reporter Geraldo Rivera exposed horrible conditions at the Willowbrook State School in New

York. His report, as well as a number of lawsuits brought by advocates and families, has led to the mandated deinstitutionalization of many individuals with DD. This process is continuing today but varies from state to state because of economic and political factors.

This recent and troublesome past for the DD community has significant implications for those who assist individuals with concurrent disabilities in achieving effective epilepsy management. Many of these have personally experienced denial of basic human rights and may be resistant to interventions that appear restrictive. Individuals with DD need to clearly understand the rationales for any therapeutic interventions. Moreover, some individuals with profound cognitive deficits are unable to act as advocates for themselves and may lack involved family members who can provide advocacy. In these cases, service providers and health care providers must advocate for the best interests of the patient.

The complex combination of epilepsy and DD issues often leads to disagreements among members of the care team as to what those best interests might be. For example, often there is the dilemma of whether to implement restrictive seizure precautions or to maintain a "normalized" environment. In such situations the team may come to an impasse, and the patient may be in the middle without receiving appropriate or consistent treatment.

As mentioned, epilepsy management in individuals with DD need not differ in intervention strategies used and expected outcomes desired from that for persons without DD. However, because of the specialized needs of the DD community, some management strategies must be utilized differently or more cautiously. What follows is a discussion of management phases, including diagnosis, medications, seizure monitoring, and long-term management aspects, and how the needs of the DD community may affect these phases.

DIAGNOSIS OF EPILEPSY

The diagnosis of epilepsy usually relies on subjective reports from clients and family, clinical observation, neurologic assessment, blood tests, CT/MRI scans, and of course, the electroencephalogram (EEG) recording. Epilepsy diagnosis is not always simple, particularly for many members of the DD community, for the following reasons.

Communication Barriers

Difficulties in communicating accounts of physical problems hampers data collection. Some individuals lack the vocabulary to adequately describe changes in sensation and movement to health professionals, particularly during interviews laden with jargon. Many lack the cognitive skills to understand the significance of reporting changes to others and therefore may not offer subjective data. Still others are nonverbal, and therefore are unable to contribute any data at all.

Unskilled Observers

Many individuals reside with caregivers who are untrained in seizure observation. Although this is also true for non-DD individuals with epilepsy, those with DD are more likely to have conditions that mimic seizures than those with epilepsy alone (Table 2). The unskilled caregiver may interpret unusual but nonseizure behaviors and movements as seizures. Conversely, the caregiver may observe true clinical seizures but consider the events a normal part of the DD condition. Still another problem faced by persons with profound DD is the unclear accountability of their caregivers. Some caregivers who provide direct assistance with activities of daily living may not consider "health issues" their responsibility and may assume that health deviations will be discovered and treated by others. Such situations may delay epilepsy evaluation and diagnosis.

Clinical Observations and Neurologic Assessment

Seizure activity rarely occurs on demand. If an individual with DD is referred to a health care professional to evaluate suspicious clinical symptoms, a thorough evaluation and history must be completed. Baseline cognitive, psychological, and mobility impairments may mask subtle signs and symptoms from the examining health professional, particularly if the professional is unfamiliar with DD. Certain clinical tools may not be well suited or easily adapted to the individual with developmental disabilities. This is particularly true of neurologic tests that evaluate cognitive status.

Burns and Snyder (1991) offer guidelines for conducting neurologic examinations of individuals with mental retardation. Their recommended adaptations are presented in Table 3.

CT/MRI Scans

These tests are used adjunctively in epilepsy diagnosis, in that they provide data about structural abnormalities that may correlate with suspected seizure

TABLE 2. *Clinical signs common in DD that can mimic seizures*

Tics
Spasms
Attention deficits
Communication difficulties
Difficulties in processing environmental stimuli
Psychotic episodes
Misdirected aggression
Hallucinations
Pseudoseizures
Somatization of emotional/psychological conflicts
Hyperactivity
Autism-like behavior

TABLE 3. *Neurologic functional abilities assessment*

Consciousness
  Awake? Able to complete tasks?
Orientation
  Person: assess by recognition of people, objects
  Place: is client able to find locations of various rooms in the house/building?
  Thing: able to identify personal possessions vs. possessions of others?
  Time: make more global—assess awareness of night/day, seasons
Memory
  Short term
    Use pictures—identify five objects in picture, then bring picture out later and ask patient to recall which items in the picture were indicated
    Use objects—select objects from a group of objects, then ask patient to indicate which objects were selected
    Ask patient to recall what was eaten at last meal, events of previous day, etc.
Long-term memory
  Ask patient to recall family members visited, trips taken, etc.
Thinking
  Ask patient to define common slang words used by patient or roommates
  Ask patient to identify objects with common textures, colors, etc.
  Use simple math, such as addition, instead of serial sevens
Language
  Assess for ability to follow commands
  Assess for ability to identify symbols, or to explain what is happening in a picture
  Ask patient to tell a simple story; assess for choice of words, grammar, flow and volume of words, intensity of speech, and emotional appropriateness
Movement
  Demonstrate first what you want when assessing motor function (e.g., demonstrate flexing your arm first).
Vision
  If unable to complete the usual vision screen, assess how well the patient moves around in the environment, how well the patient identifies objects of different size, or have the patient trace letters with a finger
Pain sensation
  Discriminating between sharp/dull requires great concentration; to assess for appropriate pain response, question patient and others on patient's historical response to cuts, scrapes, bruises, etc.
Hearing
  Client may not cooperate with test with tuning fork; assess ability to follow verbal commands; does patient turn head to sudden noises or to his/her name?
Coping
  Emotions observed in a clinic setting often not characteristic; observe behavior and emotions in patient's normal environment; assess how he/she deals with conflict with others, carries out assigned duties, behaviors during a variety of social situations

Adapted from Burns et al., 1991.

foci. The successful scan requires physical and behavioral cooperation from the individual being tested. Many of those with DD are unable to provide this cooperation because they cannot understand instructions, cannot understand abstractions such as time ("OK, lie still for just 5 more minutes"), or cannot maintain muscle control because of spasms. Sedation with diazepam or other drugs may be helpful but is often not effective in individuals with moderate to severe cognitive and/or muscle control impairments.

Electroencephalography

The EEG is, of course, the gold standard in epilepsy diagnosis. As with CT/ MRI scans, cooperation is needed from the individual being tested. Although pretest sedation can be used, sedatives may hamper the interpretation of the EEG because the sedation may mask epilepsy correlates on the EEG. In addition, if sedation is required, a natural and baseline sleep and awake EEG cannot be performed. Some physicians prefer to have an EEG completed under sedation rather than to have no EEG at all. Staff may find it helpful to have patients rehearse or visit the EEG laboratory before the test is scheduled so that they can become acclimated to the test and the surroundings.

Because of these difficulties in obtaining EEG recordings, many individuals with DD historically have been diagnosed with epilepsy without EEG data. Unfortunately, once the diagnosis of epilepsy is made in individuals with DD, the diagnosis is not always revised or withdrawn. To ensure correct diagnosis in patients with mental retardation, Coulter (unpublished data, 1989) developed quality assurance criteria. These criteria state that:

1. The seizure events must be described in detail.
2. The seizure type should be classified according to the International Classification of Epileptic Seizures
3. All seizures must be recorded in a seizure record.
4. An EEG must have been performed within the past 5 years.
5. EEGs and scans should be performed within 1 month of the request (if seizure etiology is not apparent).
6. The etiology of the epilepsy must be indicated.

Although these criteria do not appear unusual, they have not been consistently followed in the DD community. Clearly, it is not appropriate to treat an individual with an antiepileptic drug (AED) for suspected epilepsy "just to be on the safe side." Coulter's diagnostic criteria are a helpful guide for team members to use for advocacy purposes.

MEDICATION

Although monotherapy is desirable for all patients with epilepsy, polypharmacy may be required for those with difficulties in seizure control (Porter, 1989). Nevertheless, overmedication in the DD community has been demonstrated (Coulter, 1988; Lannon, 1990). Lannon reported that 46% of all patients admitted to an epilepsy unit for the mentally retarded were receiving three or more AEDs. It is suggested that many individuals with DD have had medications added to their profile without clear diagnostic rationales. Lannon states that drug rationalization (assessing the appropriateness of drug profiles) is necessary because it improves seizure control and overall functioning. Through drug rationalization, Lannon reported that 76% of the patients studied achieved better seizure control.

In addition to polypharmacy, the kinds of AED combinations observed in DD individuals have caused problems. Lannon reports that 58% of her patients were admitted with combinations of phenytoin, phenobarbital, and benzodiazepines, 18% of whom were taking all three. Such drug combinations often cause sedation to a degree that significantly impairs learning and functional skills. Coulter (1988) strongly advocates striving for monotherapy in this population and recommends that sedating drugs be withdrawn from the drug profile. He also states that the withdrawal of sedating drugs is safe, and found in his study that 35 of 44 patients experienced no decrease in seizure control when sedating drugs were withdrawn.

The sedative properties of AEDs are not the only problem faced by these individuals. Some medications produce adverse effects of dizziness or gait disturbances (although these effects are often dose-related). Such effects can pose serious safety problems in persons with baseline judgment and mobility impairments.

Some DD individuals have psychiatric or behavioral control problems in addition to epilepsy. Many drugs prescribed for concurrent problems have negative interactions with AEDs. It is imperative that all prescribing health professionals have current and complete medication profiles. Moreover, professionals must be aware that because of the communication impairments of these individuals and the possibility of unskilled caretakers, toxicity from AEDs often goes unnoticed. Coulter (unpublished data, 1989) developed criteria for the medical management of individuals with epilepsy and developmental disabilities. These are:

Neurologic consultation is obtained at least annually.

The AEDs prescribed are indicated for the seizure type that the patient experiences.

No more than *two* AEDs are prescribed.

Inappropriate drug combinations are not used.

AED levels are measured every 6 months.[1]

AED levels are recorded on the medication profile.

Appropriate adjustments will be made when AED levels lie outside of the patient's therapeutic range.

Efforts are made to identify adverse drug effects.

Actions are taken for any adverse drug effects present.

Medications are administered (taken) accurately.

Appropriate action is taken for refusal of medication.[2]

The following case study illustrates some of the problems just discussed.

---

[1] Some drugs, such as gabapentin, may not need this.

[2] Appropriate action is determined in light of the individual's self-care ability, residential setting, and medical status.

Case Study 1

Donald is a 65-year-old man with profound mental retardation, a behavioral disorder characterized by self-injurious behavior, and a suspected seizure disorder. He resides in a community home with two other mentally retarded roommates. Caregivers staff the home 24 h per day.

At the age of 17 months Donald developed scarlet fever. After this illness he was described as a hyperactive child, prone to self-injurious behavior. As a child, he attended no schools or habilitation programs. He lived with his parents until they died when he was 45 years old. At this time he was institutionalized in a facility for mentally retarded adults.

When Donald was 56 years old, while still living in an institution, he experienced an event his nonmedical caregiver described as a grand mal seizure. The consulting physician placed Donald on phenobarbital. Two weeks after starting phenobarbital he experienced another event. At that time the physician added phenytoin to Donald's profile. No neurologic consultation or EEG was obtained, Donald's events ceased, and he was diagnosed as having a seizure disorder. He experienced no other events identified as seizures while institutionalized. At the age of 60, Donald was discharged from the institution to a group home in the community. He received a medical examination by a general practitioner on admission to the community program. The physician continued his phenobarbital and phenytoin.

At the age of 61, staff at Donald's day habitation program reported ongoing daytime somnolence. The registered nurse for the program reviewed his records and sleep patterns. Medication dosing was changed to a bedtime schedule, but his somnolence did not greatly improve. In reviewing Donald's seizure records, the nurse noted that he had been seizure-free for 5 years. The nurse approached Donald's physician and requested that the phenobarbital be discontinued. The physician was opposed to this measure, but after much discussion agreed to a neurologic consultation.

Donald was referred to a neurology clinic at a large teaching hospital. The neurologist agreed to a slow taper and discontinuation of the phenobarbital. Donald completed the taper within 6 weeks without incident. Staff noted increased alertness and interactivity shortly after the taper was completed. They also noted an increase in self-injurious behavior, which required a revision of Donald's behavior management plan.

At the age of 65, after receiving phenytoin for 7 years, Donald remained free of any observable seizures. There was much discussion at Donald's interdisciplinary team meetings about the need for continuing phenytoin. Some team members felt that he had the right to be free of unnecessary medication. Others felt that the phenytoin was keeping him seizure-free. The team agreed to request that Donald's physician make a referral for an EEG and consultation with an epileptologist.

Donald's EEG showed no epileptiform data but did show a generalized slowing.

Although the diagnosis of epilepsy could not be confirmed, the epileptologist recommended that Donald continue to take his phenytoin because of "his profound mental retardation." At this time, at the age of 66, Donald remains seizure-free on phenytoin 200 mg per day. The team continues to debate the need for continuing the phenytoin. At present they are seeking a second opinion.

SEIZURE OBSERVATION AND SEIZURE SAFETY

The best way to determine medication efficacy and seizure control is to maintain accurate and complete seizure records, in which observed seizures are described and recorded. However, these records are only as good as the persons who maintain them. Lannon (1990) states that when a diagnosis of epilepsy is made in a patient with DD, any unusual behavior or movement may be labeled as a seizure. There are two primary reasons for this. First, unskilled caregivers are unable to adequately assess and describe their observations. As discussed earlier, many events mimic seizures but are in reality a manifestation of some other process. Second, when persons with DD are informed that the event they just experienced was a seizure, they learn to mislabel future events.

Lannon reports that seizure documentation can be enhanced by using a seizure calendar that labels predetermined events. For example, the patient or caregiver describes an event that is identified as a seizure. This event is given a label (such as "Seizure 1" or "Seizure A"). Each time this event occurs, the label is recorded on the calendar. This system allows for multiple types of "events" or seizures. A health care professional who later reviews the calendar, will know exactly how many of which kinds of events have occurred as opposed to a simple accounting of seizures. Many service providers utilize seizure forms or flowsheets similar to those used in many hospitals. These flowsheets contain a list of descriptors, on which staff indicate which clinical sign occurred during a seizure. Again, these flowsheets are only as accurate as the staffperson completing the form. All caregivers and staff who work with these individuals should have training in basic seizure recognition and first aid. In addition, Coulter (1988) recommends these safety principles:

All direct care staff should be trained in CPR and first aid.
First aid equipment should be available and in good working order in the patient's environment.
All seizure-related injuries should be noted.
Injury prevention practices should be implemented.
No procedures that put the patient at risk for serious injury should be performed.
Protective devices should be in good working condition and should be checked regularly.
Injuries should not be caused by wearing of protective devices.
All protective devices should be capable of quick removal in an emergency.

These recommendations are well-suited for settings such as vocational centers, habilitation centers, schools, and inpatient/residential facilities. Any restrictive protective device should not significantly impair the independence of the individual, nor should it violate basic human rights. Home settings may require additional safety practices. However, staff should be aware that home settings must strive toward the ideal of a normalized (noninstitutional) appearance without compromising safety. For more details on safety and injury prevention, see Chap. 16.

LONG-TERM MANAGEMENT ISSUES

Long-term management of epilepsy in general is described in other chapters of this book. All concepts of long-term management apply to the DD community as well. However, some key points should be made.

The role of stress in precipitating seizures is becoming a more common topic in discussions of management. Many health care providers and advocacy groups are assisting individuals with epilepsy to reduce stress by use of specific stress-reduction procedures. However, many persons with DD lack the cognitive or physical ability to utilize techniques such as meditation, imagery, relaxation therapy, and regular exercise, and emotional stress and anxiety may be pronounced in the lives of DD individuals with epilepsy.

Caregivers can assist by supporting and providing daytime "quiet times" during which the person being cared for is free to disengage, relax, or nap. If behavioral control is an issue, caregivers should intervene with actions to help the person regain control when maladaptive behaviors escalate. Such actions may include "time outs," distraction, physical activity, or reorientation. Such actions should be individualized and should be approved by members of the health care team.

Caregivers who administer medications should verify the accuracy of medication procedures and should be well versed in the possible adverse effects for the person's drug profile. Caregivers must also be diligent in assessing acute problems, because the person's ability to communicate may be limited. In addition, they should understand how to avoid medication-related problems. For example, one common problem leading to drug toxicity is dehydration. Individuals who depend on others to administer fluids often cannot communicate thirst. Even mild dehydration can lead to elevation of serum AED levels. Unlicensed, nonfamily personnel assigned to administer medications should be supervised by appropriate licensed personnel in accordance with local regulations and laws.

Education is a key factor in assisting people with epilepsy to self-manage. Self-management includes the person with epilepsy as a member of the team, provides empowerment, and may enhance compliance with management strategies. Unfortunately, many individuals are denied the opportunity to learn self-management skills because health professionals underestimate their capacity to learn.

Everyone confronts barriers to learning (Table 4). However, patients with DD and cognitive impairments often have greater difficulty in overcoming these barriers. Caregivers and providers can employ strategies to assist these people. These strategies include avoidance of jargon, making teaching content more concrete, relying on greater use of visual teaching techniques, involving the individual in the teaching process, shortening teaching sessions, and frequent repetition. Lannon (1990), using appropriate teaching strategies, reported that 80% of patients were able to fill weekly drug containers by using visual cue cards.

Effective long-term management includes periodic reassessment of management strategies, including medication. As mentioned, Coulter (unpublished data, 1989) recommends annual neurologic consultation for patients with DD. If seizure control or medication issues are not satisfactory or become worse, more frequent and more rigorous reevaluation may be necessary. Unfortunately, many health professionals do not reevaluate appropriately, partially because of patients' lack of cooperation. Health professionals sometimes do not act until strong complaints are made about the problem or there is a clear concern for safety.

Another reason why many individuals with DD do not receive appropriate and periodic assessments is lack of access to health services. Many people rely upon public assistance programs for such services. As economic and political pressures affect these programs, many individuals are denied access to specialists. Increasingly, public assistance programs are being administered under a managed care format, in which the primary physician must refer to specialists. Some primary physicians may not fully understand the complex issues involved. Anecdotally, a primary physician had said, "Well if he's not having any seizures, then the medications he is taking must be appropriate, so he doesn't need a neurologic consultation."

Much research today is focused on identifying better medical and psychosocial interventions for management of epilepsy. However, many people with mental retardation are excluded from these studies. Researchers often find that mental retardation presents too many confounding variables for their studies. In addition, many research review boards find the mentally retarded a vulnerable population and may limit researchers' access to them. Therefore, the efficacy of interventions for the DD community is not always well known before the interventions are

TABLE 4. *Barriers to learning*

Inability to abstract
Limited opportunities for environmental interactions
Poor self-concept
Short memory span
Inability to generalize
Limited learning capacity
Processing deficits
Short attention span
Difficulty understanding cause-and-effect relationships
Outward-directed locus of control

From McGwin, 1988.

utilized. Interventions implemented in the DD community may not be tailored to address the community's unique needs, thereby impairing fair trial and evaluation of specific interventions.

For many persons with DD, quality of life determinations are made by others. Although most team members consider all variables in measuring and promoting an optimal quality of life, their efforts are limited without subjective input from the patient. Unfortunately, too many professionals consider the quality of life for persons in the DD community as poor, with no chance for significant improvement because of the severity and chronicity of a particular condition.

Individuals with DD should have the same service and treatment options available to them as for the non-DD epilepsy community. Although few people would disagree with this, the concept is not universally implemented. Treatment programs that provide assistance to people with epilepsy often operate with limited resources. Treatment and services may sometimes be given to those who are most readily able to self-advocate or who can demonstrate the greatest perceived improvement in their quality of life. In addition, medical and surgical treatment options are often more available to those with private medical insurance. For example, should epilepsy surgery be offered preferentially to the non-DD individual who will return to gainful employment rather than to the equally impaired DD individual who will return to a day habilitation program? Quality of life issues are complex and require strong advocacy, which is sometimes lacking in situations involving persons with DD. Caregivers and providers should sharpen their advocacy skills so that they can assist the DD community in achieving optimal quality of life.

PSEUDOSEIZURES

A number of authors have determined that a significant number of patients with intractable epilepsy have pseudoseizures or pseudoseizures in conjunction with epileptic seizures (Gates, 1987; Meierkord et al., 1991; Walker and Rowan, 1993). However, patients who are referred to epilepsy centers for video-EEG monitoring are an uncharacteristic sample of people with epilepsy in general. It is unclear how prevalent pseudoseizures are in the DD/epilepsy community.

Pseudoseizures are epilepsy-like events that exhibit no EEG changes consistent with epileptic seizures. They usually stem from psychiatric conflict. Pseudoseizures often arise as a sign of post-traumatic stress (particularly from sexual or physical abuse), somatization of repressed anger or anxiety, attention seeking, or from efforts at obtaining secondary gain (e.g., work avoidance, financial gain). Pseudoseizures are almost three times as common in females as in males, although the explanation for this is not clear (Walker and Rowan, 1993). Some may anticipate the prevalence of pseudoseizures to be higher in the DD community than in the non-DD community because this population often has decreased cognitive skills, which are needed for effective coping and adaptation to environmental changes.

Clearly, some persons with DD are unable to appropriately cope with stress and frustrations and therefore "act out" their emotions behaviorally. Some of these behaviors can mimic seizures. Patients with genuine epileptic seizures may learn that positive attention is given to them when seizures occur and may seek that attention at other times. However, some patients with DD may report that they have experienced a seizure because someone had mislabeled a previous similar event as a seizure.

Pseudoseizures have created many negative attitudes on the part of caregivers and health providers. Many feel that the patient who experiences the pseudoseizure is in control of the event and is deliberately bringing the event forward. However, many events are generated on the subconscious level. Some patients with DD may have learned that a pseudoseizure is the most effective way to have their needs met (which is actually an effective, albeit inappropriate, adaptive mechanism). Lannon (unpublished data, 1992) presented a list of questions for health care professionals to ask themselves to help clarify their own attitudes about pseudoseizures and the persons who experience them. These questions are listed in Table 5.

Although Gates (1987) and others have described some clinical observations that are consistent with pseudoseizures, many of these nonepileptic events appear very similar to genuine epileptic seizures. Therefore, caregivers should be very cautious about assuming that an event is nonepileptic, especially when the patient does have epilepsy. Pseudoseizures can cause great injury to the patient. First aid measures and close observation should always be part of monitoring these events.

In providing assistance to a patient with DD who experiences a pseudoseizure, the following guidelines should be observed:

Protect the person from injury.

Maintain the person's dignity; never scold or ridicule; turn away bystanders to maintain privacy.

Take the event seriously; the pseudoseizure is a sign of a problem, albeit a nonepileptic problem.

TABLE 5. *Have you ever said or thought or done?*

She is only faking it.
He's only doing it for attention.
They're wasting my time. I have really sick people to take care of.
He needs to be on a psychiatric unit.
This isn't a real seizure.
If you're going to fake it, you can do better than that.
Refused to respond when someone said they were having a seizure.
Left the person alone during a non-epileptic event.
Shown by your tone of voice or body language that you were uncomfortable or rejecting the person.

From Lannon, 1992, unpublished data

Restrictive interventions and nonintervention must have clear rationales and should be consistent with the team's plan.
Document all pseudoseizures, especially antecedents to the event.

If pseudoseizures are correctly diagnosed, treatment for patients with DD is available. Gates (1987) reports success with behavioral modification and psychotherapy for patients with mental retardation. Reassurance and relaxation may be helpful for those who misinterpret unusual body sensations as seizures.

Antipsychotic medication may be indicated for patients whose pseudoseizures arise from clinical psychoses. The patient who experiences pseudoseizures often presents a complicated profile to health professionals. When DD is added to the profile, additional challenges are presented. Prognosis for pseudoseizures may not be overly encouraging, as the following case study indicates.

Case Study 2

Antoinette is a 24-year-old woman with mild mental retardation, epilepsy, and conversion disorder/disassociative seizures. The etiology for Antoinette's mental retardation and epilepsy is unclear but may be associated with low birth weight. As an infant, she lived with her single mother. She moved in with her grandmother and step-grandfather as a toddler when her mother was incarcerated on drug-related offenses. From the ages of 4 to 16 Antoinette was sexually abused by her step-grandfather and possibly by others as well. At the age of 16, the abuse was discovered by state officials, and Antoinette was placed in foster homes.

Antoinette was diagnosed with a generalized seizure disorder as a child and was placed on a variety of medication combinations. By the age of 16 she was taking phenobarbital, lorazepam, and valproate. However, she was reported to have multiple generalized seizures per week. At age 17, Antoinette began psychotherapy after some reported self-injurious behavior.

At the age of 18 Antoinette was moved to a group home for retarded adults. Her seizures and antiepileptic medication did not change. Six months later, she suffered second- and third-degree burns while in the shower and was hospitalized. Despite her cognitive impairments and inaccessibility to the hot water heater, the group home claimed that it was a suicide attempt. An investigation into the possible negligence of the group home provider began. While Antoinette was hospitalized, the provider refused to take her back after discharge, claiming that she was "too much of a liability." She was discharged to a respite home.

Within a month, Antoinette was admitted to a comprehensive epilepsy center for evaluation of her seizures and medications. She was diagnosed with pseudoseizures and was transferred to an inpatient psychiatric unit for 2 weeks. Her medications were changed to phenytoin and valproate. She was discharged to a group home owned by a different provider. At this point, many of Antoinette's historical records were lost.

Over the next 18 months, Antoinette was admitted several times for reevaluation of her seizures, her behavioral program, and psychiatric interventions. During this time, staff at the group home changed frequently, various behavioral programs were implemented, and different medications were prescribed. Eventually, she was placed on valproate, carbamazepine, lorazepam for seizures, and sertraline hydrochloride (Zoloft) for depression. Her behavioral plan recommended confrontation and nonintervention when she started pseudoseizures. Staff at her residential program (group home) and staff at her day habilitation program were often confused as to which plan and regimen were current. Antoinette received widely inconsistent intervention during this time.

At the age of 24, Antoinette was admitted to a neurobehavioral unit at a large university hospital associated with a comprehensive epilepsy center. She remained there for more than 3 months while her pseudoseizures were carefully studied, and a variety of interventions were implemented and evaluated. Her medication profile was also examined. On discharge, staff at the neurobehavioral unit presented an extensive plan for intervention. Unfortunately, the plan was developed without input from Antoinette's residential and day habilitation programs. Many interventions recommended in the plan were not feasible (because of environmental and staffing realities) to implement after discharge, so Antoinette returned to the same intervention strategies she had before her stay in the neurobehavioral unit. She was discharged on valproate, carbamazepine, lorazepam, and lamotrigine for seizures and propranolol for behavior management. Three weeks after discharge, the lamotrigine was discontinued because of lack of clinical improvement.

At this time Antoinette continues to have approximately one generalized epileptic seizure per week and multiple pseudoseizures per day. Her pseudoseizures are often brought on by stress, particularly stress resulting from changes in her daily routine. As her psychiatric/neurobehavioral staff are connected with a teaching hospital, staff personnel have changed because interns have graduated or moved on. Antoinette's residential provider may be shut down by the state because of some licensing violations. Staff at Antoinette's day habilitation program have noticed generalized fatigue/lethargy since propranolol was added to her medication profile. They are not certain who should be approached about reevaluation of the propranolol's effectiveness. Staff also report no significant improvement in Antoinette's seizures. Her future living arrangements and her medical and psychosocial prognoses remain unclear.

CONCLUSIONS

Persons with DD present a wide range of cognitive and functional abilities. Epilepsy is significantly more common in this community than in the non-DD community. Although epilepsy management strategies are similar in both communities, individuals with DD often present with special needs, which may require strategies to be carefully tailored.

Historically, the DD community has been misunderstood and, as a consequence, inappropriately diagnosed because of challenges in communication, challenges in successfully completing diagnostic tests, reliance on subjective data from unskilled caregivers, and the DD community's difficulty in accessing health professionals. As mandated, deinstitutionalization continues, and as the DD community is mainstreamed into general society, more health care professionals and service providers will be dealing with these individuals. An enhanced understanding by health care providers of this community's needs in the setting of epilepsy management will enable the care providers to better assist DD individuals in achieving an optimal quality of life.

REFERENCES

American Association on Mental Retardation. *Mental retardation: definition, classification, and systems of support,* 9th edition. Washington, DC, 1992.

Burns KR, Snyder MS. Neurological assessment: adaptations for special populations with mental retardation. *J Neurosci Nurs* 1991;23:107–10.

Commission on Classification and Terminology of the International League Against Epilepsy. Proposal for revised classification of epilepsies and epileptic syndromes. *Epilepsia* 1989;30:389–99.

Coulter DL. Withdrawal of sedative anticonvulsant drugs from mentally retarded persons: development of guidelines. *J Epilepsy* 1988;1:67–70.

Ellis CR. Nursing assessment and intervention for the patient experiencing seizures: a structured approach. *Clin Nurs Prac Epilepsy* 1993;1:4–7.

Frank J. The role of the nurse in seizure management. In: Roth SP, Morse JS, eds. *A life-span approach to nursing care for individuals with developmental disabilities.* Baltimore: Paul H. Brookes Publishing, 1994:219–48.

Freeman JM, Vining EPG, Pillas DJ. *Seizures and epilepsy in childhood: a guide for parents.* Baltimore: Johns Hopkins University Press, 1990.

Gates JR. Psychogenic seizures. *Merritt Putnam Q* 1987;4:3–15.

Hauser WA, Hesdorffer DC. *Epilepsy: frequency, causes and consequences.* New York: Demos Publications, 1990.

Lannon SL. Assessing seizure activity in mentally disabled adults. *J Neurosci Nurs* 1990;22:294–301.

Leis AR, Ross MA, Summers AK. Psychogenic seizures: ictal characteristics and diagnostic pitfalls. *Neurology* 1992;42:95–9.

Lelliott PT, Fenwick P. Cerebral pathology in pseudoseizures. *Acta Neurol Scan* 1991;83:129–32.

McGwin K. Learning characteristics of people who are mentally retarded. Videotape produced by Bethesda Lutheran Homes and Services, Inc., Watertown, WI, 1988.

Meierkord H, Will B, Fish D, Shorvon S. The clinical features and prognosis of pseudoseizures diagnosed using video-EEG telemetry. *Neurology* 1991;41:1643–6.

Morse JS. An overview of developmental disabilities nursing. In: Roth SP, Morse JS, eds. *A life-span approach to nursing care for individuals with developmental disabilities.* Baltimore: Paul H. Brookes Publishing, 1994:19–58.

Nehring WM. A history of nursing in developmental disabilities in America. In: Roth SP, Morse JS, eds. *A life-span approach to nursing care for individuals with developmental disabilities.* Baltimore: Paul H. Brookes Publishing, 1994:1–18.

Porter RJ. *Epilepsy: 100 elementary principles.* Philadelphia: WB Saunders, 1989.

United States House of Representatives. Conference report: Comprehensive rehabilitation services amendments of 1978 (Report No. 95-1780, pp. 51–52). Washington, DC: U.S. Government Printing Office, 1978.

Walker J, Rowan J. *Issues in epilepsy and quality of life: nonepileptic (pseudoepileptic) seizures (NES).* Landover, MD: Epilepsy Foundation of America, 1993.

Managing Seizure Disorders: A Handbook for
Health Care Professionals, edited by N. Santilli,
Lippincott-Raven Publishers, Philadelphia, 1996.
© 1996 Epilepsy Foundation of America.

10

Issues for Women with Epilepsy

Mimi Callanan and Nancy Stalland

Women with epilepsy have special concerns that become evident during the childbearing years. These include the effect of hormones on seizures and issues surrounding contraception, fertility, and sexuality. Although small, there is an increased risk to the mother and fetus during pregnancy. This may be because of the antiepilepsy drugs (AEDs) and the epilepsy itself (Morrell, 1995). Parenting may also be a problem for some women with uncontrolled seizures.

Hormones can affect seizure threshold by altering the excitability of the neurons. In experimental animal models, estrogen increases and progesterone decreases neuronal excitability and the chance that a seizure may occur (Morrell, 1992). Many women complain that seizures tend to increase just before or during menses and ovulation, a time when estrogen is high and progesterone is low. These seizures are commonly referred to as catamenial seizures. Other possible causes for catamenial seizures may be related to changes in body weight and water and fluctuations in AED levels (Morrell, 1992).

Women should be instructed to chart seizures on a calendar in relation to the menstrual cycle and/or ovulation if they see a trend for seizures to occur at that time. This information should then be presented to the health care provider. Some women may benefit from adjunctive hormonal therapy, such as oral, vaginal, or intramuscular progesterone or clomiphene, a estrogen antagonist.

Many hormonal changes occur during puberty and may affect seizure control. Puberty is a time when some epilepsies remit, others worsen, and some are unaffected (Morrell, 1992). It is a difficult time for adolescents, both emotionally and socially, and this may also exacerbate seizures.

Menopause is a time when the ovarian hormones estrogen and progesterone drop. Unfortunately, the effect of menopause on epilepsy is unknown. Rosciszwska (1987) studied women in menopause and found that seizure frequency was more likely to improve if seizures were associated with the menstrual cycle, if seizures began later in life, and if they were well controlled. No other studies have been reported.

Hormonal replacement during menopause is controversial and is somewhat more complicated in women with epilepsy. It is unclear whether hormonal replacement may improve, worsen, or have no effect on seizure control. The risk for osteoporosis is also greater once a woman reaches menopause. Some of the AEDs may impair vitamin D metabolism. Calcium and vitamin D supplements should be discussed. Weight-bearing exercises should be encouraged to prevent osteoporosis. Women should be encouraged to discuss all of these issues with a physician so that decisions regarding treatment are based on factual information.

Sexual dysfunction has been reported in both men and women with epilepsy (Herzog et al., 1991; Morrell 1991). This may be related to the epilepsy, to AEDs, or to psychosocial factors. Sexual dysfunction can present as a decrease in desire and arousal and occurs in at least 30% of men and women with epilepsy (Blumer and Walker, 1967).

Problems with low self-esteem and poor self-image are seen in patients with uncontrolled seizures and may lead to social isolation, resulting in less experience with intimate relationships. Fear of having a seizure during intimate moments or past experiences of seizures during intimacy may also have an impact on sexual function.

Health care providers should recognize that this may be a big concern for many people with epilepsy and should be part of every assessment. It may be uncomfortable to ask questions regarding sexuality, but patients will be relieved to know that their sexual problems might be a result of AEDs or epilepsy and are not necessarily psychological.

Fertility may be adversely affected because of the higher risk for reproductive endocrine disorders, such as menstrual abnormalities, polycystic ovaries, oligomenorrhea and amenorrhea (Herzog et al., 1982). Cummings et al. (1995) found a higher incidence of anovulation in women with temporal lobe epilepsy compared to those with primary generalized epilepsy and controls. Patients should be referred to a gynecologist who has an understanding of the special issues of epilepsy or should be agreeable to working closely with the neurologist. Assessment may include hormone levels and ultrasonography.

AEDs, which induce the hepatic microsomal enzyme system, lower the effectiveness of birth control pills in many women (Fiol et al., 1983). Therefore, either a higher-dose "pill" of estrogen and/or progesterone (estrogen >50 μg) or alternative methods of birth control should be used (e.g., foam, condoms, diaphragm, IUD). Norplant may also be metabolized faster, for the same reasons as oral contraceptives. Information is not yet available on DepoProvera and women taking AEDs. Patients should be referred to a gynecologist for further counseling on birth control methods.

The obvious result of contraceptive failure is pregnancy. All women of childbearing potential who have epilepsy should be counseled about pregnancy and the possible risks to the mother and child. This includes adolescents. Any woman of childbearing age who is capable of becoming pregnant should be instructed to take prenatal vitamins with folic acid or a folic acid supplement prior to pregnancy. Some AEDs have been shown to act as folic acid antagonists, thus lowering folic acid levels. Low maternal folic acid levels have been associated with an increased risk for malformations, particularly neural tube defects (MRC Study, 1991).

It is essential for a woman with epilepsy to plan the pregnancy. She should discuss her plans with her treating physician approximately 6 months to 1 year before conception to minimize any potential problems. Ideally, she should have an obstetrician and neurologist who can work together and consult each other throughout the pregnancy. The woman should take responsibility for discussing her epilepsy, AEDs, and other concerns, including a family history of birth defects, with both the obstetrician and neurologist at various points throughout the pregnancy.

The health care professionals may be called on to review these issues with the pregnant woman and her significant other. They can ensure that factual information is available to the parents, to minimize their fears and give them the confidence to counter any misconceptions and untoward comments made by well-meaning relatives and friends. It is important to emphasize the fact that at least 90% of women with epilepsy have normal pregnancies and normal children, and that the 10% or lower risk of an adverse outcome can be minimized.

In 53% of the cases studied there was no change in seizure frequency during a pregnancy (Andermann et al., 1985). Seizures decreased in frequency in 22% and increased in 24% of the pregnancies. The increase in seizures occurred at the end of the first trimester and the start of the second trimester (due to estrogen changes associated with pregnancy) in 50% of cases. There is some indication that seizure frequency before pregnancy can be used to predict changes during pregnancy. If seizures occur less than once a month before pregnancy, there will probably be no change in frequency during pregnancy. If seizures occur once a month before pregnancy, seizures may increase during pregnancy. Poor seizure control during pregnancy may also be due to anxiety, sleep loss, and poor medication compliance. Medication noncompliance may be related to fear of the effects of the medication on the fetus.

The incidence of birth defects is 2–3% higher in women with epilepsy than in the general population. The major malformations seen are cleft lip and palate and heart defects, specifically ventricular septal defects. All of the commonly used AEDs appear to pose similar risks for the development of congenital malformations. In the past, a "fetal hydantoin syndrome" that included growth deficiency, abnormalities of the nails and fingers, and small head size has been described but has more recently been recognized in association with epilepsy itself as well as with other AEDs (Delgado-Escueta and Janz, 1992). These minor malformations consistent with dysmorphic features of the face and digits occur in approximately 5–40% of infants born to women with epilepsy (Kallen, 1986).

Women taking valproate (Depakene, Depakote) or carbamazepine (Tegretol) during the first trimester may have an increased risk for having a child with a neural tube defect (spina bifida). The risk with valproic acid is 1–2% (Lindhout, 1992) and 0.5–1% with carbamazepine (Rosa, 1991). A serum or amniotic α-fetoprotein level and a level II ultrasound can determine with 95% confidence if a neural tube defect is present.

Certain medications appear more likely to cause problems but are infrequently prescribed today. Trimethadione (Tridione) and paramethadione (Paradione) are more likely to cause severe congenital malformations, as are phenobarbital, valproate, and carbamazepine when taken in combination. If she is being treated with these medications, a woman should probably avoid pregnancy or discuss changing to another medication before pregnancy.

There is an increase in the rate of congenital malformations with the new medications, although this information is limited and is still being gathered.

Complex partial seizures without loss of consciousness have no known problems associated with fetal development. Generalized tonic–clonic (GTC) seizures, particularly during labor, may lead to anoxia and cause brain damage to the infant. Earlier in the pregnancy, GTC seizures may result in miscarriage or other malformations (Yerby and McCormick, 1987). GTC and complex partial seizures may be associated with falls and injury to the mother and fetus. Women with epilepsy are also at greater risk for anemia, hyperemesis gravidarum, bleeding, abruptio placenta, preeclampsia, toxemia, and premature labor (Delgado-Escueta and Janz, 1992; Yerby, 1993).

Because pregnancy is a time of many bodily changes, AED blood levels in the pregnant woman also change frequently. These changes may result from increased maternal metabolism, decreased absorption, alteration in kidney function resulting in increased clearance, increased volume of distribution, and changes in protein binding due to a decrease in albumin (Andermann et al., 1985). Therefore, more frequent monitoring of AED blood levels, both bound and unbound (free), with appropriate changes in medication dosage during pregnancy, may prevent unnecessary increases in seizures. Unbound or free levels should be followed throughout the pregnancy to avoid unnecessary increases in AEDs.

A neonatal hemorrhagic disorder may be seen in the first 24 h after delivery in infants born to women with epilepsy (Bleyer, 1976). This disorder is caused by a deficiency in Vitamin K–dependent clotting factors II, VII, IX, and X. It is recommended that women receive vitamin K_1 10–20 mg every day during the week before delivery. Because no one can predict this period, it is given 1 month before the anticipated delivery date.

Because labor and delivery are physically stressful events and because there are vast maternal hormonal changes immediately after delivery, there is an increased chance for seizures during this time. Therefore, the cooperation of the neurologist and obstetrician is especially important. It is wise to discourage a woman with epilepsy from having her child delivered at home because of the potential risks. AED levels of the mother should be checked before labor, immediately after delivery, and at frequent intervals thereafter (e.g., at 1 week, 2 weeks, 1 month, and 2 months postpartum). If AEDs were increased during pregnancy, side effects may occur during the postpartum period. Therefore, women should be educated about potential side effects and what to do if they occur.

The pregnant woman with epilepsy can reduce the risks of adverse outcomes by: (a) planning the pregnancy; (b) obtaining early prenatal care and close neurologic follow-up; (c) complying with her medication regimen; (d) taking as few combinations of AEDs as possible (monotherapy is the preferred treatment whenever possible, but this should be achieved before pregnancy); (e) taking the lowest possible dose of AEDs to prevent seizures; and (f) taking prenatal vitamins that contain folic acid (it is recommended that vitamins be started before conception).

Breast-feeding should not be discouraged because the mother is taking AEDs. Only trace amounts of carbamazepine and phenytoin are found in maternal breast milk. Phenobarbital and primidone appear in higher concentrations; therefore, the clinical status of the infant exposed to these drugs can determine the need to continue or discontinue breast-feeding (McCormick, 1987). Breast-feeding may have to be avoided by mothers who take ethosuximide, as neonatal drug levels can be high (Kuhnz et al., 1984). If the parents and clinicians are concerned about fetal exposure to AEDs, supplementary feedings with formula may be considered. To enhance the success of this, the breast milk supply must be adequately established.

Although breast-feeding is now considered an acceptable option for most mothers taking AEDs, some mothers may choose not to breast-feed their babies. It may be prudent to have the father provide nighttime feedings by bottle so that the mother can avoid the possibility of sleep-deprivation seizures. Bottle feeding and feeding of solid foods can usually be safely performed by a woman whose seizures are not controlled if she uses a table-top chair or high chair into which the baby can be securely strapped.

It is important to remember that approximately 90% of the women with epilepsy will have a normal, healthy infant. However, careful review of the above issues both before and during a pregnancy can assuage many of the often unspoken fears and concerns of prospective parents. There are times when the expectant couple appears to be fixated on all the possible negative outcomes of pregnancy. If this occurs, the health care professionals may decide to focus the conversations with the parents on planning for the future and developing more positive coping strategies. In a few cases, referral to a counselor or psychologist who is well versed in the issues of epilepsy may be warranted.

Family and friends are sometimes more concerned about the ability of a person with epilepsy to care for an infant than is the person with epilepsy. An easy way to dispel the concerns of others and instill greater confidence in prospective parents is to develop a concrete plan for child care that takes into account the parent's current seizure type and frequency as well as the potential for more frequent and/or severe seizures. The professionals can help in development of this plan during the final months of pregnancy and review it with the parents immediately before birth. The plan should include procedures for diaper changing, bathing, carrying the child, and medication storage (see Chap. 16).

Women with epilepsy face many issues. As health care providers, it is our role to provide education and support to women so that they can be their own advocates and make informed decisions about their care.

REFERENCES

Andermann E, Ramsay RE, Stalland N. Epilepsy: sex, marriage, and pregnancy. Presented at the Epilepsy Foundation of America National Conference, Baltimore, October 27, 1985.

Bleyer, WA, Skinnae AL. Fatal neonatal hemorrhage after maternal anticonvulsant therapy. *JAMA* 1976;235:626–7.

Blumer D, Walker AE. Sexual behavior in temporal lobe epilepsy. *Arch Neurol* 1967;16:37–43.

Cummings L, Giudice L, Morrell M. Ovulatory function in epilepsy. *Epilepsia* 1995;36:355–9.

Delgado-Escueta AV, Janz D. Consensus guidelines: preconception counseling, management, and care of the pregnant woman with epilepsy. *Neurology* 1992;42(suppl 5):149–60.

Epilepsy and Parenting (brochure). Lorain, OH 44053. Epilepsy Foundation of NE Ohio, 5609 W. Erie Avenue, 1985.

Fiol M, Leppik I, Gates J. Epilepsy and oral contraceptives: a therapeutic dilemma. *Minnesota Med* 1983;Sept:551–2.

Herzog AG, Levesque L, Drislane F, et al. Phenytoin-induced elevation of serum estradiol and reproductive dysfunction in men with epilepsy. *Epilepsia* 1991;32:550–3.

Herzog AG, Russell V, Vaitukaitis JL, Geschwind N. Neuroendocrine dysfunction in temporal lobe epilepsy. *Arch Neurol* 1982;39:133–5.

Kallen B. Maternal epilepsy, antiepileptic drugs and birth defects. *Pathologica* 1986;78:757–68.

Kuhnz W, et al. Ethosuximide in epileptic women during pregnancy and lactation period. Placental transfer serum concentrations in nursed infants and clinical status. *Br J Clin Pharmacol* 1984;18:671–7.

Lindhout, D, Julliette, GC, Omtzigt, JG, et al. Spectrum of neural-tube defects in 34 infants prenatally exposed to antiepileptic drugs. *Neurology* 1992;42(suppl 5):111–118.

McCormick KB. Pregnancy and epilepsy: nursing implications. *J Neurosci Nurs* 1987;19:66–76.

Morrell M. Sexual dysfunction in epilepsy. *Epilepsia* 1991;32(suppl 6):S38–45.

Morrell M. Hormones and epilepsy through the lifetime. *Epilepsia* 1992;33(suppl 4):S49–61.

Morrell M. Antiepileptic drugs, seizures, and birth defects. *Int Pediatr (J Miami Children's Hosp)* 1995;10(suppl 1):58–65.

MRC Vitamin Study Research Group (Nicolas Wald). Prevention of neural-tube defects: results of the Medical Research Council vitamin study. *Lancet* 1991;338:131–7.

Rosa FW. Spina bifida in infants of women treated with carbamazepine during pregnancy. *N Engl J Med* 1991;324:674–7.

Rosciszwska, D. Epilepsy and menstruation. In: Hopkins A, ed. *Epilepsy.* London: Chapman and Hall, 1987:373–81.

Yerby M. Treatment of epilepsy during pregnancy. In: Wyllie E, ed. *The treatment of epilepsy: principle and practices.* Philadelphia: Lea & Febiger, 1993:844–57.

Yerby MS, McCormick KB. Pregnancy and epilepsy: an information pamphlet for women with epilepsy who are planning a family. Minneapolis: Minnesota Comprehensive Epilepsy Program, 1987.

Managing Seizure Disorders: A Handbook for Health Care Professionals, edited by N. Santilli, Lippincott-Raven Publishers, Philadelphia, 1996.
© 1996 Epilepsy Foundation of America.

11

Epilepsy in the Elderly

Fritz E. Dreifuss

An increasing proportion of the population of the United States is reaching senior citizen status. This state of affairs is occurring in all developed countries and is contributed to by increasing longevity and a decrease in birth rates over the past 25 years. Simultaneously, it has become apparent that whereas it used to be thought that the early age group had the highest prevalence of epilepsy, in fact there is an upsurge in prevalence after age 65. Modern methods of investigation, including MRI scanning and CT, have revealed that cerebral vascular disease, which used to be considered a relatively uncommon cause of late-onset epilepsy, does contribute significantly to this increase in epilepsy prevalence in the senior citizen age group (Hauser and Hesdorffer, 1990).

Identification becomes a little more difficult in the elderly because some epilepsies exhibited by this population are atypical. For example, spike-and-wave stupor in the elderly, presenting as episodes of confused behavior, is relatively common. Nonketotic hyperglycemia with a hyperosmolar state may present with multifocal simple partial or complex partial seizures and a less than flagrant epilepsia partialis continua, but also may escape early diagnosis. Medical attention in nursing homes is frequently sufficiently pragmatic to constitute a further handicap to early recognition of the episodic behavioral aberrations of the afflicted patient. Cerebral infarctions frequently go undiagnosed. This is particularly true in the older age groups, in which small strokes are responsible for a stepwise or episodic downhill progression in neurologic capability. Each of these might go unrecognized until there is sufficient summation of difficulties or until a more obtrusive disability leading to a motor disturbance brings the problem into the open. However, at any stage, epilepsy might supervene as a complicating factor.

A further complication in the elderly population is the tendency to falls. Many older people are receiving chronic medication and their tolerance for medication may be impaired. This is particularly true of antiepileptic drugs (AEDs) and antihypertensive drugs, the former leading to unrecognized episodes of intoxication and the latter to postural hypotension. Postural hypotension in the elderly also may occur spontaneously. These are all reasons why such a person may fall. Impaired vision, impairment of balance, and difficulty in regaining a center of gravity once lost, as is seen in the parkinsonian states, all contribute to frequent falls. Such persons frequently have unexplained bruises because they may have amnesia for the event that caused them. It is therefore not surprising that many episodes of head trauma, such as subdural hematomas, occur. These episodes all have implications for prevention.

A further problem in nursing home and retirement communities is the number of patients receiving medications for unknown and undocumented reasons. For example, many patients take phenytoin and/or phenobarbital, and have done so for many years, for reasons that are entirely undocumented. This is particularly true when there is discontinuity of medical care of many years and the initial records are lost in the midst of antiquity. In many instances this can be almost as large a problem as the unrecognized population with epilepsy, as these represent persons who do not require medications and whose medications may be contributory to motor and intellectual disturbance.

An identification project was conducted in a series of institutions for the mentally retarded (O'Neill et al., 1977) that can be used by clinicians and other health resource facilities for development of a coordinated approach to the institutionalized person with epilepsy. A vital component was the presence of a designated person in the institution with a special interest in the identification of epilepsy. Special epilepsy clinics were established for management of patients with uncontrolled seizures, and outcome measures were developed to evaluate the results of intervention. Definite effects on health care of the residents were demonstrated, with reduction in seizure frequency, incidence of status epilepticus, seizure-related deaths, and AED toxicity. The majority of the identification and management of patients with epilepsy can be performed by a nurse responsible for the day-to-day coordination of client services, data collection, data analysis, and nursing staff education. The availability of neurologic consultation is critical to the dispatch with which acute problems in epilepsy can be managed. In the project under discussion, changes in seizure control over time, the reduction in toxicity and in complications of epilepsy, and the reduction in the number of AEDs employed provided tangible evidence of the improvement that could be achieved through heightened awareness of epilepsy among this underserved population.

Syncope usually presents little difficulty in diagnosis if a careful history can be obtained. Confusion with epilepsy arises in the presence of unusually prominent or prolonged premonitory symptoms, such as may occur with tachyarrhythmias. A feeling of light-headedness, slowed response times, a drugged or detached feeling, and fading of sight and sounds may superficially resemble the psychic phenomena of a complex partial seizure. If the hypoxia associated with complete loss of consciousness is severe enough, tonic posturing or clonic jerks of the limbs may occur (convulsive syncope) and can further contribute to the diagnostic dilemma.

Important differential points for all forms of syncope include a predisposing setting, the absence of automatisms, absence of a typical tonic–clonic sequence, absence of incontinence (with micturition syncope, the question of which event came first may occasionally be difficult to sort out historically), and the absence of a true postictal phase. With more severe syncopal attacks, the patient may awaken feeling weak, uncomfortable, and uncertain about what happened, but there is none of the significant confusion, lethargy, and amnesia that follow generalized convulsive and complex partial seizures. The presence of some premonitory symptoms, typically light-headedness, and the usual swooning quality to the loss of consciousness help to differentiate fainting spells from atonic seizures.

Transient global amnesia is a syndrome manifested by sudden unexplained memory loss lasting for minutes to hours, typically occurring in the fifth to eighth decades. Although an epileptic substrate for transient global amnesia has been postulated, this is unlikely. Memory loss as the sole manifestation of epilepsy is rare. In addition, the patient's age, lack of prior seizures, low incidence of recurrence, and absence of automatisms, alterations of consciousness, or other symptoms more typical of epilepsy argue against this hypothesis. The most reasonable pathogenetic explanation relates transient global amnesia to cerebrovascular disease and bilateral ischemia of the mesial temporal lobe or thalamus.[1]

The following vignettes represent patients who are regular attenders in an epilepsy clinic. They do not represent rare or arcane disorders but are everyday examples of specific problems faced by persons in nursing homes and in retirement communities.

Clara D. was a 75-year-old woman who had had seizures for approximately 12 years. She lived with her almost blind husband in a mobile home, and despite the fact that the welfare department tried to find more supervised living conditions, the couple was fiercely independent. They maintained their own living quarters with the help of a nephew and occasional visits from a public health nurse who looked after their various needs, including the husband's glaucoma eye drops. Over the years Mrs. D. would come to the neurologic clinic quite intermittently, usually showing some evidence of bruising from various falls sustained during seizures. Her blood levels showed a rather variable degree of compliance with the prescribed medication regimen. The independence ended when Mr. D. fell and broke his hip.

The plight of this older couple is not at all unusual. Mr. D. continued to drive his ancient car despite his poor vision, kept the household supplied with groceries and medications, and managed to turn a deaf ear to his wife's ever-increasing confused denunciations.

Dolly W. was 78 years old and had been in a nursing home for approximately 5 years. The family physician of many years had retired because of ill health and a new physician attended the nursing home. On reviewing Dolly's medications, he noted that she had been receiving phenytoin and phenobarbital for at least 15 years. It was not clear why she was taking these drugs, as there was no record of a seizure disorder. Apart from Alzheimer's disease, no specific neurologic features were noted. An EEG did not reveal any evidence of a seizure disorder. The phenytoin and phenobarbital were gradually discontinued.

---

[1] Portions of this chapter are modified from Pedley TA, Hauser WA. Classification and differential diagnosis of seizures and epilepsy. In: Hauser WA, ed. *Current trends in epilepsy: a self-study course for physicians.* Unit I. Landover, MD: Epilepsy Foundation of America, 1988:8.

Nettie T. had had a seizure disorder for many years and had suffered from chronic schizophrenia since her twenties. She was now 62 years old. She had been in a state hospital for many years, but when deinstitutionalization became the vogue she was discharged. Her antipsychotic drugs were continued on an outpatient basis from the local mental health clinic and she was referred to the neurologic clinic for her AEDs.

During her hospitalization in the state hospital, she had lost most of her family support systems through the attrition of age and mortality. At the time she was living in a boarding situation and was fortunate in having someone supervise her day-to-day activities, such as cleanliness and nutrition.

Her medication regimen was kept as simple as possible because she was not going to be able to take advantage of the more sophisticated AEDs that required several times a day dosing. Even so, her blood levels were quite inconsistent.

These three vignettes illustrate some poignant examples of the problems of the elderly in which the epilepsy represented the entry point into our sphere of interest. The first case represented epilepsy as a damaging, injury-causing illness, contributed to by relative isolation and a gradual diminution in competence on the part of the patient and her husband. In the second case, an elderly person was "warehoused" in a nursing home and given AEDs as an old routine for no good reason. The third case illustrated the problems of the deinstitutionalized person who was relatively lucky in finding a comparatively supportive milieu. Many such cases are found among the street people in our larger cities.

Epilepsy in the elderly frequently complicates other problems of aging and a more complex series of needs than those of a more self-reliant generation. Multisystem disorders of aging require a more comprehensive approach.

REFERENCES

Hauser WA, Hesdorffer DC. *Epilepsy: frequency, causes and consequences.* New York: Demos, 1990.
O'Neill BP, Ladon B, Harris LM, Riley HL III, Dreifuss FE. A comprehensive, interdisciplinary approach to the care of the institutionalized person with epilepsy. *Epilepsia* 1977;18:243–50.

Managing Seizure Disorders: A Handbook for Health Care Professionals, edited by N. Santilli, Lippincott-Raven Publishers, Philadelphia, 1996.
© 1996 Epilepsy Foundation of America.

12

Educating Patients and Families to Manage a Seizure Disorder Successfully

Jean T. Shope

The majority of people with epilepsy live in the community and are treated for the most part as outpatients by clinicians in primary care settings. After the appropriate diagnosis and seizure classification have been determined and the best drug chosen and prescribed, the patient and family assume the day-to-day management of the seizure disorder and its attendant problems. Health care professionals can do much to ensure that patients and their families are adequately prepared to do their part in managing the epilepsy and to achieve the treatment goal of reduced seizure frequency and severity. This chapter discusses the necessity and importance of patients' and families' ability to manage the seizure disorder, what they need to know, what attitudes and beliefs are most beneficial, what skills are essential, what behaviors are necessary, suggested educational interventions, how to choose the intervention, and how to monitor and evaluate the educational efforts.

SELF-MANAGEMENT OF THE SEIZURE DISORDER

Because most seizure patients are ambulatory and living in their communities, they and their families or significant others must take a major role in the care and management of the seizure disorder. The patient or family are involved full-time, whereas the health care professional is only consulted occasionally. The same clinician may not always be available to a patient over the many years of a chronic seizure disorder. To a great extent, it is the patient's decision when and why consultation with a health care professional may be needed. Patients and families are required daily to make independent decisions relating to medications (e.g., what to do about running out or forgetting), the effect of various activities on their seizure disorder, or the effect of the seizure disorder on their life (e.g., career decisions, parenting). The professionai's and patient's mutual goal of good seizure control is severely threatened when patients do not know and understand what they should or should not do and follow these recommendations on a daily basis. Medication noncompliance, for example, is a major cause of seizures and status epilepticus among treated patients. Noncompliance with prescribed treatment regimens is not a problem unique to epilepsy. It has been noted in many treatment settings, as has patients' lack of understanding, knowledge, or memory of what a health care professional may have advised them.

It is, however, quite possible to ensure patients' comprehension of medical information, to improve medication compliance (taking medication as prescribed), and therefore to improve seizure control. Health care professionals can structure their interactions with patients and families in such a way that patients are helped to manage their seizure disorder successfully. The effectiveness of such endeavors depends on certain qualities of the health care professional–patient interaction and on the patient education approach.

CARE PROVIDER–PATIENT INTERACTION

One of the most critical components of the health care delivery process is the interaction between the care provider and the patient and family. If this interaction goes well, patients are satisfied and know how to manage their health problem. When the provider–patient interaction does not go well, patients may seek care elsewhere, submit to further diagnostic procedures, or not follow medical advice and therefore continue to have seizures. Because of the nature of treatment for seizure disorders (trying one drug at a time and adjusting the dosage), patients may not experience improvement quickly. A health care professional who explains this process to patients and is open and approachable for questions to be asked will find that patients understand the process better and are more able to carry out their role in treatment.

Several studies have looked specifically at aspects of professional–patient interaction and their impact on patient medication compliance. Compliance is more likely with medication that has been prescribed by a patient's regular physician. Moreover, in studies that have assessed the compliance of the patients of more than one physician, some physicians' patients are significantly better compliers than others. The explanation for this difference may lie in the way medication is prescribed or in characteristics of the physicians' interaction styles.

When the prescribed dosage of medication is inadequate, or when the diagnosis and/or the prescribed treatment are inaccurate, compliance with the medication is reduced. Several aspects of the prescribed medication itself have also been shown to be related to compliance. Tablets are more often taken as prescribed than are liquid medications. Compliance is also better when a smaller number of medications is prescribed and when no other treatments are recommended. Compliance often decreases over the duration of medication administration. Side effects have sometimes been shown to be associated with a decrease in medication compliance. Providers should consider all these factors when prescribing and adjusting patients' antiepileptic drugs (AEDs).

Compliance with prescribed treatment is also better when certain characteristics of the provider–patient interaction are present, i.e., when the clinician truly understands the patient's and family's concerns and when the family's expectations for the encounter with the provider are met (e.g., diagnosis made, medication prescribed). Compliance is better when explanations and instructions are clearly given and understood. The patient's and family's agreement with the professional on the diagnosis and necessity for follow-up visits is also associated with compliance. When the health care provider is perceived as warm and friendly and when patients and families feel that they are respected, medication compliance is better. In one study, physicians used positive adjectives to describe patients who were later identified as compliers, even though the physicians could not successfully predict who would comply. Provider–patient interaction that is more recent and more frequent also results in better compliance. Health outcomes are better when the professional–patient interaction is oriented to consider the patient as an active participant in the treatment process rather than as a passive, obedient recipient of care. The extent to which patients view their care as offering them an "active patient orientation" has been shown to relate to adherence to a prescribed treatment regimen. Services are considered to afford an active patient orientation to the extent that they contain the following qualities:

Attitudes and expectations communicated to patients by health professionals are supportive of patients' motivations and abilities to contribute to the treatment process (within the medical facility) and to understand and carry out treatment recommendations, with active participation reinforced through such means as praise and graphic display of clinical progress

Illness management is conducted as a collaborative process between patient and health professional, involving two-way communication and joint decision-making. Patient input is actively encouraged through direct solicitation of information/opinions and responsiveness to questions

Medical resources are provided in such a way as to ensure their usefulness to the patient, i.e., explanations are full and clear, instructions are explicitly operationalized, and skill training and technical aids are made available to assist self-care activities (Schulman, 1979)

PATIENT EDUCATION APPROACH

In the past, patient education efforts were often limited to providing patients with information about their condition through some type of class or in a simple pamphlet. Well-intended though these efforts were, patient education that provides information or knowledge alone does not produce behavior change, the desired outcome. Skills must also be taught. Research in the area of compliance has also revealed several affective factors, such as beliefs and attitudes, that appear to be correlated with patients' ability to follow prescribed regimens.

From this background, the components of a comprehensive patient education approach are identified: knowledge, attitudes, skills, and behavior. These components are each necessary, but alone not sufficient, to produce desired behavior change. In seizure disorders, for example, the desired health outcome is reduced frequency and severity of seizures. The usual behavior to achieve that outcome is the taking of daily AED. However, experience has shown that not all patients take their medication properly just because it has been recommended by their physician. If one focuses on the patient and on what changes or steps must take place for the patient to be able and willing to manage his or her own seizure disorder, one can see why education that is limited to information is not adequate. The components of a comprehensive patient education approach should be thought of as a sequence of educational objectives: (a) knowledge of what is necessary to do; (b) belief or attitudes that make it possible to carry out the behavior; (c) skills in carrying out the behavior; and (d) the actual performance of the behavior (for seizure disorders, medication on a daily basis). Each of the four types of educational objectives is discussed below in terms of specific knowledge, attitudes, skills, and behavior that patients must achieve to manage their seizure disorder on a daily basis.

Although health care professionals may already be "educated" in the sense that they themselves have the appropriate knowledge, attitude, and skills for daily AEDs compliance, it is a giant step to assume the patient's perspective and to be sensitive to what patients need to know, believe, and be able to do so that they can carry out the health care professional's recommendations. The way to arrive at such educational objectives is first to determine what the desired health outcome is, then to list the behaviors necessary to achieve that outcome, and then the knowledge, attitudes, and skills necessary to perform the behavior. It is best to limit the objectives attempted to only the most important ones for seizure management. Methods of reaching these objectives (educational interventions) and ways to assess patients' achievement of the objectives will be discussed later.

KNOWLEDGE

There are several basic facts that patients must know to manage their seizure disorder. These facts are limited in number and are considered essential to carrying out the recommended behaviors. Research has shown that lengthy medical explanations about a patient's disease (anatomy, physiology, pathology) are not what most patients need or want and do not necessarily lead to appropriate management behaviors. Instead, the information given should be limited to that which is necessary for patients and families to follow the medical advice and thus to manage their condition. Of course, if patients seek more information and ask questions, it is appropriate to provide that information.

The knowledge that seizure patients and families need is summarized in Table 1, and falls into four categories: knowledge about seizures, medication, medical

TABLE 1. *Educational objectives for self-management of a seizure disorder*

Knowledge	Attitudes	Skills	Behavior
Seizures What they are Can occur anytime Status epilepticus What to report to physician	Agreement with diagnosis Belief in susceptibility Belief in severity	How to provide care How to get medical help if needed How to report to physician	Provide proper care Get help when necessary Report seizures as appropriate
Medication Name and strength Appearance Times/day Therapeutic blood level Problems to report	Belief that efficacy of medication outweighs its costs/barriers Self-efficacy Internal locus of control	How to schedule How to remember doses How to manage missed dose How to maintain supply How to report problems	Follow schedule Take as prescribed Manage missed dose Maintain supply Report problems
Medical care Medical follow-up Physician EEG ADL Medical information available at all times	Belief that effectiveness of medical follow up, EEG, and ADL outweighs costs/barriers Self-efficacy Internal locus of control	How to keep appointments: EEG ADL monitoring Physician follow-up How to have medical information available	Keep physician and laboratory appointments Carry/wear medical information
Lifestyle Healthy lifestyle advice (e.g., diet, rest, stress) Potential problems Family Psychosocial Educational Vocational	Belief that effectiveness outweighs costs/barriers Self-efficacy Internal locus of control	How to get help How to follow lifestyle advice How to solve problems	Follow lifestyle advice Work on solving problems

care, and lifestyle. Patients should know that a seizure is the symptom of temporarily uncontrolled electrical activity in the brain. They should also know what type(s) of seizure they have and its characteristics (e.g., staring, falling, muscle contractions). Patients should know that their seizures can occur at any time. Even though some patients may tend to have an aura and others may identify a typical time of day, month, or even year for their seizures, they should realize that the potential exists for a seizure at any time. They also need to know the possibility of status epilepticus occurring and that if convulsive seizures continue for more than 5 min, emergency medical help is required. Finally, patients should know to report any change in type or increase in frequency of seizures to their health care provider.

Patients need to know that medication is the best way to control seizures, that the goal is the best control possible with the fewest side effects, and that it may take time and medication adjustment to achieve this goal. Specific medication knowledge that patients need includes the following: the name, strength, and appearance of their prescribed medication and the number of times per day they are to take it. It is essential that they understand the concept of therapeutic blood level of medication: that a protective level is essential at all times, that it takes a few weeks to build up to this level, that daily medication is required to maintain this level, and that they must not stop their medication abruptly because seizures could result. Patients also need to know what problems of their particular medication, such as side effects and toxic effects, should be reported. They also need certain knowledge about what is involved in their continuing medical care. The health care provider should tell them when they should be seen again for follow-up and when they should report for AED level monitoring and EEG. Patients should be told the purpose of these tests: that the AED blood level will determine if enough medication is in the blood to prevent seizures and that the EEG will determine if the brain's electrical activity is under normal control. They also need to know that their medical information (diagnosis of seizure disorder and current therapy) should be available to anyone who might find them needing help so that only appropriate assistance is given to them. This can be done by using a medical information tag or wallet card or simply by carrying a card stating that they are under a doctor's care with the care provider's telephone number.

Finally, patients need to know how their lifestyle may affect their seizures and how their seizures may affect their lives. Certain patients may discover activities that trigger their seizures and should therefore plan to avoid such activities as much as possible. Alcohol use is not usually recommended. Advice that is good for everyone to promote a healthy lifestyle is probably especially useful for seizure patients: adequate rest, exercise, diet, and stress management. Patients will vary in the extent to which changes in the lifestyle area are necessary or recommended. Patients should also know that in trying to manage their lives and seizure disorders they may encounter psychosocial, educational/vocational, or family problems and that appropriate help is available if and when they need it.

ATTITUDES

In the affective area, several attitudes, beliefs, and personality characteristics that have been found empirically to be related to patient compliance are desirable objectives of a patient education approach (see Table 1). Attitudes are hard to change in and of themselves and are highly related to the necessary information, skills, and behavior. As the other objectives are met, sometimes the appropriate attitudes also are achieved. Several of the beliefs mentioned below are from the Health Belief Model, a theoretical framework that has been tested with seizure patients.

In the first content area of seizures, patients need to agree with the seizure diagnosis in order to be able to follow the recommended advice. They also need to understand that they are susceptible to seizures, i.e., that there is a substantial likelihood that they will have another seizure. Belief in severity of the seizure disorder is also essential—not whether that each seizure is "hard" or not but rather that having the condition is something serious and that the seizures themselves are worth preventing for whatever harm they may cause. Certain attitudes and beliefs about the medications are also important for patients' success in self-management. Patients need to believe that the medication is or will be effective in controlling their seizures, reducing either the frequency, severity, or both. But there are "costs" and barriers associated with taking medication: it costs money; patients have to arrange to get it; it's a nuisance to remember; it may be embarrassing to have to take it; patients may be afraid of taking medication. Patients' belief in the medication's efficacy must outweigh the perceived costs and barriers for patients to carry out the tasks associated with following a prescribed medication regimen. Patients also should believe in their own self-efficacy, i.e., their ability to carry out the medication regimen as prescribed. They need to believe that they can be responsible enough and devise a good system for remembering their medication. A personality characteristic considered important in following medical advice is an internal vs. an external, locus of control. Persons with an internal locus of control feel that they have greater control over their life and health than do persons with an external locus of control, who feel that fate or luck exert more control than they do.

In the medical care content area, many of the same attitudes are important. Patients need to believe that the efficacy of medical follow-up, EEG, and AED blood level monitoring outweighs the various barriers they may perceive (e.g., out-of-pocket costs, time away from job, physical discomfort, hassles of making appointments, finding transportation). Patients also need to believe in their own self-efficacy to follow up on their medical care (e.g., that they can surmount the various hurdles, get time off from work, get a babysitter, get a ride) to do their part in monitoring their seizure disorder. Again, an internal locus of control will help patients feel that doing these things can make a difference in their outcome.

In the area of lifestyle advice, attitudes are also important and, again, they are much the same as in the other content areas. Patients' beliefs that following the advice will help (and that it is worthwhile compared to the nuisance or cost or deprivation required) are essential to following the recommendations. Here also, patients need belief in self-efficacy, e.g., the belief that indeed they can avoid alcohol, and manage stress. Finally, internal locus of control is helpful because patients who feel that they have control over events in their lives are much more likely to take actions on their own behalf.

SKILLS

Knowing what to do (knowledge) and feeling that is important (attitude) are necessary but not sufficient ingredients of a patient education approach. To carry out medical advice, patients must know how to do each activity, i.e., they must be equipped with the required skills. The teaching of skills should include practice in performing the skill, not merely information.

In the seizure content area (see Table 1), patients and their families must know how to provide care for the seizures. Although patients may not be able to provide their own seizure care, they should know how to tell others what they will need done in case of a seizure. They also need to know how to get medical help if needed and how to contact their health care provider to report a seizure.

In the medication content area, there are several important activities patients must know how to do. They must know how to schedule their medication as prescribed, also scheduling it to be both convenient and easy to remember. They must devise methods for remembering their medication that will work for them, whether they keep their medication in a special place (e.g., near their toothbrush), or use a pill dispenser for each day's supply, or record their doses on a calendar. They must also know how to manage a missed dose—whether to make it up or not, and when. Patients must also know how to maintain their medication supply, how and when to get refills and how to get medication if they have lost theirs or are out of town without any. They must also know how to report any problems with the medication.

In the medical care area, patients obviously need to know how to keep their medical and laboratory appointments and how to cancel appointments if necessary. They also need to know how to obtain a medical emergency tag or card and how to complete the information needed.

Lifestyle advice can be a very difficult area in which to acquire skills. For example, a health care professional's advice to a patient to "avoid stress" is very incomplete without learning and practicing the stress management techniques taught in workshops designed for that purpose. The same comment can be made about diet and exercise changes or even avoiding the use of alcohol, which may be an established habit pattern that requires several skills to be learned in order to produce the desired change. Knowing how to get help and resources available for lifestyle changes as well as problem-solving is important. When problems are identified (e.g., family, psychosocial), learning how to deal with them, work on them, and solve them is crucial.

BEHAVIOR

The knowledge, attitudes, and skills objectives just discussed form the foundation for the behaviors listed in Table 1, the principal objectives of the patient education approach. When behaviors in all the areas are performed, the best possible seizure control will be achieved. These behaviors must be carried out on a regular basis for patients and families to be successful in managing the seizure disorder. The skills described earlier match each behavior and provide the necessary "know how," but the behavioral objective of patient education is the regular, routine (daily or as necessary) performance of these same skills over time. In the seizure area, patients and families must provide proper care for seizures as they occur. If medical or other help is required, they must get it, and they should report the seizures to the provider as requested at the next visit or before (e.g., number, type, change in type, time of day).

In the medication area, patients and families must acquire and maintain their medication supply, remember to take it as prescribed, manage missed doses as they have been advised, and report specified medication problems to their health care professional. They must perform these behaviors day in and day out regardless of holidays, vacations, or working.

In regard to their medical care, patients must make and keep appointments with the provider and EEG and blood level monitoring laboratories at the recommended intervals. They should have their basic emergency medical information with them at all times.

Finally, patients should maintain a lifestyle that reduces their seizure problems as much as possible. Over the months and years, adaptations may become necessary. Various problems may evolve, but patients and families must deal with them. If the patient education approach has been successful, patients and families will be well equipped to manage the seizure disorder, having the appropriate knowledge, attitudes, and skills to maintain the recommended behaviors over time. Various ways to achieve these objectives are discussed below.

EDUCATIONAL INTERVENTIONS

Now that the educational objectives, the *what* to teach, have been spelled out, one can turn to *how* to teach it or what type of educational intervention to use. Interventions should be appropriate to the situation (office practice, hospital setting, school, home health care, voluntary agency) and to the needs of the patients and families involved. The first aspect to consider is exactly who will be receiving the patient education. Will the targeted group be adults, children, or patients and their families? Are they inpatients or outpatients? Do enough individuals need to be educated at once on the same topics to make groups of similar people possible? Are there certain individuals with special needs to be addressed, such as those who are often noncompliant with medication, or alcoholic patients? Determination of who will be receiving the education and describing their specific characteristics is a necessary first step.

The second factor to consider in choosing educational interventions is who is available and capable to do the educating. Will it be the nurse, social worker, psychologist, teacher, or another staff person? Is there a local voluntary agency or hospital with an educational program in place or the wherewithal to develop one? Is there a patient advocate or a strong group of patients who can form a self-help group? Patients may be referred to another group or setting to meet some of the educational objectives, whereas you may choose to meet others.

A third factor is the choice of educational methods to be used and whether the patient education program is formal or informal. One might want to choose to use a lecture, explanation, film, or videotape (either to individuals or groups) to express certain information (knowledge objectives), but allow time for essential discussion or questions to be answered. Providing the same information in a take-home written version is very helpful. Attitudinal objectives may best be attained by utilizing discussion among groups of patients or a self-help group. Hearing from other patients and families what their experience has taught them to believe (e.g., that the medication is effective) can be very useful. Including the family or others in the teaching and building of the patient's social support system is especially useful. Contracting for behavioral change (such as taking medication as prescribed), involving a written agreement between the patient and health care provider, is an approach that has shown some success. The methods of education chosen must be appropriate for the type of objective and the patients or families who will receive it.

A fourth factor to consider is the material (e.g., handouts, videos) being used in patient education. Many materials are available from voluntary agencies, such as EFA affiliates, as well as from commercial organizations. One should evaluate the material for how well it fits each objective. Does it cover the point adequately and accurately but not too extensively? Is the information written or stated clearly and at the appropriate reading or vocabulary level? Has all medical terminology been explained in lay terms? Even excellent pamphlets and other materials are rarely adequate in and of themselves, but used in conjunction with other educational methods can be very helpful.

A fifth and final aspect of educational interventions is perhaps the most important and involves several principles that should apply no matter who the target group or educators are or what methods and materials are used. The educational intervention should start with determining what level of understanding the learners have (what they know and do not know). Objectives should be prioritized and the most important ones addressed first rather than trying to teach everything at once. The intervention may also need to be individualized to some extent, with some patients needing more or less attention in certain areas or specific details than other patients. Patients need repetition of information over time in an ongoing process as their understanding, experience, and situation change. Feedback from patients is essential so that the educator can determine if they have learned and understood the knowledge and skills being taught and are understanding and using work terms appropriately. As positive behavior change takes place and is maintained, it is important that it be reinforced by the provider's recognition, praise, and encouragement. Reinforcement of positive behaviors must be monitored and is discussed below.

MONITORING PATIENT EDUCATION EFFECTIVENESS

The effort involved in good patient education should be equally matched by efforts to determine how well the patient education is working: is it being done, and is it doing any good? Documentation in the client's record of health teaching activities is very useful. Even a simple checklist can serve as a record of what objectives have been taught and what feedback has been obtained. Such a system makes it possible to examine data from a group of individuals periodically to determine what methods are working well. To determine effectiveness, one needs to learn the degree to which the behavioral objectives are being met, e.g., are individuals performing the desired behaviors on a regular basis? For people with seizures, the provider can determine if the individual and families have appropriately reported problems with seizures and if they have obtained help when necessary. Families can be questioned to determine the type of care they provide when a seizure occurs.

In the medication area, health care professionals can ask patients how they are doing following their schedule, remembering to take all their doses, and knowing what to do when a missed dose is discovered. The professional should also be aware from interactions with patients whether medication problems are reported and whether the patient maintains an adequate supply of medication or tends to run out and require prescriptions at odd times. Indicators of medication noncompliance might be seizures or even status epilepticus, but by far the most useful (although not perfect) indicator and reinforcer of medication compliance is the AED level. When the AED level is used as an indicator of compliance, the prescribed amount must be considered in relation to the level. When several serial levels are available under the same conditions (steady state), variability among the levels can indicate noncompliance.

In the medical care area, appointment keeping is the behavioral outcome and can be monitored to some extent in the patient's medical record. Patients can be asked to show the medical information they carry.

In the lifestyle area, the health care professional should inquire about any problems and how patients are managing to follow the recommendations. Are they following through on referrals? Have problems improved? In the monitoring of each of these areas of behavioral objectives, when the outcomes are less than optimal it is important to determine why the objectives have not been achieved and to do something about it. Perhaps the individual did not experience the educational effort and plans for that process must be made. Or perhaps the person's situation has changed, making new learning essential (an adolescent, for example, may be living away from home for the first time). The patient should have an opportunity for active input in determining the best course of action to achieve the mutual goals of himself and care provider. Perhaps individual counseling is in order if there are problems to be solved that interfere with the responsible performance of self-management. Monitoring of behavioral outcomes should be a continuous process, with the health care professional showing active interest, obtaining feedback from patients, maintaining good communication and interaction, and following up any areas requiring change.

CONCLUSION

People with epilepsy and their families must carry a large responsibility for the day-to-day management of the seizure disorder. Successful self-management can occur when health care professionals expect patients to be active and responsible and when these professionals have positive interactions with their patients. A patient education approach should be aimed at the achievement of knowledge, attitude, skill, and behavioral objectives in the general areas of seizures, medication, medical care, and lifestyle. The way patients are educated should be appropriate to their needs and can be done in a variety of ways. The outcome of education, successful self-management of the seizure disorder (achieving objectives in each area), should be monitored and reinforced throughout the course of treatment. A variety of print and video materials are presently available to support these efforts. Refer to Appendix D, "EFA Resources."

REFERENCES

Schulman BA. Active patient orientation and outcomes in hypertensive treatment: application of a socio-organizational perspective. *Med Care* 1979;17;267–80.

Managing Seizure Disorders: A Handbook for Health Care Professionals, edited by N. Santilli, Lippincott-Raven Publishers, Philadelphia, 1996.
© 1996 Epilepsy Foundation of America.

13

Understanding Compliance and Areas for Intervention

Mimi Callanan, Joyce Cramer, and Patricia Osborne Shafer

Compliance, or adherence to a planned treatment regimen, is important to maintaining health and preventing complications. In turn, noncompliance is viewed as any deviation from a planned course of therapy, whether purposeful or not. Noncompliance is widespread and is a major reason for failed therapy.

Cramer et al. (1988) used a novel electronic monitoring system to assess medication compliance rates and to show that patients with epilepsy take an average of 73% of medication as prescribed, whereas other compliance studies indicate that at least 15% of all patients, with the average being 50%, are noncompliant (Black et al., 1982; Browne and Feldman, 1983). No psychosocial or other factors could be used to predict who would be a poor complier (Browne and Feldman, 1983). In a study using microelectronic monitors, compliance rates were highest 5 days before and 5 days after a clinic visit, with a significant drop in compliance 1 month later (Cramer et al., 1990). In disorders such as epilepsy, compliance with prescribed treatment plans may mean complete control of seizures. However, because the disorder is difficult to see and is bothersome only when a seizure occurs, people with epilepsy may believe that medication can be taken sporadically.

All medical practitioners must accept the presence of noncompliance with various aspects of the treatment provided to patients. Patient defaulting can occur either early during the first exposure to the treatment plan or later during chronic treatment. Epilepsy, once diagnosed, may require life-long medical attention, making it an ideal focus for the study of compliance. Seizure disorders occur in all age groups, from pediatric to geriatric. Nevertheless, health care professionals can probably use similar strategies to develop patterns for adherence to therapeutic plans by all patients. During the first exposure to the need for antiepileptic drugs (AEDs), patients are dealing with acceptance of the diagnosis as well as their need to take medication. Development of tolerance to side effects complicates the early treatment stage because the patient often experiences negative feedback from the prescribed treatment. As seizures come under control, the patient experiences a second opportunity to establish a long-term adherence behavior pattern. The larger problem occurs in long-term treatment when patients occasionally miss doses and go on to test the need for medication because seizures do not reoccur immediately.

In understanding and assessing compliance, one must focus on the reasons for not complying with specific treatment plans. The following reasons for non-compliance have been identified:

Financial difficulties
Misunderstanding instructions
Lack of information
Inconvenience of medication time
Side effects
Running out of medication
Not knowing what to do when a dose of medication is missed
Doing well and therefore feeling that medication is no longer needed
Poor family support
Denial
Forgetfulness
Memory problems
Fear of seizure control
Dependency
Powerlessness
Embarrassment
Poor patient/doctor relationship
Patient's health belief

In addition, some reasons for noncompliance in the elderly and individuals with multiple handicaps include:

Decreased muscle strength
Decreased visual acuity
Decreased or declining memory
Hearing loss
Swallowing difficulties
Many medications to remember

This list may not be all-inclusive but by taking time, developing a trusting relationship with the patient, and asking specific questions, the health care professional should be able to identify reasons for noncompliance and begin to implement interventions to change this pattern. Setting realistic goals with the patient may obviate future complications.

One of the first steps to increasing compliance is education. Explanations should be simple to understand and given in nonscientific language. Epilepsy is a disorder that can be controlled with medication. Emphasis on this fact may help the patient to understand the importance of taking medication at the specified time and dose. A brief understanding of steady-state levels and half-lives of the medication may help the patient develop a greater awareness of how medications work, why they must be taken at specific times throughout the day, and why they must be taken regularly. Medication side effects should be addressed, as well as how the patient and health care professional should handle the patient's complaints. Depending on the side effects, many suggestions can be given, e.g., taking medication after meals. Discussion of side effects will also emphasize the importance of having laboratory tests conducted on a routine basis.

Detailed instructions should be given on how to take medications (e.g., t.i.d., after meals), what to do if a dose is forgotten, how to refill medications, how to contact the physician and/or nurse, and the dangers of stopping medication abruptly. For those using elixirs, explain the need to shake the bottle thoroughly and to use an accurate measuring spoon, cup, or syringe. Each patient will have specific needs that should be addressed individually. Encouragement is beneficial to increase patients' active participation in their care. Written instructions, no matter how minor the changes, are also very important.

Elderly patients have special needs. For example, elderly patients may need large print or magnifying glasses to read instructions. Calendars, color-coded bottles, or schedules with the medication attached may be necessary. In addition, elixirs or chewable tablets may be needed for those with swallowing difficulties. Easy flip-top containers are available for those who have weakness or manual dexterity problems. Inconvenient scheduling, memory problems (especially in the elderly), denial of illness, and fear of losing independence are several reasons why patients forget to take medication. Denial and feelings of dependency must be dealt with through counseling. Patient participation may obviate dosing problems. Suggested interventions dealing with poor memory include daily and/or weekly medication containers, medication instructions placed in a convenient and readily available place (refrigerator), scheduling medication at times that are easy to remember (meals and bedtime), and a watch that beeps at medication times.

Typical strategies to aid in adherence to a medical regimen include education, dosing, scheduling, and monitoring issues that are pertinent to all types of patients experiencing a variety of medical problems. Cramer and Russell (1988) discuss the types of strategies that can be used to enhance adherence to a medical regimen. A brief overview is outlined in Fig. 1. They developed a new program for adherence counseling primarily to avoid losing patients who were at high risk to drop out of a treatment program after the initial diagnosis of epilepsy. The adherence counseling program should be generally applicable to all types of health care issues because it concentrates on the individual rather than the disease state.

This counseling program was developed into a systematic adherence documentation checklist for epilepsy patients which addresses the 14 typical adherence problems and the 23 types of adherence strategies that can be used to resolve these problems (Tables 1 and 2). The health care team can select a strategy to solve the patient's primary adherence problem. It would not be unusual for

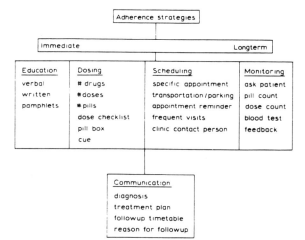

FIG. 1. Brief overview of the major strategies. (From Cramer and Russell, 1988.)

individual professionals to prefer a few intervention strategies and to use them repeatedly. However, the broad scope of strategies listed are reminders of other techniques that might be useful.

The core of the adherence counseling process is engagement of the patient in discussions. Didactic education about epilepsy and the need for medication to prevent seizures often is not absorbed during the brief visit with a physician. Long-term follow-up tends to focus on current side effects and seizures that had occurred during the last interval. Therefore, when the patient reports no side

TABLE 1. *Adherence problems*

Psychological
    Nonacceptance
    Emotions
    Other priorities
    Social criticism
    Decision to omit doses
    Negative thoughts
Planning
    Forgot regular schedule
    Forgot disrupted schedule
    No medication
    Lacked information
Medical
    Side effects
    Illness
    Testing efficacy
Other
    Not yet known
    Other adherence problem

From Cramer and Russell, 1988.

TABLE 2. *Adherence strategies*

Provide information
    Education about treatment
    Education about disease
    Understand adherence problem
Increase motivation
    Persuasion
    Help with other problems
    Reduce negative consequences
Collect information from patient
    More data at visit
    Plan to collect data
    Plan telephone contact
Modify schedule
    Psychological support
    Plan cue
    Plan how to cope
    Dose schedule change
    Stepwise dose increase
Change contingencies
    Discuss adherence failure
    Reduce negative consequences
    Reduce side effects
    Plan contact
    Use specific reinforcement
    Plan positive consequence
Refer patient for
    Discussion with physician
    Additional medical treatment
    Psychological support
    Social service help
Other items
    Other strategy

From Cramer and Russell, 1988.

effects or seizures the interview is over quickly without using the opportunity to refocus on the therapeutic goal. Specific questioning about medication-taking habits, reasons for missed doses, and discussion of drug serum concentrations re-engages the patient in the treatment plan. Providing follow-up care, convenient appointments, and pill boxes for medications are helpful tools for patients who want to use these as cues for their routines. However, all of these are passive approaches that can be left unused by the passive patient. The cost of taking time to discuss adherence problems and to attempt to provide assistance aimed at these specific problems may be high for many physicians. In a health maintenance organization the cost of physician time or nurse time must be weighed against the cost of emergency care for the patient who has a breakthrough seizure because of inadequate treatment.

Physicians are trained to explain diagnoses and the need for medication or other treatment but often do not convey this information in a manner that is easily understandable, acceptable, or remembered by the patient. Further assistance by the nurse and other medical staff, including physician's assistants, pharmacists, and clinic assistants, often is used to increase patient education in the hopes of avoiding misunderstandings and misapprehensions that lead to poor compliance. These staff members can easily be trained to use specific compliance strategies to address particular needs of individual patients in a modest amount of time. Patient information booklets and pill boxes cannot replace the need for direct communication with the patient by the nurse or a physician.

Teaching and counseling about safety and daily living activities do not ensure that a person with epilepsy will follow prescribed treatment or recommendations. In addition to the foregoing teaching and counseling suggestions, the Health Belief Model is a helpful framework from which to develop an educational program for an individual with epilepsy.

The model consists of four basic health beliefs that influence a person's likelihood of taking a health action:

Perceived susceptibility to disorder, i.e., susceptibility to recurring seizures and behavioral or cognitive changes

Perceived severity of disorder, i.e., how epilepsy affects the person's life

Perceived alternatives of treatment, i.e., effects of medications, surgery, and lifestyle modifications

Perceived benefits vs. risks, i.e., benefits of seizure control and control of the effects of epilepsy vs. risks for recurring seizures, side effects, cost of treatment, and epilepsy controlling one's life

The premise of this model is that a person must work through one belief before progressing to the next. In this model each patient must believe that if seizures are affecting daily life or safety, alternatives can be chosen to treat seizures and to control their effects on daily life. The patient must also believe the benefits of these choices outweigh the risks and that the choices can be carried out successfully. The Health Belief Model can be utilized to conceptualize how a patient—or in the case of a child or dependent, the parent or guardian—works through this process of making decisions regarding care, to assess what beliefs and knowledge may affect this process, and to develop a care plan for teaching and counseling. The following sections present information relating to each of these beliefs about safety. For more information on safety, see Chaps. 12 and 16.

PERCEIVED SUSCEPTIBILITY TO EPILEPSY

The diagnosis of epilepsy and the need take AEDs do not ensure a person's belief of susceptibility to recurring seizures. Often a lack of understanding about susceptibility and/or beliefs regarding the diagnosis contribute to a person's indifference toward or rejection of safety needs or denial of the effect of seizures on daily living. Many factors about a person's seizures and behavior can also influence perceptions of susceptibility.

An adolescent who has had seizures since childhood may feel susceptible to recurring seizures because he has experienced them or lived with the fear of seizures longer than an adolescent newly diagnosed with seizures. However, in children who have always been told "you'll outgrow them in adolescence" this may not be true. As these children reach adolescence, they may take more risks and deny or disregard daily living effects in their belief that their seizures have ceased or will cease and that there is nothing for them to worry about.

Seizure type is another factor affecting a person's belief of susceptibility. Large "visible" seizures (i.e., generalized tonic–clonic) are more disruptive to daily life and increase the risk for injury. These seizures are also harder to deny than partial or absence seizures, and a person's perceptions regarding susceptibility may therefore be more acute. Less obtrusive seizures, such as absence (petit mal) or partial seizures, are frequently not diagnosed or are misdiagnosed as behavioral or psychiatric problems, so individuals with these may not even be aware that they have seizures. Even if these seizures are diagnosed correctly, they are often more frightful or more embarrassing to the person who experiences them, as the behavior is less acceptable to others. Persons with these types of seizures, particularly complex partial seizures, may try to deny or hide the seizures from others, further removing from them the belief that they are susceptible to recurring seizures.

Seizure frequency may influence a person's perception of susceptibility. Although there may be problems for someone with frequent seizures to confront, that person may be more aware of susceptibility and therefore amenable to teaching and counseling. Persons with less frequent seizures, however, may be more likely not to worry about them or may deny that they have epilepsy. Such people are more prone to noncompliance and to safety and daily living problems. They may feel less inclined to modify activities to prevent injury or decrease precipitants of seizures.

Understanding whether and how a person perceives susceptibility to seizures is the first step in assessing issues of safety in daily living. If inadequate knowledge or misbeliefs are present, the person may have an inappropriate or distorted perception of how the seizures affect his or her life and the need to take any action. Teaching and counseling must address the basics of epilepsy, including the possible behavioral manifestations and triggers of seizures. The risks for seizures must be addressed, not only the potential for physical injury but also the potential for status epilepticus and more uncontrolled seizures.

SEVERITY OF DISORDER: EFFECT ON DAILY LIFE

How epilepsy affects daily life and safety depends on seizure and behavior variables, support systems (quantity, quality, and attitudes), and the individual's emotional reactions and coping behaviors. McCorkle and Benoliel's Social Enforced Dependency Scale can be used to help categorize the effect of epilepsy on a person's abilities and independence in areas of self-care, mobility, and social activities. Self-care and mobility are the most relevant aspects pertaining to effect of seizures on daily life. Self-care may be impaired by chronic physical deficits associated with epilepsy, intermittent deficits, such as postictal hemiparesis or confusion, injuries sustained during seizures, or poor coordination or difficulty in walking because of drug toxicity. At times, supervision or assistance may be needed for a person to perform even the most basic self-care. If seizures are frequent, i.e., many times per day, dependence on other people for self-care increases. For some people behavior or cognitive problems may have the greatest impact on self-care. Problems such as distractibility, impaired memory, poor insight and judgment, impaired visuospatial or language skills, and impulsive or uninhibited behavior can all affect self-care in different ways. For example, a distractible child or adolescent may have difficulty in completing activities such as bathing and dressing without the help of structure or cues from a parent. Impaired visuospatial skills may cause problems with bathing or grooming. Poor insight and judgment may limit the person's awareness of the need for basic activities of daily living or may lead to poor habits.

Depending on seizure behavior and frequency, mobility may be affected. A person may need to restrict certain activities to decrease the risk for injury or exacerbation of seizures. Medications may limit mobility because of their adverse effects. A person's functional abilities, such as activity and exercise tolerance, sleep patterns, nutritional status, sexuality, cognitive and perceptual abilities, coping issues, and self-image are also important to assess. A review of this information yields important data on how a person perceives the effects of seizures and may identify lifestyle areas that may have an impact on seizures. This information can then be utilized as a basis for teaching lifestyle modifications and management of seizure triggers as part of the treatment plan. Objective data obtained from neuropsychological and educational testing is also important to help validate the person's concerns, to identify actual or potential problem areas not perceived by the patient, and to help providers plan appropriate interventions. If cognitive deficits such as impaired insight and judgment are found, the health care professional must focus more heavily on helping the person to weigh risks of injury and need for safety precautions, as the patient may be unable to do this alone.

Teaching and counseling about the severity of epilepsy should start with the need for seizure observation, care, and safety precautions. Increasing the person's awareness and knowledge about the type and frequency of seizures, appropriate first aid, and the need for safety precautions may help to dispel fears and promote appropriate beliefs.

ALTERNATIVES OF TREATMENT

Side effects of medications may increase a person's risk for injury. Excessive sedation or poor coordination from toxic levels of medications may contribute to falling, bumping into objects, or getting burned. Sedation, inattention, or impaired memory may hinder the person's awareness of the environment and the need for safety precautions. Sometimes side effects are related to the type of medication and at other times they may be related to the dosage or dosage schedule. For the former, if side effects are causing injury or impairing daily living skills, a change of medications should be considered if possible. For dose-related side effects, the first step is to alter the dosage schedule in an effort to reduce the untoward side effect. Giving larger dosages at bedtime, redistributing the dosage amounts, or more frequently dosing may resolve the problem. If not, the next step is to reduce the dosage until the side effects resolve or decrease to acceptable levels. If seizures increase as a result, the physician may have to consider medication changes or, if this is not possible, to weigh the benefits of seizure control vs. the risks for side effects.

When side effects occur, the patient's initial reaction is often to stop the medication. In many cases this is most harmful, as the risk for status epilepticus is high with abrupt withdrawal of medications. Impulsive behavior in adolescents and young adults, in conjunction with a need for control and independence may enhance the tendency to stop medications in this age group. It is also important to remember that medications are usually the only visual reminder of a person's epilepsy and dependence. Therefore, psychological reactions to the epilepsy may be misdirected to the medications.

Changes in daily life are often necessary to maintain safety and decrease factors that might precipitate seizures. If these changes are perceived by a person as restrictions or dictums for change, the likelihood that they will be followed is lessened. Restrictions may be perceived as another loss of control, especially if it makes people feel different from their peers. If a lot of change is required in daily life or if no positive benefit can be easily visualized, the chance of successful change is also limited. *Modifying* rather than restricting lifestyle to cope with the effects of seizures on safety and daily life is the preferred method of teaching changes. The goal of lifestyle modifications should be focused on helping the patient to feel more in control of the epilepsy. Outcome criteria that are easily attainable and visible must be established. Changes must be addressed slowly, focusing on one or two aspects of behavior at a time so that the amount of change is not overwhelming and the patient can see the benefits of each change. Utilizing a tool to evaluate the effects of a change is helpful. Having a patient complete seizure calendars, recording seizure frequency and type as well as the targeted behavior for change for a month or so before the change and then for a month or so after a change in lifestyle, is a very useful self-monitoring tool.

Types of lifestyle modifications can be categorized into two groups: compensatory measures and trigger management. *Compensatory measures* consist of retraining or reaching alternative approaches to cope with cognitive or behavioral deficits. A neuropsychologist may be extremely helpful in this area. Environmental changes or safety aids to decrease the risk for injury are another method of compensatory changes. *Trigger management* includes identifying factors that may precipitate seizures and making changes to decrease their chance of occurrence. It is not possible or advisable for any person to avoid all possible precipitants. It *is* possible to identify the most likely precipitants and the person's "high risk" time. The goal is to limit the number of precipitants that can increase susceptibility to seizures at any point in time.

RISKS VERSUS BENEFITS

Once a person has worked through beliefs and understanding regarding susceptibility to seizures, severity of the disorder, and alternatives of treatment, the risks vs. benefits of various health actions must be weighed. Providers, parents, or significant others may make recommendations or prescriptions, but it is the individual's responsibility to carry out these activities. If a patient decides against prescribed treatment or recommendations, the health care professional must then question whether this decision was based on informed reasoning, anger, resentment, or impulsive behavior. The parents or legal guardians of children and adolescents may try to force them to adhere to safety precautions or lifestyle modifications, although forced treatments will not help alter their beliefs or knowledge. Counseling should be encouraged to address feelings and to teach more about epilepsy and its treatments.

The benefits of pursuing treatment for epilepsy are better control of seizures and control of the disorder itself, with improved psychosocial functioning and independence. The risks of treatment may include side effects from medications, costs of treatment, severe alterations in daily life, or feelings of dependence on medications. Risks of nontreatment may be worsened seizure control, behavior, and psychosocial function.

Understanding the spectrum of compliance or self-efficacy is an important concept. Age, lifestyle, changes, geographic relocation, and concurrent illness, are only a few of the factors that require reassessment in this area. The health care professional plays a key role in supporting the patient and family through this dynamic process.

REFERENCES

Black RB, Hermann BP, Shope JS. *Nursing management of epilepsy.* London: Aspen, 1982.
Browne TR, Feldman RG. *Epilepsy diagnosis and management.* Boston: Little, Brown, 1983.
Cramer JA, Prevey ML, Ouellette VL, Mattson RH, Scheyer RD. How often is medication taken as prescribed? A novel assessment technique. *JAMA* 1988;261:3273-7.
Cramer JA, Russell ML. Strategies to enhance adherence to a medical regimen. In: Schmidt D, Leppik IE, eds. *Compliance in epilepsy.* Amsterdam: Elsevier, 1988:163-5.
Cramer JA, Scheyer RD, Mattson RH. Compliance declines between clinic visits. *Arch Intern Med* 1990;150:1509-10.

Managing Seizure Disorders: A Handbook for Health Care Professionals, edited by N. Santilli, Lippincott-Raven Publishers, Philadelphia, 1996.
© 1996 Epilepsy Foundation of America.

14

Parenting the Child with Epilepsy

Joan Kessner Austin

This section describes how epilepsy in a child affects parents and the stages that parents commonly experience in their response to the epilepsy. Included is a description of how epilepsy can make parenting more difficult. Suggestions for assessment and intervention are given, with examples.

IMPACT ON PARENTS

Parents in general desire children who are healthy and who fit into the American cultural values of conformity, independence, and competition. Consequently, children who do not possess these qualities may be devalued by our society (Goldin and Margolin, 1975). Parents of children with epilepsy are confronted with having a child who is considered less than perfect. In addition, the characteristics of epilepsy, such as unpredictable episodes of loss of control over functioning, often subject the child to negative social responses (Goldin and Margolin, 1975).

That the onset of childhood epilepsy is stressful to parents is well documented in the literature. Both direct interviews with parents and reports of parental reaction from health care professionals indicate that parents go through an unsettled period after diagnosis. Parental reaction to epilepsy is similar to the chronic grief process described by Olshansky (1962) in depicting the grief reaction of parents to a mentally defective child. Parents of children with epilepsy can be seen as grieving for the loss of a healthy child or at least the loss of a seizure-free child. Although reactions of parents vary and a multitude of reactions are seen, families do appear to go through stages. Austin (1979) identified four stages in adaptation to epilepsy. These four stages are disbelief, anger, demystification, and conditional acceptance. A description of each follows.

Disbelief

The initial parental reaction is usually one of disbelief. Parents often report feelings of shock and a sensation that the seizure really did not happen. Disbelief

145

is not an unusual response to a completely unexpected event. Seizures are rarely expected, especially in an otherwise healthy child.

Disbelief may also take the form of ignoring the seizure completely. For example, parents may explain some seizures as the child "being in a fantasy world" or "having a nervous reaction." In this stage, parents simply do not believe that their child really has epilepsy.

Anger

Once disbelief subsides, parents become aware of the ramifications of epilepsy on their lives and their children's lives. The consequences of epilepsy include financial expense of medical treatment, worry about how well the seizures will be controlled, dread of witnessing future seizures, and worry about effects of antiepileptic medication (AEDs). As parents become aware of the ramifications of epilepsy, the stage of anger usually begins.

In this stage, parents often experience strong feelings of guilt, depression, and anxiety. Parents also might be embarrassed that their child has a disorder to which a stigma is attached and, at the same time, they feel guilty about being embarrassed.

Anger makes sense because the epilepsy has disrupted the status quo of the family, and parents are confronted with the need to cope with both the epilepsy and the disruption. In this stage, irritability often occurs in family members, which can lead to even more family disruption. Dealing with the emotions that arise in this stage is stressful for the entire family.

Demystification

The stage of demystification is marked by active seeking of information about epilepsy. Because there are so many myths surrounding epilepsy, parents usually feel more comfortable as they learn the facts about this condition.

During this stage, parents also learn that the prognosis for epilepsy is not always predictable and that it is difficult to postulate an outcome for any specific case. Uncertainty is something with which parents must learn to deal. They can also begin to put epilepsy in perspective as they realize that many other chronic physical disorders could be more disruptive to the health of their child.

Conditional Acceptance

This final stage occurs when the family gains a sense of control over the epilepsy and becomes able to live fairly comfortably with the disease and its ramifications. It is possible for parents to have a sense of control even when the seizures themselves are not controlled, by developing plans for how to handle them when they occur. In this stage, parents are more comfortable about allowing their children to be as independent as is appropriate for their situation.

IMPACT ON PARENTING

Parenting a child free of chronic illness or disability is not without problems. Therefore, the presence of a chronic physical disorder presents an additional problem. Kessler (1979) points out that parents of children with chronic physical conditions are confused about how and when to discipline, their feelings of sympathy for the child, their desire to protect the child, and their own frustrations of dealing with a child with a chronic medical condition on a daily basis. They often find themselves either ignoring behavior they should not overlook or becoming overstrict. Parents may also be more indulgent with a child to help compensate for the child's epilepsy (Austin, 1979).

Epilepsy presents unique problems in parenting because of its characteristics. The unpredictability of the seizures can cause both parents and child to lose a sense of control. Therefore, the parents often react by overcontrolling or by failing to exert any control at all (Ziegler, 1979). Because epilepsy is not visible to others and carries a social stigma, parents can worry about whether to disclose the condition to others. Parents fear that disclosure may result in segregation of the child, yet hiding it may lead to anxiety and fear of a seizure in public (Goldin and Margolin, 1975). Affected children are also fearful about their seizures. Austin (1993) found them to be worried both about their own health (e.g., fear of dying) and about how others would respond to seizures. Some children feared that they would be rejected by their peers. As a consequence, parents are faced not only with dealing with their own concerns about stigma but with helping their child to deal with the responses of others.

Parents also are confronted with learning how to manage a chronic illness. Many parents have little experience in dealing with complex health care settings and find the experience intimidating. Parents and children often have many fears and concerns about the epilepsy, which may add to their stress in dealing with health care professionals. Moreover, parents are confronted with the need to become skillful in handling future seizures and their treatment. For example, they must learn how to handle future seizures, when to call the nurse or physician, when to go to the emergency room, how to administer medications, and how to recognize side effects of medications. Austin et al. (1995) found that parents have many concerns about being able to manage this new parenting role.

CLINICAL IMPLICATIONS

Beliefs

In general, people act in accordance with their beliefs. Therefore, it is important to know what parents believe about their children's epilepsy because it affects how they act as parents. A comprehensive assessment of beliefs should include information on parents' beliefs about the cause or etiology of seizures, their attitudes about the child's epilepsy, and their knowledge about epilepsy and its treatment. It is especially important to assess for fears of unlikely causes (e.g., brain tumors) and eventualities (e.g., death and loss of intelligence).

An assessment of parent attributions about possible causes of epilepsy is important because sometimes parents harbor unspoken fears that they may have caused their child's epilepsy. These fears may have been generated by the physician asking about a family history of epilepsy, a description of labor and delivery, and any fall that could have resulted in a head injury to help determine the etiology of epilepsy. A common reaction to the onset of epilepsy is to search for causes (Austin et al., 1995; Ziegler, 1979). Parents may try to determine causes by examining the child's past. Some parents blame themselves and feel burdened with guilt; other parents blame each other, which can lead to more family disruption and marital stress.

Parental attitudes towards epilepsy have long been reported as affecting parent and child adaptation to this condition. Bagley (1971) proposes that parents have negative attitudes toward epilepsy because of the stigma associated with it. Negative attitudes are proposed to lead to poor parental adjustment. In turn, the poor parental adjustment leads to behavior problems in children with epilepsy (Austin et al., 1984; Austin and McDermott, 1988). Therefore, parental attitudes about their children's epilepsy should be assessed on a regular basis.

One way to assess attitudes is to use the Fishbein Model as described by Austin and colleagues (Austin et al., 1984; Austin and McDermott, 1988). The Fishbein Model proposes that attitudes are made up of beliefs and feelings associated with those beliefs. Assessment of attitudes is carried out in two steps: eliciting beliefs about epilepsy and identifying feelings associated with those beliefs. Parents are asked to list beliefs or the things they associate with their child's epilepsy. For example, they may view epilepsy as being frightening to others and therefore have a negative feeling associated with that belief. Parents also might report that dealing with epilepsy has brought the family closer and that they have positive feelings associated with the closeness. The use of this method provides the opportunity to assess parents' unique beliefs and concerns about their child's epilepsy.

Parental knowledge about epilepsy and its treatment should also be assessed to identify gaps and inaccuracies. Often parents are given a lot of information when the child is first diagnosed and they do not remember all of it. Those who are in the stage of disbelief may not pay full attention to the information because they do not believe that they will need the information. They may also receive inaccurate information from neighbors and friends. Therefore, it is important for health care professionals to assess the parents' knowledge about epilepsy, administering medication, side effects of medications, first aid for seizures, and events that need prompt attention, such as status epilepticus. It is important for a health care professional to be available to answer questions in between visits.

In addition, parents should have opportunities to talk to health care professionals without the child present (Austin et al., 1995).

The health care provider should base interventions on the assessment of parents' beliefs. The goal of interventions should be to make sure that these beliefs are based on accurate information. Fears and guilts should be explored and information provided to clear up misconceptions. The professional should make sure that parental attitudes are as positive as possible, and should provide information and challenge negative beliefs. For example, if a parent believes that epilepsy causes children to be more prone to later drug addiction, the parent should be taught about the difference between therapeutic drug levels and emotional dependency on a drug.

Parental Coping and Adaptation

It is important to assess parental coping and adaptation on a regular basis. Coping consists of the behaviors used by a parent to help deal with the stress associated with epilepsy. Adaptation refers to how well the parent is functioning or the outcome of the coping. A comprehensive assessment would include information on aspects of epilepsy that are stressful, coping behaviors the parent is using to deal with stress, and how well the parent is functioning. To guide the assessment, it is important to identify which stage of adaptation the parent is in.

Stressors can be identified by asking parents about problems being experienced. Often it is helpful to tell parents what other parents have found to be successful, such as fears about seizures causing brain damage or death and worries about how to handle sibling jealousies. Mentioning common concerns lets parents know that they are no different from other parents and should help them to feel comfortable in talking about things that are stressful to them. Common areas of parental concern include fears about the effects of seizures and medication, how to handle seizures at school, how to tell grandparents, neighbors, and babysitters about seizures, how to help the child deal with teasing and rejection from peers, and how to discipline.

Coping patterns can be assessed through open-ended questions in an interview or by use of self-report questionnaires. Interview questions should focus on what the parent is doing to deal with stressors. For example, the parent could be asked questions such as, "What do you do that makes you feel better?" "What do you do when you are worried about your child's epilepsy?" "What kinds of things do you do just for you?" and "Does it help to read books about epilepsy?"

There are several self-report questionnaires available for assessment of family coping and adaptation. Table 1 lists self-report questionnaires that measure parent coping, family resources, family functioning, and family relationships. All of them can be used to assess families in the clinical setting.

How well the parent is functioning should be assessed within the context of stages in response to epilepsy. For example, denial right after diagnosis would

TABLE 1. *Instruments for assessment of family coping and adaptation*

Target	Instrument	Description	Source
Parent coping behaviors	Coping Health Inventory for Parents	45-item scale to assess three coping patterns	McCubbin and Thompson, 1991
Family resources	Family Resource Scale	31-time scale to assess eight family resources	Dunst et al., 1988
	Family Inventory for Resources for Management	69-item scale to assess four family strengths	McCubbin and Thompson, 1991
	Family Hardiness Index	20-item scale to assess four aspects of family hardiness	McCubbin and Thompson, 1991
	Family Support Scale	18-item scale identifying people who are helpful	Dunst et al., 1988
Family functioning	Family Functioning Index	15-item scale to assess six areas of functioning	Pless and Satterwhite, 1973
	Family Functioning Style Scale	26-item scale to assess two areas of family strength	Dunst et al., 1988
Family relationships	Family APGAR	5-item scale to assess satisfaction in five areas of family relationships	Smilkstein, 1978
	Family Relationships Index	27-item scale that assesses three areas of family environment	Moos, 1986

be appropriate. Denial a year later, however, would be an indication of poor adaptation. Parents should be assessed for stress on the marital relationship and symptoms such as inability to sleep, feelings of sadness, and feelings of inadequacy.

Interventions should be aimed at reducing stressors and negative coping strategies, identifying resources, and facilitating positive coping strategies. Often stressors are reduced by providing information that counteracts irrational fears and worries about epilepsy. Other stressors, such as the unpredictability of seizures, can be addressed by helping parents to develop a plan for dealing with seizures regardless of when and where they occur, which should provide a sense of control over epilepsy. See Chap. 19 for more information on stress management.

Health care professionals should encourage parents to join a support group where they can learn how other parents deal with common problems associated with epilepsy. They can be referred to the Epilepsy Foundation of America (1-800-EFA-1000; Internet: postmaster@efa.org) for help in finding a local affiliate in their area. Many of these affiliates have parent telephone networks that enable parents to provide support to each other (Epilepsy Foundation of America, 1989).

Some parents exhibit poor adaptation and require counseling from mental health professionals. For example, those who are experiencing symptoms of depression should be encouraged to seek counseling from a therapist who is knowledgeable about parental adaptation to a chronic physical disorder in a child. With counseling, these parents can be helped to learn new adaptive coping strategies to replace maladaptive ones and can be helped to express feelings and to work through problems instead of withdrawing from the family.

REFERENCES

Austin JK. Stages in a family's reaction to epilepsy in a child. Psychosocial aspects of epilepsy. *Indiana State Nurses' Assoc Bull* 1979;5:1–3. (Available from National Epilepsy Library, Epilepsy Foundation of America, 4351 Garden City Drive, Suite 406, Landover, MD 20785.)

Austin JK. Concerns and fears of children with seizures. *Clin Nurs Pract Epilepsy* 1993;4:4–6.

Austin JK, McBride AB, Davis HW. Parental attitude and adjustment to childhood epilepsy. *Nurs Res* 1984;33:92–6.

Austin JK, McDermott N. Parental attitude and coping behaviors in families of children with epilepsy. *J Neurosci Nurs* 1988;20:174–9.

Austin JK, Oruche UM, Dunn DW, Levstek DA. New-onset childhood seizures: parents' concerns and needs. *Clin Nurs Pract Epilepsy* 1995;2:8–10.

Bagley C. *The social psychology of the child with epilepsy.* London: Rouledge and Kegan Paul, 1971.

Dunst C, Trivette C, Deal A. *Enabling and empowering families: principles and guidelines for practice.* Cambridge, MA: Brookline Books, 1988.

Epilepsy Foundation of America. *Epilepsy parent and family networks resource materials.* Landover, MD, 1989.

Goldin GJ, Margolin RS. The psychosocial aspect of epilepsy. In: Wright GN, ed. *Epilepsy rehabilitation.* Boston: Little, Brown, 1975:66–80.

Kessler JW. Parenting the handicapped child. *Pediatr Ann* 1987;6:654–61.

McCubbin NI, Thompson AI, eds. *Family assessment inventories for research and practice.* Madison, WI: University of Wisconsin Press, 1991.

Moos RH. *Manual for the Family Environment Scales, 2nd ed.* Palo Alto, CA: Consulting Psychologists Press, 1986.

Olshansky S. Chronic sorrow: a response to having a mental defective child. *Social Casework* 1962;8: 106–21.

Pless IB, Satterwhite B. A measure of family functioning and its application. *Soc Sci Med* 1973;7: 613–21.

Smilkstein G. The family APGAR: a proposal for a family function test and behavior. *J Fam Pract* 1978;6:1231–9.

Ziegler RG. Psychologic vulnerability in epileptic patients. *Psychosomatics* 1979;20:145–8.

ADDITIONAL READING

Freeman JM, Vining EPG, Pillas DJ. *Seizures and epilepsy in childhood: a guide for parents.* Baltimore: The Johns Hopkins University Press, 1991.

Jan JE, Ziegler RG, Erba G. *Does your child have epilepsy?* 2nd Ed. Baltimore, MD: University Park Press, 1992.

McCollum AT. *The chronically ill child: a guide for parents and professionals.* New Haven: Yale University Press, 1981.

Ozuna J. Psychosocial aspects of epilepsy. *J Neurosurg Nurs* 1979;11:243–6.

Managing Seizure Disorders: A Handbook for Health Care Professionals, edited by N. Santilli, Lippincott-Raven Publishers, Philadelphia, 1996. © 1996 Epilepsy Foundation of America.

15

The Student with Epilepsy in an Educational Framework[1]

Nancy Santilli, W. Edwin Dodson, Ann V. Walton, Barbara Flock, and Judith Harrigan

ROLE OF SCHOOL HEALTH PROFESSIONAL AS CASE MANAGER AND EDUCATOR

The knowledgeable school health professional can make a great difference for the child with epilepsy. The school nurse, social worker, or guidance counselor is often the single, constant health professional who has the opportunity to assess, interact, and encourage the child and family throughout these critical years of development. Armed with the facts about epilepsy, they can develop with the child, family, and school personnel long-range plans that will afford the child every opportunity to acquire the intellectual, emotional, and occupational skills necessary for life.

Generally speaking, the following can be said about students with epilepsy[2]:

Psychosocial function may be impaired among people with epilepsy, although studies have tended to evaluate patients with poor seizure control.

Psychosocial impairment may be greater in those with many seizures compared with those with only a few seizures.

The occurrence of status epilepticus is an even more important predictor of psychosocial impairment than seizure frequency.

Cognitive function may be impaired by antiepileptic drugs. This is explained, in part, by slowed motor responses.

Many children receiving phenobarbital in doses sufficient to achieve "therapeutic" blood levels (15 μg/ml or more) will experience hyperactivity.

Learning disabilities are more common among children with epilepsy than in the general population and may benefit from early identification and treatment.

Children with epilepsy are more likely to have impairment of self-concept and behavior than children with asthma.

---

[1]This chapter is copyrighted by the Epilepsy Foundation of America but may be duplicated for use by nurses and others in their efforts to educate school personnel.
[2]Adapted from Hauser and Hesdorffer, 1990.

There is no evidence that organized, directed ictal aggression occurs in people with epilepsy.

The student with no prior history of epilepsy or seizure disorder who suffers a seizure in the school setting creates a challenge for the school. After dispensing first aid and performing a thorough assessment of the student, the school nurse or designee must collect all vital data to share with the parent and the clinician.

It is important to obtain an accurate description of the events preceding the seizure as well as the seizure itself. The school health professional must gain input from all the staff members who witnessed the event or who had suspicions of previous events. This information is valuable for the clinician in evaluating the student's medical problem.

Included below are some pertinent questions that must be asked of the staff:

Were any specific problems and/or behaviors noted before the seizure?
Were specific movements/tremors of any extremities noted?
What time of day did the seizure occur?
How long did the seizure last?
Was the student incontinent?
Did the student become cyanotic?
Were there any other physical data?
Does the student remember any preceding events?

In addition to collecting information about the possible seizures, the school health professional should notify the student's parents as soon as possible. Often a designated staff member can use the student's emergency data card to contact the parent, especially if the child's condition requires the school health professional to remain with the child. It is important for the parents to be advised to have their child examined by a physician. A child who is coherent and able to walk can be transported by the parent. Otherwise, the child should be transported via ambulance to the closest medical facility. Staff should encourage the parents to share their child's early medical history with the physician. A written summary of the seizure activity should be sent with the parent for the physician, because the parent is often overwhelmed during this time and may be unable to comprehend all the pertinent information. Requesting that the parent have the physician send a report of the medical evaluation to the school enables the school health professional to clarify the seizure activity and workup to the staff.

A complete documentation of the incident should be charted in the student's health record. This information should include the staff observations and the physical assessment data. Many school districts require the school nurse or health professional to complete a district accident form and/or incident report that can be placed in the student's cumulative record.

After care has been rendered and the situation has been discussed with the parent, attention should be focused toward the staff. Staff members may feel upset and concerned by a perceived inability to care properly for the student.

Many teachers have never witnessed an actual seizure, and their apprehension is a normal phenomenon. Reassurance is a valuable first step but should be followed with an in-service program about epilepsy and its management.

The following steps are recommended for establishing an in-service program:

Explain the need for the program to the principal (to gain cooperation and permission).

Emphasize that the program should be scheduled soon after the event.

Collect information sheets or brochures on seizure disorders. These are available from the Epilepsy Foundation of America (EFA) or its local affiliates. Refer to Appendix D, EFA Resources.

Request a speaker from a local medical center or contact the local chapter of EFA for materials or speaker, if the school health professional feels that an outside speaker will be more effective.

Ensure that information about first aid of seizures be included in the program (see Appendix C, Seizure Recognition and First Aid.

An in-service program is a perfect opportunity to discuss other forms of epilepsy that may occur in a school population. For example, the student who appears to daydream or is unable to follow specific directions may be having absence (petit mal) seizures. The teacher can play a major role in removing the stigma of epilepsy by recognizing potential medical problems and by educating students about a classmate's seizure disorder.

When the student who has had a seizure returns to school, the school health professional should inform the staff of the problem and the medical evaluation with a written memo. The memo should include the diagnosis, any specific restrictions, type of seizure medication, whether medication will be given during school hours, side effects that may affect academic performance or fine or gross motor ability, and the suggestion to discuss specific questions or problems with the school nurse, treating health care professional, guidance counselor, or other appropriate individual.

Most people have a very vivid memory of the first seizure they ever saw and know exactly how they felt about it. It can be a very dramatic event, and the fact that it is extremely sudden and unexpected makes it all the more startling. Even for those who have never seen a seizure, there is enough misunderstanding about epilepsy that they may be afraid of the possibility of seeing one.

When the Individuals with Disabilities Education Act, Public Law 94-142 (formerly titled the Education for All Handicapped Children Act), was first passed, school personnel were faced with the possibility of having students with uncontrolled seizures in their classrooms. This was a frightening concept for many of them who had never seen a seizure and were hesitant about the possibility of such an experience in the classroom. Unfortunately, teachers at that time were not trained to deal with students with any sort of disability. Now, many years later, college courses are available to teach the prospective teacher about different debilitating conditions and how to work with students who have chronic conditions. Frequently, however, only those interested in special education take the courses. This means that many teachers are still unprepared to deal with the child who experiences a seizure in the classroom.

Teachers' attitudes and expectations have been implicated as a possible negative source of influence on the academic performance of children with epilepsy (Holdsworth and Whitmore, 1974). Unfortunately, school personnel may be unaware of the effects the seizures and the medications may have on the child's academic, behavioral, and social achievement. To support the child with epilepsy and to foster the development of the child's potential, school personnel need accurate information about the following: (a) seizure recognition, causes for behavior exhibited during seizures, the spectrum of the disorder, and appropriate first aid; (b) how the seizure disorder may be affecting the student academically, behaviorally, and psychosocially; (c) what, if any, limitations are necessary for the student; and (d) how to assist peers to understand and accept the student with seizures.

The school health professional has a unique opportunity to provide the information necessary for school personnel to feel confident about having a child with epilepsy in the classroom. Given sufficient and pertinent information, all school personnel will be better prepared to assist the child during a seizure and to make appropriate adjustments to the educational program. Once trained about seizure disorders, they will be in a better position to provide psychological assistance by accepting the student as a normal healthy person who occasionally may have seizures. This will bolster self-esteem for the child and will serve as a role model for other children. The well-informed teacher may be able to strike the balance necessary to tip the scales in favor of the student's developing into an independent, socially adept individual.

It is extremely helpful to start with the perceptions and feelings that teachers may have about persons with epilepsy. In describing the first seizure they ever saw, they will soon realize that they may share a common fear. This is a fear that can be diminished by understanding of what a seizure is and how to assist the student, as well as the rest of the class, when a seizure occurs.

Knowing what type of seizures a student has, whether or not the seizures are controlled, how the seizures are manifested, how often they occur, and what time of day they are most likely to occur is valuable for the teacher and can make a great deal of difference in the teacher's level of confidence in working with the student. For the child who continues to have seizures, knowing that the seizure activity is time-limited and that it will usually resolve by itself is reassuring.

Knowledge of absence seizures is extremely important for all teachers because they can frequently be case-finders. Seizures of this type can cause serious problems with the child's attention span and concentration, as illustrated in the following scenario.

Sue has been having difficulty with paying attention in class. There are times when she simply seems to be staring into space. When the teacher calls her, she seemingly hesitates for a moment and then responds. However, she is not able to give an accurate answer to the teacher's question. At other times she is apparently attentive but still has difficulty in responding appropriately to the teacher's questions.

Because absence seizures are subtle and typically last only for a few seconds, they can go undetected. A child such as Sue may be having as many as 50 or more of these seizures each day. Although all students have periods of staring or daydreaming, the difference with absence seizures is the lack of facial emotion associated with these episodes.

Tim, when called on to read out loud, frequently loses his place. He reads several lines ahead of himself. Likewise, during a spelling test he will miss three or four words in a row, but later can spell them correctly.

Possible indicators of absence seizures are evident in scholastic performance and in physical activities; examples may include the following:

Scholastic performance: difficulty following spoken directions, skipping or repeating lines of words while reading aloud, difficulty with reading or inattentiveness

Physical activities: brief spells, a few seconds of acting strange or doing unusual things such as rolling the eyes, blinking rapidly, or other unusual eye movements, staring into space, or seeming to be in a daze (Santilli and Tonelson, 1982)

Early recognition and treatment may limit the extent of scholastic problems that might develop. Although 10 s may not seem like a long time, several gaps in attention and concentration during a teacher's explanation of a math problem may make the difference between the student understanding or not understanding the process. If this happens many times a day, which is typical in absence seizures, the frustration level of the child, teacher, and family rises and can cause the child to withdraw or to become resentful and act out behaviorally. A positive response in recognizing and treating the seizure is a major factor in protecting the child's self-esteem. Steps in dealing with the problem are: (a) early detection and accurate diagnosis; (b) appropriate medication to control the seizures; and (c) patience on the part of the teacher and fellow students, who must be willing to respond positively when asked to repeat what they just said.

When a teacher recognizes that a child is having problems like those described above, it is important to inform the parents. Of course, no teacher can make a diagnosis of epilepsy, but the teacher should alert the parent to the behavior being observed and to the fact that the child may be having learning problems, possibly as a result. The teacher and school health professional should also encourage the parents to report the teacher's observations to the child's clinician promptly. In turn, the clinician will be in a position to determine if the child is having absence seizures.

Tonic–clonic convulsions are the most dramatic seizure type.

Bob has always been a very active boy. Although he has had some difficulty academically in school, he is popular with the students and very successful in sports.

> While waiting in the cafeteria line one day he suddenly let out a strange cry and fell to the floor. He stiffened for a moment and then began to convulse. He turned blue and was incontinent. The event lasted approximately 2 min and was very upsetting for all who witnessed it. Bob was embarrassed by the circle of astonished and wide-eyed faces that surrounded him when he recovered consciousness.

With this type of seizure the student is perfectly normal one minute and convulsing the next. A seizure of this type usually causes disruption in the classroom and evokes fear, revulsion, and panic among students and the teacher. On regaining consciousness, the student who had the seizure must cope with the physical exhaustion and aches of a seizure, the undesirable position of being the center of attention, the possible embarrassment of soiled clothing, lack of understanding of what has happened, and the anger and frustration of having had the seizure.

The result is often a decrease in self-esteem, with the possibility for social withdrawal or behavioral problems. The teacher should understand that although the seizure looks frightening, it is usually very brief and the first aid for it is quite simple. Unfortunately, many teachers still believe that it is necessary to place a tongue depressor or other object in the mouth of the person experiencing a tonic–clonic seizure. This does no good, and may even cause damage. Inform the teacher that the student is *not* going to swallow the tongue. The student should be turned on his or her side with the head positioned gently to provide the best airway and also to allow secretions to drain (see Appendix C, Seizure Recognition and First Aid).

Usually it is not necessary to send the child home after a seizure unless the seizure has been unusually severe or the child was injured in some way. The best course of action is to allow the student to rest as needed and then return to normal classroom activity. Optimally, the student should remain with classmates. This also helps other students to become more comfortable with seizures. Social isolation makes the epilepsy more mysterious and supports the idea that a student with seizures is "different."

Partial seizures are frequently unrecognized by the general public, including school personnel, and this seizure type is often misunderstood.

> On several occasions, Karen has exhibited some odd behavior in the classroom that has been disruptive to the class. Each time it happens she will stand up with a dazed look on her face, and wander around the room while mumbling incoherently. She will pull at the sleeve of her sweater as if trying to remove it. When the teacher asks her to sit down she does not respond. After a couple of moments Karen seems to "come to" and sits down with a confused and perplexed look. The students consider her somewhat "crazy," but the teacher wonders if she has been taking some sort of drugs.

The most common features of the complex partial seizure include a decreased awareness of the environment, a dazed look, and purposeless activity such as wandering about, mumbling incoherently or talking nonsensically, lip smacking, picking at clothes, and automatic repetition of some movement. Unfortunately, observers often judge this behavior to be caused by alcohol or drug abuse. It is therefore particularly important for school personnel to recognize this seizure type. First aid for complex partial seizures consists of simply seeing that the student is protected and not interfered with until reorientation takes place after the seizure.

For a child with complex partial seizures, control of the seizures is important not only from the medical standpoint but also because of the impact that continued seizures may have on both scholastic and social development. The odd behavior during the seizure leads to misinterpretation and misjudgment by school personnel, classmates, and family. The adverse reaction of observers can lead to ostracism or can make the student so confused and embarrassed as to cause withdrawal, anger, or behavioral problems.

> Andy has had a seizure disorder for approximately 4 years and still has an occasional seizure in school. He has many friends and gets along with his classmates. Academically he is doing well in school. He participates in class discussions and his grades are consistently in the upper range. He is involved in sports and is on the school's basketball team.

Many children with epilepsy, like Andy, have no academic or social adjustment problems. However, children with seizures are children at risk. "We know quite conclusively that seizures in children are, at times, correlated with learning and achievement difficulties, behavioral problems and a broad range of psychosocial outcomes" (Ferrari, 1989).

As indicated earlier, the functional status of children with seizures may fall into one of three categories: the uncomplicated, the compromised, and the devastated. Because the uncomplicated, like Andy, will rarely have difficulty in school, and because those who are devastated are typically in special education classes, the main focus here is on the compromised student. Although free of serious mental and motor problems, the compromised student frequently experiences a variety of social, emotional, and educational problems.

The primary task of the teacher is education of students. Therefore, the focus is on factors that help or hinder the student during the educational process. The school nurse plays a major role in assisting teachers to understand the medical problems that may affect the child.

In determining what information and assistance school personnel need, it is helpful to ascertain their expectations about students with epilepsy. The knowledge base differs from one teacher to the next and may be based on misinformation or on previous experiences that were less than satisfactory. Teachers should have access to the most current information. Specifically, they need to know how a medical condition and its treatment may affect the student.

The school health professional must identify children who are at risk in the educational setting and must provide specific information about each individual. This equips the teacher with enough knowledge to develop an appropriate educational plan for the student. The goal of this plan is to assist the child in developing effective educational, social, and vocational skills, thereby increasing the chances for a normal life.

> Jimmy has had a seizure problem for 3 years. He is diagnosed as having tonic–clonic seizures and has been on medication. Although his seizures are well controlled, he tends to be hyperactive in the classroom and frequently is disruptive. The other students shun him and frequently make fun of him. Although he has an average IQ, he is not doing well in school. He does not like school and is frequently absent for no apparent reason.

> Tina has been diagnosed as having absence seizures and is on medication. Before starting the medication she was often observed staring into space and being unable to respond accurately when asked a question. Since beginning medication she seldom stares into space but still appears to have difficulty paying attention in class. She seems to be attentive but fails to respond to the teacher when asked a question, or her response seems inappropriate to the question asked.

> Mike has complex partial seizures with a focus in the right temporal lobe. His seizures are controlled with medication. He is not doing well in school because he cannot remember what he has learned from one day to the next. He has become aggressive and belligerent. When the teacher confers with the parents, they tend to become defensive and insist that Mike is not disruptive at home. They blame the teacher for any difficulties in school, saying that she simply does not understand Mike.

Jimmy, Tina, and Mike are experiencing problems that are detrimental to their scholastic success and social development. They are compromised to various degrees by their epilepsy, although their seizures are usually controlled. Underlying manifestations of the disorder may affect a student academically as in the case of Tina and Mike, or behaviorally, as in the case of Jimmy and Mike, or socially, as in the case of Jimmy. Unfortunately, the task of the school health professional in providing appropriate information and assistance to the school personnel is complicated.

Determining what is causing a student to have academic difficulties can be challenging. Nevertheless, it is essential for school personnel to be aware of the types of factors that may be involved and how they interact so that appropriate intervention strategies can be developed. The problem may be the result of a multiplicity of factors, such as side effects of medications, neurologic deficits affecting the memory, and lowered family expectations. These factors are summarized in Table 1.

Demographic Factors

Demographic factors such as social class and ethnic background are important factors that interact with epilepsy and antiepileptic drug therapy to influence attitudes toward the disorder, attitudes about learning, and measurements of cognitive ability and academic performance. For example, although many variables can affect IQ, most of the determinants of IQ cannot be defined in large-

TABLE 1. *Factors that may influence cognitive functioning, behavior, and psychosocial adjustment in epilepsy*

Demographic	Biologic	Psychosocial	Medication
Education	Age	Family/social support	Number of
Ethnic and cultural	Sex	Locus of control	medications
background	Type of epilepsy	Stigma	Medication type
Socioeconomic	Etiology	Discrimination	AED levels
background	Duration of epilepsy	Social exclusion	Compliance
	Seizure frequency	Negative life events	
	Number of episodes		
	of status		
	epilepticus		
	Age at onset		
	Related		
	neuropsychological		
	deficits		
	Temperament		

Adapted from Hermann et al., 1988.

scale investigations. Furthermore, the variables that are usually considered are interrelated.

In the National Collaborative Perinatal Project (NCPP) the relationship between various factors and IQ measured at up to the age of 7 was evaluated. Overall, the strongest determinants of intellect were socioeconomic factors. However, considering all predictor variables, the investigators could account for only 25–28% of the variance in IQ among whites and 15–17% among African-Americans (Broman et al., 1975). The highest correlation ($r = 0.38$) was found between socioeconomic index and IQ. The correlation between maternal nonverbal IQ and the child's IQ was lower ($r = 0.28$). This value yields a coefficient of determination of approximately 8%. The effects of socioeconomic factors are manifest in various ways. Whereas 20.2% of children from families who had the lowest socioeconomic index failed a test of language comprehension at age 8 years, only 2% from the highest social stratum failed (Broman et al., 1975). Most studies of children with epilepsy do not allow for these types of socioeconomic effects.

Ethnic and cultural values also have a strong impact on the way families react to epilepsy and on how they value education and learning. Fear, misunderstanding, and stigma about epilepsy are more prevalent among some ethnic and minority groups, making adjustment to the diagnosis an even greater challenge for the family. These perceptions influence the way various ethnic groups label and recognize seizure symptoms and access medical care. They also influence the groups' interactions with the medical system, compliance with treatment, and the use of traditional health practices (for more details see Chap 20).

Epilepsy is more common among certain ethnic and racial groups. The rate is 1.3–2.2 times greater for nonwhite than for white males and 1.4–1.7 times greater for nonwhite than for white females. The interpretation of racial differences must be made with caution as nonwhite populations are biased toward lower socioeconomic groups. Socioeconomic class is a confounder of these types of results, i.e., the higher prevalence in certain groups probably reflects socioeconomic factors rather than ethnicity (Hauser and Hesdorffer, 1990).

Biologic Factors

Biologic factors also contribute to learning problems among children with epilepsy. As a group, children with epilepsy have more than their share of developmental disabilities. Approximately 9% have IQs below 70, a percentage that is three times greater than the general population (Fig. 1). Learning disabilities and certain psychiatric conditions, such as depression and behavioral disorders, are also more common among people with epilepsy, although these are more difficult to quantify. In most cases the learning impairment is the result of an antecedent neurologic injury that also caused the epilepsy. Of course, seizures per se can cause interruptions of awareness and thereby impair cognitive function. When this occurs, controlling the seizures usually restores learning cognitive ability. Rarely, epilepsy heralds a progressive brain disorder that also causes dementia.

Many other potentially disabling conditions are associated with an increased risk for epilepsy. For example, one-third of children with cerebral palsy and almost half of those who are severely mentally retarded also have epilepsy. How to properly plan for these children's education can be complex. However, being

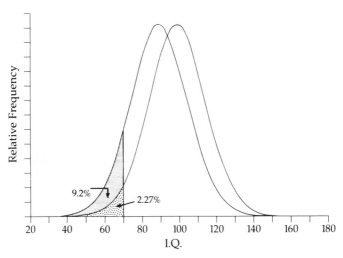

FIG. 1. The student with epilepsy in an educational framework. (From Dodson and Pellock, 1993.)

aware of potential problems and starting the planning early can help to avoid pitfalls.

Even children with epilepsy who do not have overt neurologic abnormalities are at increased risk for academic underachievement, particularly in the basic skills of reading, language skills, and arithmetic. Many of them are significantly behind their peers in academic achievement levels (Seidenberg, 1989). The factors that underlie these problems have yet to be clearly identified. There is increasing evidence to suggest that deficits in attention and memory are important contributors to the high incidence of learning problems in students with epilepsy (Marshall and Cupoli, 1986). This may be a problem intrinsic to the child or it may be a side effect of AEDs. If there is a consistent problem, the parents should be alerted so that information can be given to the child's physician. Reevaluation and possible adjustment in medication may be necessary. Seizures that interfere with consciousness, such as generalized seizures, also interfere with attention, reaction time, and concentration.

It is helpful to examine the data from yearly standardized achievement tests given in the school system to identify underachievers. If a significant problem is found, then the child should be referred for a thorough neuropsychological evaluation. Such an evaluation can identify areas of cognitive and behavioral strength, as well as deficits (Seidenberg, 1989). This information is critical for planning.

Independent of epilepsy, boys have more academic problems than girls. This difference is also seen in children with epilepsy. For example, reading skills are poorer among boys with epilepsy than among girls with epilepsy (Stores and Hart, 1976). However, all children with epilepsy are at increased risk for reading problems. The Isle of Wight study indicated that the problem was in reading comprehension (Rutter et al., 1970), whereas the Oxford study indicated that it was in reading accuracy (Stores and Hart, 1976). Seidenberg concluded that students with epilepsy, regardless of seizures type, tend to be 1 year behind their peers in reading (Seidenberg, 1989). They also underachieve in spelling and arithmetic. This academic vulnerability is based on specific cognitive deficiencies rather than on subnormal intellect. The underachievers are distinctly impaired on measures of auditory-perceptual and language-processing abilities. Areas not distinctly impaired included visuospatial reasoning and problem-solving skills, gross motor skills, and nonverbal learning and memory.

Children with signs of academic problems should be assessed. The assessment process can help to identify the student's strengths and weaknesses and can provide critical information about the student's learning style. The knowledge gained provides the student, parents, and school counselor with valuable information to develop strategic plans to build on individual strengths. Table 2 itemizes skills that may need to be assessed initially by the nurse and then in greater depth by these professionals. This list is meant to be a guide; other professionals should be consulted as needed or as available.

TABLE 2. *Areas of development to be assessed and professionals responsible for each*

Area	Skills assessed	Specialist
Speech/language	Articulation, pronunciation, verbal abilities, vocabulary, understanding, and following directions	Teacher/nurse/ speech pathologist
Gross motor skills	Using large muscles; walking, skipping, running, throwing, balance, and coordination	Teacher/nurse/ physical therapist
Fine motor skills	Using small muscles: handwriting, buttoning, puzzles, eye tracking, feeding, hand dominance, hand sewing, soldering, or playing a musical instrument	Teacher/nurse/ occupational therapist
Perceptual/ sensory processing	Visual perception, design copying, planning of body movements, and such skills as toleration of touch and movement in space necessary for sensorimotor development	Teacher/nurse/ occupational therapist
Cognitive/learning	IQ, learning styles, achievement, thinking, reasoning, understanding, work habits, attention, tolerance of distraction, adaptive behaviors, areas of interest	Teacher/nurse/ special educator/ psychologist/ educational diagnostician
Hearing	Auditory abilities	Nurse/teacher/ audiologist
Vision	Visual and sensory abilities	Nurse/teacher/ ophthalmologist/ physician
Nutrition	Caloric intake, habits, variety of food, growth, nutritional status	Nurse/teacher/ registered dietician/ nutritionist
Medical	Brain maturation, related conditions, physical development	Nurse/teacher/ pediatrician/ developmental pediatrician/ neurologic pediatrician/ epileptologist
Social/emotional self-help	Family functioning, stresses, coping, dressing, feeding, sleeping, behaviors, peer interactions	Nurse/teacher/family worker/social worker/visiting teachers

continued

TABLE 2. *Continued.*

Area	Skills assessed	Specialist
Medication	Sensory, perceptual and motor planning, detailed evaluation of effects on attention, memory, cognitive learning skills, and sensory processing related to antiepileptic drugs, toxicity	Nurse/teacher/ physician/ educational diagnostician/ neuropsychologist

Adapted from Quinn, 1988.

Psychosocial Factors

Psychosocial factors can affect behavior and adjustment among children with epilepsy. The word "epileptic" still carries a great deal of stigma. The negative social attitudes regarding epilepsy are difficult to reverse. Health care professionals such as the school nurse, social worker, or school counselor are frequently able to help children with epilepsy and also should be aware of these prejudices.

For many parents, seeing the child have a seizure is the most frightening experience in their lives. The diagnosis of epilepsy affects the individual and the entire family. Many families undergo a vulnerable and unsettled period after their child is diagnosed with epilepsy. Feelings of guilt, anger, isolation, and frustration are common. Hopes for a healthy, perfect child are challenged. Although responses vary, all families experience some sense of loss and grief. Families appear to go through four stages in coping with a child's epilepsy: denial or disbelief, anger, demystification, and conditional acceptance.

The confusion, fear, and sense of guilt that many parents feel may lead to overprotection of the child. Parents' fears about their child's seizures often lead them to make fewer demands on the child. They worry that the child may have more seizures when emotionally upset and seek to avoid such situations. Overprotection can lead to isolation of the child, lower expectations for the child, and potentially to lowering of the child's self-concept and self-esteem. It is important for school personnel to be sure that they do not fall prey to the same response pattern.

A common problem for children with epilepsy is significantly lower self-esteem. This is more common than for other chronic disorders, such as diabetes and asthma, or for other neurologic disorders (Hauser and Hesdorffer, 1990). Parents know the child best and can provide important information on the child's developmental patterns and problems. To build self-esteem, children with epilepsy need to take chances and succeed. To foster this type of growth it helps to assess the child's strengths and weaknesses. When children succeed they should be praised. The school health professional plays a unique role in starting the process to help both teachers and students understand and accept the person with epilepsy as a normal human being with some weaknesses and many strengths. Emphasizing strengths and success can help the person with epilepsy to build self-esteem.

Medication Effects

Toxicity limits the suitability of all the AEDs. At best, each drug is tolerated by only 60% of individuals (Mattson et al., 1985). At low doses, AEDs cause few effects on learning and behavior, but at high doses and concentrations all AEDs are toxic. Reducing the number of drugs or reducing drug doses and levels decreases toxicity and improves performance (Trimble, 1987). The major problems occur among patients who require high drug levels for seizure control.

It is important to emphasize that despite adverse drug effects, seizure control abets neuropsychological performance (Seidenberg et al., 1981). Measurements that improve include the overall IQ plus improvements on both verbal and performance subtests.

The behavioral affects of AEDs have been recognized for years (Table 3). In some cases these changes are striking and easy to recognize. For example, when

TABLE 3. *Behavioral side effects that have been attributed to antiepileptic drugs*

Phenobarbital
  Transient drowsiness
  Excitement
  Irritability
  Tearfulness
  Aggression
  Hyperkinetic syndrome
  Impaired vigilance
Benzodiazepines (Klonopin, Valium, Tranxene, Ativan)
  Hostility
  Disinhibited behavior
Ethosuximide (Zarontin)
  Mood changes
  Lethargy
  Euphoria
  Psychosis
Primidone (Mysoline)
  Same as phenobarbital
  Idiosyncratic confusional state
  Mood swings
  Paranoid psychosis
  Personality deterioration
Phenytoin (Dilantin)
  Psychomotor slowing
  Intellectual deterioration
  Psychiatric illness
  Personality change
Carbamazepine (Tegretol)
  Transient drowsiness
  Psychosis

From Stores, 1975.

a previously well-behaved child becomes hyperactive, impulsive, and mean, the diagnosis of behavioral toxicity is easy. On the other hand when a male toddler becomes more active, inquisitive, and negative, one may be dealing with a normal phase of development.

The adverse effects of AEDs on learning are difficult to detect. Only rarely are they identifiable by standard IQ testing. Specialized tests of attention, memory, and specific academic abilities are necessary, but even here results are difficult to interpret. Relatively few differences are found in these types of studies, and the magnitude of the differences is usually small. Because this is such a difficult area methodologically, most studies have been performed in older children or in adults.

The adverse cognitive effects of AEDs selectively involve specific aspects of mental processing. Mental speed, motor speed, motor performance, short-term memory, and attention are mentioned more often than the ability to retrieve and use information in solving problems. Drugs such as phenobarbital, primidone, and phenytoin do less well compared with carbamazepine or valproate.

Phenobarbital is a good example of how an AED can interfere with academic performance. Phenobarbital affects motor performance tasks that require sustained effort, concentration, and memory (Macleod et al., 1978). Higher concentrations cause more problems than low concentrations. In children, phenobarbital also adversely affects neuropsychological measures that are influenced by speed and memory (Camfield, 1979).

Among the AEDs, phenobarbital and the benzodiazepines diazepam and clonazepam cause the most problems. These drugs are sedative and cause behavior disturbances in children, including depression (Robertson et al., 1987). Children with epilepsy who take barbiturates have more behavior problems at school. They are also more likely to exhibit excess worry, self-destructive behavior, and complaints of persecution (Ferrari et al., 1983). In one study of children who took phenobarbital daily for prevention of febrile seizures, 42% developed a behavior disturbance compared to 18% of children with febrile seizures who were not medicated (Wolf and Forsyth, 1978). When there was a prior behavior disturbance, 80% became worse on phenobarbital. The most common complaint was hyperactivity. When phenobarbital causes negative, defiant, disruptive behavior in the classroom, the child usually should be switched to another medication.

For years phenytoin was judged to have few or no adverse neuropsychological effects. Compared to barbiturates it was nonsedating and did not cause hyperactivity. Most patients who developed cognitive difficulties had overt signs of phenytoin intoxication. In the 1970s, however, reports began to appear suggesting an association between phenytoin and assorted behavioral and mental problems, although no single problem stands out (Andrewes et al., 1986). High levels of phenytoin reduce the performance IQ of adults, but this results from slowed motor performance and not from changes in the verbal IQ. Trimble (1987) has reported concentration-related adverse effects of phenytoin on memory.

Carbamazepine has relatively few behavioral and cognitive side effects when administered to normal volunteers in low or moderate doses (Trimble, 1987). It does, however, have concentration-related effects on cognitive performance. Compared to children with low carbamazepine levels, children with moderate levels have an increased error rate on tests of hand dexterity and speed. Some studies have suggested that carbamazepine increases mental speed for arithmetic. When this is modest, overall performance can improve. However, if the effect is marked, careless mistakes increase.

Comparative studies of carbamazepine vs. phenytoin indicate that both have advantages on different measures. Among adults with seizures controlled on monotherapy with either phenytoin or carbamazepine, Andrewes et al. compared learning. Two of 22 measures favored carbamazepine. Other comparisons of phenytoin vs. carbamazepine indicate superior performance for either drug, depending on the specific test item. In a recent review, carbamazepine was superior on nine subtests vs. three for phenytoin (Trimble, 1987). Comparative studies of carbamazepine vs. phenobarbital usually indicate either no differences or advantages for carbamazepine (Robertson et al., 1987).

Although valproate has fewer troublesome cognitive and behavioral side effects than older drugs, it is not trouble-free. Similar to the situation with phenytoin, individuals who take higher doses of valproate do less well on certain test items than individuals who take lower doses. Valproate (compared to placebo) decreases motor performance on several measures when it is administered as an add-on medication.

Valproate, like carbamazepine, has slight advantages over phenobarbital and phenytoin in certain situations. Among mentally retarded children with epilepsy, valproate has fewer adverse effects on learning and behavior than phenytoin or phenobarbital (Gay, 1984). In a recent investigation that compared valproate vs. phenobarbital in children with mild epilepsy, four of 33 cognitive measures favored valproate to a statistically significant degree. Significant differences were also found on three of 48 behavioral measurements. These differences are small, and group members vary widely in these abilities or behaviors. In these types of studies, the investigators cannot tell which drug a particular child is taking. These issues are therefore difficult to define and resolve in individual children.

During the past several years, three new AEDs have been approved for use: felbamate, neurontin, and lamotrigine. Felbamate, although an effective agent for the atonic seizures seen in the Lennox–Gastaut syndrome, carries a high risk for aplastic anemia and hepatic toxicity. Its usage is therefore limited. Neurontin and lamotrigine have been approved as adjunctive therapy for partial seizures. The long-term effects of these agents on cognition and behavior are yet to be defined. A number of materials are available to assist in educating the school community about seizure disorders. EFA's "Count Me In" program has a school nurse manual, two videos for elementary and secondary schools on basic information about epilepsy and appropriate first aid, and "Spider-Man Battles the Myth Monster" comic book. In addition, there is a variety of print and video material for teachers, students and counselors. *School Planning, a Guide for Parents of Children with Seizure Disorders* is a comprehensive guide available to assist parents in working effectively with the school community on behalf of their child. All of these materials are available through EFA (see appendix D, EFA Resources).

Although the effects of AEDs on learning and behavior are complex, several conclusions can be drawn. Multiple-drug therapy and high levels of any AED are likely to cause cognitive and behavioral side effects. However, cognitive side effects of AEDs are not reliably detected by standard IQ tests. Specialized tests are required to detect the subtle effects of these drugs on mental speed, short-term memory, and motor performance. The differences on neuropsychological tests that are attributed to drug effects are typically small, resulting in a high degree of overlap among the different drug treatment groups. When compared in groups of individuals, certain AEDs, especially barbiturates, benzodiazepines, and phenytoin, are associated with behavioral and cognitive abnormalities more frequently than carbamazepine and valproate. For this reason, selection of the right drug and the right dose for an individual child often involves trial and error.

REFERENCES

Andrewes DG, Bullen JG, Tomlinson L, Elwes RD, Reynolds EH. A comparative study of the cognitive effects of phenytoin and carbamazepine in new referrals with epilepsy. *Epilepsia* 1986;27: 128–34.

Broman SH, Nichols PL, Kennedy WA. *Preschool I.Q. prenatal and early developmental correlates.* Hillsdale, NJ: Lawrence Erlbaum Associates, 1975.

Camfield CS, Chaplin S, Doyle AB, et al. Side effects of phenobarbital in toddlers; behavioral and cognitive side aspects. *Can J Pediatr* 1979;95:361–5.

Dodson WE, Pollock J. *Pediatric epilepsy.* New York: Demos, 1993.

Ferrari M. Epilepsy and its effects on the family. In: Hermann B, Seidenberg M, eds. *Childhood epilepsies: neuropsychological, psychosocial and intervention aspects.* New York: John Wiley & Sons, 1989:159–72.

Ferrari M, Barabas G, Matthews WS. Psychologic and behavioral disturbance among epileptic children treated with barbiturate anticonvulsants. *Am J Psychiatry* 1983;140:112–3.

Gay PE. Effects of antiepileptic drugs and seizure type on operant responding in mentally retarded persons. *Epilepsia* 1984;25:377–86.

Hauser WA, Hesdorffer DC. *Epilepsy: frequency, causes and consequences.* New York: Demos, 1990.

Hermann B, Whitman S, Dell J. Correlates of behavior problems and social competence in children with epilepsy aged 6-11. In: Hermann B, Seidenberg N, eds. *Childhood epilepsies: neuropsychological, psychosocial and intervention aspects.* New York: John Wiley & Sons, 1988:143–57.

Holdsworth L, Whitmore K. A study of children attending ordinary school: I. Their seizure patterns, progress and behavior in school. *Dev Med Child Neurol* 1974;16:746–58.

Macleod CM, Dekaban AS, Hunt E. Memory impairment in epileptics: selective effects of phenobarbital concentration. *Science* 1978;202:1102–4.

Marshall RM, Cupoli JM. Epilepsy and education: the pediatrician's expanding role. *Adv Pediatr* 1986;33:159–80.

Mattson RH, Cramer JA, Collins JF, et al. Comparison of carbamazepine, phenobarbital, phenytoin, and primidone in partial and secondarily generalized tonic-clonic seizures. *N Engl J Med* 1985;313: 145–51.

Quinn P. When epilepsy is not the only problem: assessing special needs. In: Reisner H, ed. *Children with epilepsy: a parents' guide.* Kensington, MD: Woodbine House, 1988:128–46.

Robertson MM, Trimble MR, Townsend HRA. Phenomenology of depression in epilepsy. *Epilepsia* 1987;28:364–72.

Rutter M, Graham P, Yule W. *A neuropsychiatric study in childhood.* Philadelphia: JB Lippincott, 1970.

Santilli N, Tonelson S. Screening for seizures. *J Pract Nurs* 1982;32:16–24.

Seidenberg M. Academic achievement and school performance of children with epilepsy. In: Hermann B, Seidenberg M, eds. *Childhood epilepsies: neuropsychological, psychosocial and intervention aspects.* New York: John Wiley & Sons, 1989:105–18.

Seidenberg M, O'Leary DS, Berent S, Boll T. Changes in seizure frequency and test-retest scores on the Wechsler Adult Intelligence Scale. *Epilepsia* 1981;22:75–83.

Stores G. Behavioral effects of anti-epileptic drugs. *Dev Med Child Neurol* 1975;17:647–58.

Stores G, Hart J. Reading skills of children with generalized or focal epilepsy attending ordinary school. *Dev Med Child Neurol* 1976;18:705–16.

Trimble MR. Anticonvulsant drugs and cognitive function: a review of the literature. *Epilepsia* 1987;28(suppl 3):S37–45.

Wolf SM, Forsyth A. Behavior disturbance, phenobarbital, and febrile seizures. *Pediatrics* 1978;61: 728–31.

Managing Seizure Disorders: A Handbook for Health Care Professionals, edited by N. Santilli, Lippincott-Raven Publishers, Philadelphia, 1996.
© 1996 Epilepsy Foundation of America.

16

Safety and Activities of Daily Living for People with Epilepsy

Patricia Osborne Shafer, David R. Austin, Mimi Callanan, and Carol Maier Clerico

Many myths and misperceptions about epilepsy remain. A recent survey of 1,000 people in the general public and 331 people with epilepsy was conducted to explore current myths and misperceptions (NFO Research, 1995). The study revealed that many people in the general public do not know what occurs during a seizure and do not know appropriate first aid. Ninety-five percent of the respondents from the general public believe that seizures are all convulsions. A majority (66%) inappropriately believe they should secure the tongue of a person during a seizure, and only 46% would know to turn the person on his or her side (NFO Research, 1995). Many problems of daily living were reported by people with uncontrolled seizures. For example, 77% expressed fear of public embarrassment, 72% had problems with memory loss, 66% expressed dependence on others and feelings of not being in control, and 60% had a fear of driving (NFO Research, 1995).

Maintaining safety and coping with the effects of seizures on daily life are vital aspects of living with seizures or epilepsy. Safety precautions can be viewed positively as a means of preventing unnecessary injury or disability while maintaining independence. They can also be viewed negatively as restrictions imposed by family, friends, employers, or governmental regulations. In the latter case, safety measures may be perceived as burdensome if they impede a person's attempt to lead a normal life. People with epilepsy and their loved ones may worry about injury or even death as a consequence of uncontrolled seizures. The unpredictability and frequency of the seizures may enhance these fears. People with seizures, particularly uncontrolled seizures, may feel their need to be in control threatened when told by health care professionals, family members, or friends not to pursue certain activities for fear of injury or of precipitating seizures. It is important for everyone, health care professionals and people with epilepsy, to accept the fact that living with seizures means living with certain risks. This also involves learning what each person can do and focusing on strengths rather than restrictions. Nurses and other professionals can support the person with epilepsy by providing education about lifestyle modifications to enhance safety, aid in seizure control, and promote independence and personal control (Shafer, 1994).

Activities of daily childcare, work, and recreational activities vary greatly with the person's age, functional ability, and seizure type and frequency. Daily activities in the environment at home, in school, or on the job can be approached with an eye, an ear, and a hand towards safety. However, it is also important to encourage children and adults with epilepsy to become as independent as possible in daily activities. A child who cannot (or will not) care for his or her own basic needs has a difficult time being accepted by peers in later years, and may grow into a dependent adult. A caregiver who cannot (or will not) help the person with seizures to develop independence may foster dependence and poor self-esteem that last throughout the person's life.

This chapter addresses daily living activities in relation to general safety management and tips, first aid, trigger management, and medication management for selected populations.

TYPES AND CAUSES OF INJURY

Available information on risks of injury with seizures is limited but indicates that the incidence of injury sustained during seizures is less than anticipated by the general public. A recent prospective Canadian study revealed that 15% of seizures presenting for medical attention caused injury or death (Kirby and Sadler, 1995). Most of the injuries were minor, such as head contusions and lacerations. Seven people died during seizures, however, emphasizing the severity of this disorder. A review of studies on risks with seizures found that: (a) people with epilepsy have a decreased risk of accidents as compared to others without seizures; (b) a small group of people with epilepsy account for the majority of injuries; (c) people with secondarily generalized epilepsy and frequent tonic–clonic seizures have the most accidents; and (d) the majority of injuries are minor and happen at home (Sonnen, 1990). In general, however, seizure-related injuries may range from cuts, bruises, falls, or burns to a variety of musculoskeletal injuries. Severe injuries and death can occur from head injuries during falls or motor vehicle accidents, or even from drowning.

Although an injury can occur during or after any type of seizure, most often seizures that alter awareness or consciousness, and those that lead to a fall, pose the greatest risks. In addition, side effects of medication may increase the risk for injury by causing sedation, blurry or double vision, incoordination, imbalance, tremors, or ataxia, to name a few. Concomitant neurologic disorders may give rise to other deficits that affect movement, sensation, mentation, communication, and other aspects of behavior.

SAFETY MANAGEMENT

The process by which people learn to live with their epilepsy to gain seizure control and to achieve a satisfactory quality of life is called self-management. Maintaining safety is one aspect of self-management and is usually accomplished by modifying lifestyle and environment to prevent injuries and enhance seizure control. However, people with epilepsy must first know how to assess their risk for injury in relation to the activities they wish to pursue. Adjusting lifestyle and environment to avoid high-risk activities when an individual is most vulnerable to seizures can then be done.

Assessing Risks

Assessing risks for each person with seizures involves considering benefits of safety and participating in desired activities with the cost of safety precautions and the risks for injury. To make informed and rational choices, people must first understand their seizures and the factors that will affect safety. The following questions can be used as a guide for people with epilepsy and their families to assess individual risks and make appropriate choices (Santilli, 1991; Santilli, 1992).

What type of seizure do I have and what occurs during and after a seizure?
Is there a pattern to my seizures? Are they predictable? How often do they occur?
What risks are involved in this activity?
Can I reduce the risks of this activity?
How important is it to me to participate in this activity?
What are the benefits of participating?
What are the costs (e.g., personal, financial) of safety measures?

Developing A Safety Management Plan

The nurse or other professional can work with a person with epilepsy to develop an individualized "safety management plan" using the information obtained from the risk assessment. This plan should include a menu of practical tips that a person can use to lessen risks and remain as independent as possible in the least restrictive environment. The individual with seizures can then decide whether to pursue a certain activity and when, what type of safety precautions to take, and how to make daily activities and environment safer.

Some limitations in daily activities are the result of physical or mental deficits that preclude task independence and can be modified or eliminated by the use of specific adaptive techniques or equipment. Others are imposed by caregivers or family members who lack safety awareness or fear injury to their loved ones.

The following safety tips may make activities of daily living easier for the child or adult with epilepsy and for caregivers. They consist of examples, both from people with epilepsy and from health care professionals, of what can be done to live safely. These tips must be individualized on the basis of age, functional status, seizure behavior, and seizure frequency. It is important for people to look at the areas in which they have a particular concern, explore which ideas may be appropriate for them, and develop their own safety management plan.

Safety Tips for Daily Living[1]

Bathing/Toileting

Always use nonskid strips or bath mat in tubs or showers.

Keep hot water temperatures low to avoid burns.

Always check water temperature with hands before stepping into tub or shower; if sensation is poor, have someone else check the water temperature first.

Use a tub seat, shower seat, or bath bench with safety straps to avoid falls, or sit in the bottom of tub and use a hand-held nozzle.

Use tub safety rails or grab bars when getting in or out of the tub or shower.

Cover all heating units with padded covers to avoid burns.

Put protective covers on faucet handles, tub spout, or nozzle.

Keep all electrical appliances out of the bathroom and away from water.

Use electric razor (in a room other than the bathroom).

Keep the bathroom well ventilated to avoid excess heat build-up.

Make sure that the tub drain works properly.

Consider installing an automatic water shut-off so that shower will turn off if the drain becomes plugged or covered.

Take showers when someone else is home; singing in the shower alerts others as to how you are doing.

Use plastic bottles and containers.

Open doors outward and don't lock doors; try hanging an "occupied" sign on the bathroom door instead.

Never leave a child alone in the bathroom.

Have two adults assist with the bath of an infant or young child or do a sponge bath if a parent has seizures.

Use a baby sponge or infant seat that supports an infant in a tub with shallow water.

Dressing

Avoid accessories or jewelry with sharp edges.

Assemble clothes in one area to avoid frequent trips back and forth.

---

[1] Adapted from Clerico, 1989, and Santilli, 1992.

If you have difficulty with attention, sorting, organizing, or other visuospatial skills, keep clothes organized by types of outfits, colors, or seasons.

Store clothes at easy-to-reach height to avoid climbing.

Use shatterproof mirrors and hang at child's height to avoid climbing.

Place infants or young children on the floor when changing diapers or clothes.

Feeding/Eating

Ensure that caregivers know how to assist someone who is choking.

Eat only when sitting up.

Use nonskid surfaces under plates and cups.

Consider a bowl or scoopdish for eating when coordination is a problem.

Avoid foods and drinks that are very hot; use a cup with a lid and spout ("commuter cup") for warm liquids and to avoid spills.

If available, use chairs with sidearms to prevent falling.

Let someone else carry food trays.

Infants and young children should be secured in an infant seat, highchair, or appropriate chair.

Check mouths of infants and young children to make sure they have swallowed everything after eating.

Do not leave infants and young children alone while eating.

Sleep

Lower the height of the bed, and put mats or carpeting beside the bed.

Advise people to avoid sleeping on a top bunk bed.

Side rails may be helpful for people who frequently experience seizures at night.

Use a crib or bed from which a child cannot climb out.

Use an intercom or nursery monitor to alert family members to a person having a seizure at night.

Avoid fatigue and sleep deprivation by resting and/or nap when possible.

Mobility

Do not drive unless you have a valid license and are not having seizures.

Use car seats or seatbelts when traveling.

Explore local dial-a-ride services and public transportation if you can't drive.

If the parent has seizures, an infant should be moved by using a stroller instead of being hand carried.

Use a stroller to move a child with severe or frequent seizures.

If falls are frequent, consider a helmet and knee and elbow pads while moving around, particularly if frequent atonic seizures occur.

When bike riding, wear helmet, knee pads, and elbow pads; if possible, ride on side roads or bike paths.

If you wander unaware during a seizure, try to travel with a friend and wear or carry medical alert identification.

Stand back from the road when waiting for a bus and from a platform edge when taking subway or train.

Consider using elevators instead of steep escalators or stairs.

The safety of taking a taxi instead of public transportation may be worthwhile if you have frequent seizures.

Go with a friend if you are traveling outside in extremely cold weather.

When traveling alone, speak to a flight attendant and explain what to expect if you have a seizure.

Homemaking and Home Safety

Keep rooms and hallways clear of clutter and avoid scatter rugs.

Pad sharp corners and edges on furniture; use carpeting and padded flooring if falling is a problem.

Use chairs with armrests and rounded armchairs when possible.

Avoid ironing alone and use an iron with an automatic shut-off.

Keep sharp utensils in an out-of-the-way spot to avoid cuts when reaching into drawers.

Remove burner controls on stove.

Use a microwave oven and microwave dishes.

Use long oven mitts to pull out shelves in a conventional oven.

Use back stove burners and potholders that cover the arm.

Use rubber gloves when washing dishes.

Use a cart to transport dishes and hot foods, or slide foods along counters to avoid carrying them.

Use vegetable choppers and food processors to avoid cutting with a knife; use precut frozen or canned fruits and vegetables.

Use a steamer, colander, or cooking basket to lift cooked foods out of hot water.

Cook with a "buddy" in the kitchen.

Store all frequently used items at accessible heights.

Use nonbreakable dishes, utensils, and plastic containers.

Keep electrical and telephone wires out of walkways.

Cover heating units and place protective shields around fireplaces, wood stoves, or kerosene heaters.

Don't carry hot fireplace ashes or lighted candles through the house.

Avoid smoking and lighting fires when alone.

Keep all cleaning agents in locked cabinets and out of the kitchen and bathroom.

Use curling irons or other appliances with automatic shut-off switches.

Do not let a child with seizures use a curling iron or other electrical appliances unattended.

Keep breakables away from children.

Be sure that any motor-driven equipment, such as a lawnmower, has a "dead-man's handle" that will stop the machine if the hand releases normal pressure.

Put automatic shut-offs on all power tools in a home workshop.

Advise neighbors what to do if a person is found wandering outside alone.

To prevent a person from wandering outside during a seizure, make sure that outside doors are securely locked; consider an alarm system on the outside door that will alert others in the house if someone tries to open it during a seizure.

Recreation

Use common sense when choosing recreational activities.

Play with a buddy and avoid activities in which you can't fall safely, or high-risk activities such as rock climbing, parachuting, skydiving, scuba diving, hang gliding, or unsupervising swimming or skiing.

Waterplay with sprinklers can be just as refreshing for children as a pool.

If falls are likely, wear a helmet with face guard and protective clothing such as elbow pads, knee pads, and protective eyewear.

Play on soft surfaces such as grass, carpet, or mats whenever possible.

Stay away from unprotected heat sources or sharp edges.

Take frequent breaks and stay cool.

Drink plenty of fluids.

Avoid tight, overcrowded spaces that are not well ventilated or free of objects.

Do exertional activities in a cool room or outdoors in the early morning or evening to avoid the hottest part of the day.

Use soft rather than hard balls.

Always wear a life jacket when swimming or boating; swim with a buddy.

Avoid open flames; sit well back from campfires and stoves.

Use a playpen or play with the child on the floor.

Limit infants and young children to safe, confined play areas.

Personal Safety

Make sure that caregivers, family members, or friends know seizure first aid.

Know first aid for choking, and make sure that family and friends do, too.

Carry an emergency medical card in a wallet or pocket, and consider medical alert jewelry.

Alert local police, rescue squad, and neighbors about seizures, especially frequent partial seizures with wandering.

Encourage family and care providers to develop a plan for emergency care of seizures, including emergency administration of medications or when to call an ambulance.

Use any auras or warning you might experience to reduce risk for further seizure activity and/or injury.

Avoid activities that are known to increase the risk for seizures.

Consider using a pillbox to help remember medicines and store them safely away from children, preferably in a locked cabinet.

Help family members, especially young children, learn what to do by having "seizure drills" that review first aid steps and how to call for help.

Infants and Children

For infants and children with seizures the same general safety tips are important to consider, as well as those specific to children or parents with seizures. In addition, childproofing the home, just as any parent would do, is extremely important for young children. Tips for the parent with epilepsy are described in Chap. 17.

Resources

Ideas for safety management are limited only by one's creativity. Some people with seizures may benefit from individualized consultation about specific safety concerns. Nurses, occupational therapists, and rehabilitation engineers can provide help for safety management and particularly for assistive devices and resources. Occupational therapists can evaluate what adaptations are needed and assist in lifestyle modifications for safety and trigger management. Rehabilitation engineers have particular expertise in designing safe and efficient environments.

WORK SAFETY

Work is an environment that may have potential for real hazards. Some individuals with uncontrolled seizures may need to have specific adaptations in their work environments or jobs until their seizures are under control. This is especially true for people with epilepsy who operate heavy equipment or who work under potentially disastrous circumstances should a seizure occur. The worker's ability to perform the following activities may need to be assessed: "climbing and working unprotected at heights, driving or operating construction vehicles, transportation jobs, working around unguarded machinery, working near fire or water, working for long periods in an isolated situation, using hand-held power tools fixed in the on position" (Privitera and Scheer, 1991). As with all activities, common sense helps guide work decisions.

Jobs can often be made safer with a few changes and employers are in many cases required by law to make reasonable accommodations. People with epilepsy should be encouraged to review any possible job-related risks with their providers and consider appropriate safety modifications. In addition, telling co-workers about the type of seizures and appropriate first aid can allay fears and dispel misconceptions. If stress aggravates seizures, it may be helpful to look at job-related stress in relation to seizure control and consider stress management techniques. The following tips are specific to workplace safety and should be individualized for each person and situation.

Avoid climbing higher than you can safely fall, especially on concrete floors.
Always use reliable safety harness, and use a hard hat or helmet.
Avoid working around dangerous machinery if you are having seizures, and use automatic shut-offs or safety guards on all machinery.
Avoid shift work changes that require long work hours without sleep.
If you are photosensitive, avoid work settings with flickering and flashing lights, or try polarized glasses to counteract the effects.
Consider wearing protective clothing such as helmet, elbow and knee pads, or protective eyewear.
Keep a small pillow tucked in a drawer so that a co-worker can place it under your head if you fall during a seizure.
Keep a change of clothes at work in case clothes become soiled during a seizure.
Consider using a personal sign-in sheet so that co-workers know you have left your desk on purpose and not during a seizure.

Fear of discrimination often obscures good work judgment. It is an unfortunate fact that some individuals with epilepsy have lost jobs or were unable to obtain employment because of their seizures. The Americans with Disabilities Act now prohibits discrimination on the basis of a disability, and people with epilepsy should be informed of their rights and responsibilities under the ADA. Educational programs are available through local Epilepsy Foundation of American affiliates or health facilities specializing in epilepsy to educate potential employers about epilepsy, employment concerns, and reasonable accommodations. For individuals who have lost jobs or are having difficulty finding work, referral to a vocational rehabilitation agency or employment program of an Epilepsy Foundation affiliate is recommended. For more information on epilepsy employment, see Chap. 18 and Appendix D, EFA Resources.

RECREATION SAFETY

A number of opinions have been expressed by physicians and therapeutic recreational specialists with regard to recreation for people with epilepsy. Some thoughts by these health professionals have been very specific, stipulating that precautions be taken with certain activities and that other activities should be avoided altogether. For example, Howe-Murphy and Charboneau (1987) believe that there should be more than normal supervision while persons who have epilepsy are swimming, and that sports where contact or falling may occur (e.g., boxing, football, ice hockey, lacrosse, wrestling, rugby, diving, and trampolining) should be avoided. Others take a more liberal position. They follow the principle that a person with epilepsy should be allowed to participate in most activities as long as a nonseizure-prone partner is present. Even those who take a more liberal stance recommend giving careful consideration to such activities as scuba diving and hang gliding, in which partners would not be able to offer help immediately (James, 1988).

Perhaps a reason for diversity in opinions is that each person is unique and should be considered individually. As suggested in the EFA's guide for camp counselors, *The Child with Epilepsy at Camp* (1981), "epilepsy is a condition which must be assessed individually and about which it is difficult to generalize." The authors of the EFA camping booklet go on to say, however, that if parents and physician feel that the child has adequate seizure control to go to camp, then the camper should be able to take part in regular camp activities without special restrictions. They believe that campers should be able to enjoy biking, riding, boating, swimming, and other sports activities. In fact, they state that research has shown that children are less likely to have seizures when participating in physical activities than when they are inactive.

There are reasonable precautions that staff should take when working with campers who have epilepsy. For example, staff should be particularly watchful when children are swimming or in any other situation where loss of consciousness might be hazardous. Polarized sunglasses may help campers with seizures triggered by flashing or bright lights, such as bright sunlight reflecting off a lake or shining through the trees. When assigning horses in riding programs, staff should consider the temperament of each horse and how it might respond to unexpected situations. As with all campers, children with epilepsy should wear protective head gear when riding or rappelling and should wear life jackets when boating or fishing (*The Child with Epilepsy at Camp,* 1981). Camp staff also should be aware that abrupt changes in sleep habits may lower the seizure threshold, as can the consumption of alcohol (James, 1988).

Common sense dictates that certain recreational activities should be avoided by seizure-prone individuals. These include activities that involve possible physical harm (e.g., boxing) and sports that are potentially dangerous if one loses consciousness (e.g., scuba diving, sky diving, hang gliding, rock climbing, and unsupervised swimming). Exercise, in general, should pose no problems for individuals with uncontrolled seizures and can be encouraged to improve health. In fact, a study of leisure and recreational habits of 44 adult inpatients with uncontrolled epilepsy revealed that the majority were sedentary, with limited social contact and poor physical fitness (Bjorholt et al., 1990). A subsequent experimental study on the effect of physical training revealed improved physical fitness, improved mental state, and more sociable behavior (Nakken et al., 1990). Individual but not significant effects of exercise were seen in relation to seizure control and AED levels.

Factors that may precipitate seizures such as fatigue, hypoxia, hypothermia, and hypoglycemia may be caused by exercise or sports, but the relationship is not clearly determined (Gates, 1993). Patients who find that their seizures are triggered by exercise may need to pace themselves by taking frequent breaks and alter their type of exercise. For example, stretching or conditioning exercises may be more appropriate than high-impact aerobic exercises.

Persons with epilepsy, like anyone, need a well-balanced lifestyle that includes leisure time. They need to take part in a variety of leisure pursuits, including social recreation, sports, hobbies, and travel. They may also profit from leisure counseling from a therapeutic recreation specialist, or other qualified professional, to become aware of their leisure attitudes and habits and to make wise decisions about their leisure activities. In doing so, they can focus on the vast number of activities available to them rather than dwell on the few activities from which they are excluded (James, 1988).

When seizures are well controlled, persons with epilepsy are no different from others who take risks and seek challenges to experience personal growth. However, certain activity limitations may be indicated for those whose seizures are frequent or severe. As a general rule, persons with epilepsy can participate in the vast majority of recreational activities by taking a few simple precautions.

DRIVING

Driving a motor vehicle is often viewed as an essential component of adult life. It offers independence and increases opportunities for employment, social activity, and recreation. All states impose a legal restriction on driving for persons with epilepsy, although details of the restriction vary from state to state. These laws attempt to protect the person with epilepsy and the public from harm. However, driving restrictions exert considerable negative influences on an individual's lifestyle, self-esteem, and self-worth. If public transportation is not available, these problems are compounded. Education about driving regulations, including the risks and benefits of complying, should be provided to each individual with epilepsy by all health professionals. In addition, options for alternative means of accessible transportation will be needed by many, e.g., discounts on public transportation, vans for the disabled or elderly, and car pooling. The EFA supports a "model driving law," which was developed at a conference on driving and which can be used for educational and legislative opportunities in individual states. See also Chap. 20 and Appendix D, EFA Resources.

FIRST AID

Educating people with epilepsy, family members, friends, and the general public about appropriate first aid for both generalized and partial seizures is a vital part of epilepsy teaching. Goals for management of a person during a seizure include preventing injury, maintaining an open airway and adequate respiratory exchange, providing reassurance and education to the patient and bystanders, recognizing emergency conditions, and knowing when to call for additional help.

Guidelines for helping a person during a generalized tonic–clonic seizure include the following.

Assist the person to a supine position as soon as possible.

Look for medical alert information.

Turn the person to one side and place a soft object (i.e., pillow, jacket) underneath the head; this allows secretions to drain from the mouth, prevents aspiration, and allows the tongue to fall forward, preventing airway occlusion. It is important to educate people with epilepsy and the general public that it is not possible to swallow the tongue during a seizure.

Do not place anything in the person's mouth during a seizure; during the initial phase of a generalized tonic–clonic seizure, jaw muscles tighten making, it impossible to open the mouth. Forcing an object into the mouth may cause damage to the jaw or teeth. Padded objects should not be used.

Loosen tight clothing.

Remove sharp objects in the immediate vicinity.

Do not restrain the person in any manner; restraint of any type may result in broken bones or bruises from the severe rigidity and contractions that occur during a seizure.

Reassure bystanders that the person will be alright after the seizure, and discourage onlookers; calmly informing individuals about a seizure can alleviate anxiety and fears.

An ambulance should be called when there is no documented evidence that the individual has epilepsy, when the seizure lasts longer than 5 min, when the individual has one seizure after another without waking up, or when serious injury has occurred; it is important that family members be instructed about when to call an ambulance.

For complex partial seizures, similar safety measures are taken. The general procedures for treating partial seizures include remaining with the individual until they are completely aware of who they are and their environment, avoiding restraints, protecting them from injury by removing potentially harmful objects, remaining calm, and offering reassurance.

During complex partial seizures, some individuals may wander or appear confused. In these situations it is best to guide the person away from harmful objects and potentially dangerous situations by using a calm voice, nonthreatening gestures, and a gentle touch. It may be necessary to lock doors or use a door alarm for people who may be alone and have frequent complex partial seizures.

Absence seizures do not require specific first aid intervention. Anyone who interacts with a person experiencing absence seizures must remember that these individuals experience a temporary lapse in alertness. Therefore, they may not be able to provide for their own safety. For children, a buddy system may work well.

Frequent atonic seizures pose the greatest risk for personal injury and may cause head, facial, and dental injuries. A protective head helmet and, when necessary, a face mask may be needed. Many people have found that Cooper hockey helmets and Danmar helmets provide good protection. Custom-fitted helmets are particularly helpful for people with skull defects. Mobility and independence can be increased for people with very severe seizure disorders by use of a wheelchair with a seatbelt or a chest restraint. Because these supports are physical evidence of a medical problem, however, some people may not want to use them. A physical therapy consultation can be obtained for appropriate fit to a wheelchair and instruction on its use.

Resource materials about first aid techniques for a variety of seizure types are listed in Appendix C, Seizure Recognition and First Aid, and can be used for educating family, friends, school personnel, co-workers, and the general public. School and work personnel should be informed that people do not have to leave school or work because of a seizure. Resting for a short while after a seizure is usually enough time to allow the person to return to previous activity.

LIFESTYLE MODIFICATIONS FOR TRIGGER MANAGEMENT

Management of triggers involves identifying factors that may precipitate seizures (Aird, 1983) and then modifying lifestyle to decrease their chance of occurrence. It is not possible or advisable for any person to avoid all possible precipitants. It is possible, however, to identify the most likely precipitants and the person's "high-risk" time. For example, in women, seizures may occur more frequently around the time of menses because of hormonal changes or reproductive disorders. If fatigue also affects a woman's seizures, she should try to modify her activities so that she is not sleep-deprived or pursuing sports that cause fatigue at the time of menses. If she can perform these activities without difficulty at other times, then she should continue to do so. The goal is to limit the number of precipitants that can increase susceptibility to seizures at any time. Examples of lifestyle modifications for commonly reported triggers are listed below.

Sensory Stimuli

Noises

Use earplugs, portable tape players, or radios with earphones, especially in noisy places such as buses, subways, and in crowds. Distraction by singing or focusing on another activity can minimize the impact of sudden noises.

Light/Dark Patterns

Wear polarized or tinted glasses; focus on distant objects when riding in a car to decrease the effect of light/dark patterns, such as flashing sunlight through trees or oncoming headlights. Avoid discos, strobe lights, or flashing bulbs on Christmas trees or decorations. Use a screen filter on computer terminals to decrease contrast glare and flickering.

Hyperventilation

Perform relaxation-breathing exercises; breathe into a paper bag; pace activities and exercise.

Alcohol/Drugs

Avoid all recreational or illicit drugs and discuss alcohol use with your doctor. Many of these substances can increase seizures or interfere with compliance and other medications. It is usually best to limit or moderate alcohol intake. Complete avoidance may be recommended if seizures are definitely associated with alcohol use or if alcohol use is a problem.

Sleep

Good sleeping habits, including a consistent schedule and getting enough sleep, are most important. Keep a record of sleep pattern, seizures, and general well-being. Trouble sleeping at night or waking tired in the morning can be caused by not enough sleep, side effects of medication, seizures, stress, or a sleep disorder.

Discuss medicine schedule with health care provider; changing times of doses may aid sleep. Limit caffeine, especially in the afternoon and evening. Avoid alcohol and nicotine before sleep. Limit work or studying late at night, and allow time for relaxation before going to bed. Exercising in the early evening may promote relaxation and sleep. Taking warm showers or back rubs before bedtime can decrease muscle tension. Try relaxation exercises or relaxing music before sleep. Limit naps in the daytime, and avoid napping in the early evening. If anxiety or worries are a problem, talking to someone or writing down feelings and problems before may help. If you are unable to fall asleep within 15 min, get up and do something else for 15 min or so. Go back to bed and try again, but don't toss and turn in bed all night. If sleep disturbances persist, consult doctor and consider a sleep evaluation.

Exercise

Pace exercise to avoid over-fatigue. Avoid exercising in mid-day during hot weather. Increase leisure and recreational activities for general physical and emotional health. See Safety Tips for Recreation, above.

Diet

Have a well-balanced diet and eat at consistent times. If appetite is poor, consider frequent small meals. If you're sensitive to certain foods or notice an association with seizures, modify your diet accordingly to limit bothersome foods. Consider nutritional counseling for weight gain or reduction.

Illness, Fever, or Trauma

Notify the doctor or nurse if you are sick with other illnesses, have a fever, injure yourself, or need other medicines, such as antibiotics or cold medicines. Some over-the-counter medications can trigger seizures or interact with AEDs. Try to limit other triggers or stress when you are sick.

Hormonal Changes

Both men and women may notice a cyclic pattern to their seizures. If this is present, record seizures and cycles on a calendar and review with your physician. Women should note the dates and time of their menses and ovulation in relation to their seizures. If these patterns are persistent and seizures are not responsive to medication, a neuroendocrine evaluation may be warranted. Women who have seizures in relation to their menses should try to modify lifestyle to limit other seizure triggers during the high-risk menstrual period. Some women benefit from changes in their medicine schedule during parts of their menstrual cycle. Consult a physician about use of birth control pills. Some of these may affect seizures and not be effective contraceptives when used in combination with AEDs.

STRESS AND COPING

Emotional stress can precipitate seizures, and problems from seizures may cause stress, anxiety, or depression. Keep a calendar of seizures in relation to your moods and stress level. During stressful times, try modifying lifestyle factors that can be changed, and consider counseling to help cope with seizures or other problems. Use a diary to write down feelings, and use "time out" periods to think out problems and ways to deal with them. Joining a group for stress management, therapy, or support may be helpful. Learn relaxation exercises to help cope with stress and prevent exacerbation of seizures by stress (Rousseau et al., 1985; Dahl et al., 1987; Relaxation Project, 1990). Discuss any emotional changes with a physician, nurse, or other health care professional, as further evaluation for counseling or medications may be needed.

These lifestyle modifications address daily living activities as they may affect seizure control. They can also be utilized to evaluate and change the detrimental effects of seizures on daily life. For a person who complains of fatigue and sedation from seizures or medications, evaluating sleep habits and other lifestyle issues that could affect sleep or cause fatigue (such as concurrent illness, stress, or diet), may be more helpful than changing medications. The added benefit is that seizures may also decrease. Ultimately, the goal of any lifestyle change is for persons with epilepsy to feel more in control of their lives and to participate actively in their care.

SUMMARY

Safety is an important part of life for everyone but has special significance for people with epilepsy. Immediate and continuous attention to all daily activities is needed to prevent injury that may occur during or between seizures. Nurses and other health care professionals can assist people with epilepsy and their families to obtain and maintain the knowledge, attitudes, skills, and behavior necessary to manage epilepsy and lead a productive and normal life. Nurses must be supportive of finding an appropriate balance between safe, healthy behaviors and the individual's personal goals and desired quality of life.

REFERENCES

Aird RB. The importance of seizure-inducing factors in the control of refractory forms of epilepsy. *Epilepsia* 1983;24:567–83.

Bjorholt PG, Nakken KO, Rohme K, Hansen H. Leisure time habits and physical fitness in adults with epilepsy. *Epilepsia* 1990;31:83–7.

Clerico CM. Occupational therapy and epilepsy. *Occu Ther Health Care* 1989;6:41–74.

Dahl J, Melin L, Lund L. Effects of a contingent relaxation treatment program on adults with refractory epileptic seizures. *Epilepsia* 1987;28:125–32.

Gates JR, Spiegel RH. Epilepsy, sports and exercise. *Sports Med* 1993;15:1–5.

Howe-Murphy R, Charboneau BG. *Therapeutic recreation intervention: an ecological perspective.* Englewood Cliffs, NJ: Prentice-Hall, 1987.

James MR. Therapeutic recreation services for individuals with convulsive disorder. Unpublished paper, 1988.

Kirby S, Sadler RM. Injury and death as a result of seizures. *Epilepsia* 1995;31:25–8.

Nakken KO, Bjorholt PG, Johannessen SI, Loyning T, Lind E. Effect of physical training on aerobic capacity, seizure occurrence and serum levels of antiepileptic drugs in adults with epilepsy. *Epilepsia* 1990;31:88–94.

NFO Research. *Myths and misperceptions about epilepsy.* Greenwich, CT: NFO Research, Inc., 1995.

Privitera MD, Scheer SJ. Vocational capacity with epilepsy. In: Scheer SJ, ed. *Medical perspectives in vocational assessment of impaired workers.* Gaithersburg, MD: Aspen, 1991:293–300.

Relaxation Project. *An eight week course in relaxation training: a tool for controlling your seizures.* Chicago: Center for Urban Affairs and Policy Research, Northwestern University, 1990.

Rousseau A, Hermann B, Whitman S. Effects of progressive relaxation on epilepsy: analysis of a series of cases. *Psychol Rep* 1985;57:1203–12.

Santilli N. Activities of daily living. In: Resor SR, Kutt H, eds; *The medical treatment of epilepsy.* New York: Marcel Dekker, 1992:539–43.

Santilli N. The patient's perspective on epilepsy. In: Lesser RP, ed. *The diagnosis and management of seizure disorders.* New York: Demos, 1991:135–50.

Shafer PO. Nursing support of epilepsy self-management. *Clin Nurs Prac Epilepsy* 1994;2:11–4.
Sonnen AEH. How to live with epilepsy. In: Dam M, Gram L, eds. *Comprehensive epileptology.* New York: Raven Press, 1990:753–67.
The child with epilepsy at camp. Landover, MD: Epilepsy Foundation of America, 1981.

ADDITIONAL READING

Betts T. Managing the person with epilepsy. In: Morgens Dam M, ed. *A practical approach to epilepsy.* New York: Pergamon Press, 1991:137–68.
Gillham RA. Refractory epilepsy: an evaluation of psychological methods in outpatient management. *Epilepsia* 1990;31:427–32.
Hauser WA, Ng SKC, Brust JCM. Alcohol, seizures, and epilepsy. *Epilepsia* 1988;29(suppl 2):566–78.
Legion V. Health education for self-management by people with epilepsy. *J Neurosci Nurs* 1991;23:300–5.
Shafer PO, Santilli N. Living safely with epilepsy. In: Schachter SC, ed. *Brainstorms companion: epilepsy in our view.* New York: Raven Press, 1995:111–29.
Ozuna J, Hawken M. Learning needs of the epilepsy patient. In: Redman B, ed. *Neurologic care: a guide for patient education.* New York: Appleton-Century-Crofts, 1982:133–51.
Snyder M. Revised epilepsy stressor inventory. *J Neurosci Nurs* 1993;25:9–13.

*Managing Seizure Disorders: A Handbook for
Health Care Professionals,* edited by N. Santilli,
Lippincott-Raven Publishers, Philadelphia, 1996.
© 1996 Epilepsy Foundation of America.

17

When the Parent Has Epilepsy

Nancy Stalland and Patricia Osborne Shafer

THE DECISION TO START A FAMILY

Concerns about being a parent with epilepsy begin much earlier than the birth of a child. For a man or woman with epilepsy, frequently even the issue of whether or not to marry is considered. Basic issues of self-esteem and self-worth are developed long before adulthood and contribute to an individual's feelings of being an attractive, "acceptable" spouse as well as a competent and capable parent. Many times unspoken fears underlie an individual's expressed desire not to marry or have children. Lechtenberg (1984) states that in the general population, 69% of men and 70% of women marry. Among people with epilepsy, only 56% of men and 69% of women marry. The frequency of marriage, however, is no different for those with epilepsy than in the general population if seizures started after the age of 20 or if they were controlled by age 12.

Subtle probing by a health care professional may reveal fears of family or friends and advice that having children "is not wise," "is too much stress," or "will aggravate seizure control." Some people also fear that having epilepsy makes one incompetent to be a parent! Acknowledging these fears and misconceptions will enable the person with epilepsy to educate family and friends about epilepsy and to explore their own feelings or fears of being a parent. Many couples, even if a prospective parent has well-controlled seizures, may fear that seizure control may worsen at a later time and affect their ability to care for their children (Lechtenberg, 1984).

GENETIC FACTORS

The incidence of epilepsy in the general population is 1–2%. Although there have been many advances in understanding the genetic aspects of epilepsy, it is still a very complex and misunderstood area. Genetic markers have been found for some forms of epilepsy; however, many couples incorrectly assume that all epilepsy is inherited. Epilepsy does often occur in families. The parents, siblings, and offspring of a person with epilepsy are more likely to have epilepsy than the general population (Hauser and Hesdorffer, 1990). About 10% of the general adult population will have a first-degree relative with epilepsy, and about 30% of the general adult population will have a first-degree relative with seizures (Hauser and Hesdorffer, 1990). The specific and individual risks of epilepsy being transmitted to a couple's child depend on a number of factors and can be discussed with an epileptologist and genetics counselor. The geneticist considers factors such as a parent seizure type, age at onset, etiology, and family history of seizures in assessing the chances of epilepsy in a couple's children. In addition, other risk factors for genetic disorders, age-related concerns, and the risks for birth defects associated with medications or with the presence of epilepsy can be explored. A genetic consultation can frequently be obtained by referral from an epilepsy specialist or obstetrician and can alleviate the fears of prospective parents and their extended family. A discussion of epilepsy and pregnancy can be found in Chap. 10, and more information on genetics is contained in Chap. 2.

NEWBORN AND INFANT CARE

Family and friends may be more concerned with the ability of a parent with epilepsy to care for an infant or newborn than the parent is. Developing a specific plan for child care that takes into consideration the parent's seizure type and frequency, as well as the potential for more frequent or severe seizures, may help to dispel the concerns of others and instill greater confidence in the prospective parents. Health care professionals, and nurses in particular, can help to develop this plan with the prospective parents during the final months of pregnancy and can review it again immediately before birth. The plan should include the need for additional supports, particularly during the early postpartum period when the parents are adjusting to the new child and the risk for seizures is greatest because of hormonal fluctuations and medication changes. Parents may need to consider using aid from friends and family members to obtain breaks during the day or a full night's sleep to prevent exacerbation of seizures by sleep deprivation. Paying close attention to the parent's health is crucial, with lifestyle modifications and medication management to enhance seizure control and prevent medication toxicity.

Safety is also a major concern, both for the parent with epilepsy and for the newborn. Prospective parents should childproof the house early, keeping in mind the safety of the child if the parent were to fall or be unconscious for a period of time. All parents should get down on the floor and see the world through a child's eyes, looking for all potential hazards. The parent with epilepsy may take additional safety precautions, such as:

Using a playpen so that the child has a safe play area
Using safety gates and locking doors to prevent a child from wandering outside
    if a parent should have a seizure

Using an "umbrella stroller" to minimize carrying the child if the parent has
   frequent seizures
Avoiding front or back infant carriers
Changing diapers on a portable changing pad either on the floor or in the
   middle of the bed, rather than on a changing table
Keeping extra sets of clothes, diapers, and toys on each level of the house to
   minimize stair climbing
Giving the infant a sponge bath when the parent with seizures is home alone
Using disposable diapers instead of pins and cloth ones
Feeding the infant while it is securely strapped into an infant seat or highchair
Keeping medications in childproof bottles and out of children's reach

FEEDING

Breast-feeding is considered an acceptable option for most mothers taking
antiepileptic drugs (AEDs). Most medications are not excreted in breast milk in
sufficiently large amounts to cause harm. However, the decision to breast-feed
or not is an individual one and is based on many factors. For example, infants
of mothers taking phenobarbital may be more sleepy than usual, hypotonic, or
irritable. If these behaviors occur breast-feeding may be contraindicated. Parents
must receive both scientific and practical information on breast-feeding while
taking AEDs so that they can make informed choices (Santilli, 1993). They
should be aware of normal infant behaviors and development, as well as adverse
symptoms indicating that AEDs are affecting infant behavior. If problems arise,
parents can consider continuing breast-feeding with supplemental formula feedings or mixing formula with breast milk to minimize adverse symptoms from
drug exposure (Santilli, 1993).

Whether the infant is breast- or bottle-fed, it may be helpful to have a partner
take over the nighttime feedings so that the mother can avoid excessive sleep
deprivation. Mothers with epilepsy who are breast-feeding can use a breast pump
to provide bottles for nighttime feedings. To prevent injury to the infant, mothers
who have seizures involving loss of consciousness or movement can breast-feed
while holding the baby in bed. If the seizures are frequent, it may be wise to
breast-feed with another adult nearby so that if a seizure occurs the infant can
be cared for during and after the seizure. Bottle feeding and feeding of solid
foods can be safely performed by using an infant seat or highchair into which
the baby can be securely strapped.

EXPLAINING SEIZURES

Parents with epilepsy often wonder when and how to tell their children about
seizures. The frequency of seizures may influence these decisions. Lechtenberg

(1984) tells of an 18-month-old boy who was aware enough of his father's seizures that he was able to imitate them perfectly.

Parents may worry that their children are too young to discuss epilepsy. However, a child of 2 or 3 years has a much better ability to comprehend than to express itself. Therefore, early discussions using simple concrete terms to explain to a child what is happening to Mommy or Daddy can be very helpful. There are many ways to explain seizures to children of any age, with age-appropriate materials available from the Epilepsy Foundation of America (EFA). For a very young child, such as a toddler, the parent may wish to state simply that when Mommy falls or "spaces out" she is having a seizure and she'll be okay in just a minute. The most important thing is to acknowledge to the child that something is happening, reassure him that he is safe and that so is the parent, and familiarize him with what to do. As children enter school they are able to handle larger, more abstract concepts. What a seizure is can be explained in a little more detail, such as describing it as a brief short circuit in the brain. Using pictures of the brain to show where seizures may come from and what happens during one can be very intriguing to a school-aged child and can make the experience more real. Encouraging children to draw what they believe happens during a seizure and even how they feel about the seizures can be very useful to see how they are coping with a parent's epilepsy.

Failure to explain a seizure may increase anxiety in the child, or the child may create her own explanations or fantasies. Children may blame themselves for the parent's seizures, be afraid to leave the parent, or worry about their safety. They also obtain information from unreliable sources, such as neighbors or peers (Lechtenberg, 1984; Lechtenberg and Ackner, 1984). The parent should be advised to explain to the child that she has not caused the seizures and that the parent is not angry. If the parent has shaking movements during the seizure (generalized tonic–clonic seizure) or walks away (complex partial seizure), this behavior is because of the seizure activity and not because a parent is angry or is trying to ignore the child. Excellent references are *Parenting and You* and *When Mom or Dad has Seizures,* both available from the EFA, which address the full spectrum of issues facing parents with epilepsy. Middleton et al. (1981) present an excellent discussion of siblings' reactions to epilepsy which pertains equally well to children of a parent with epilepsy. The literature for children with epilepsy can be easily adapted to explaining seizures in a parent and is written and illustrated at age-appropriate levels. Important issues to address with young children include the following:

Mom or Dad will be okay, in some cases even stating that they will not die when a seizure occurs

Just because Mom or Dad has seizures does not mean that they too, will, have seizures; the parent might explain that when the child is angry and walks away from someone or pretends that he is not listening, this is not the same as the seizure he sees in Mom or Dad

The children did not cause the seizure to occur, and seizures are not their fault

Mom or Dad still loves them and won't "go away" or abandon them when seizures happen

In many cases the parent is the best source for teaching the child about seizures. A child's capabilities, developmental level, learning needs, and adaptation can be more easily assessed by the parents. In other situations a parent may be too close to the children to talk about the seizures, or the children may not want to disclose their fears or fantasies to the parent. A close family member, a friend, or a health care professional, such as a nurse or social worker, can provide basic seizure information. It can also be very helpful for children to meet their parent's doctor or nurse so that they know that the parent is being taken care of, that there is someone for them to call, and can feel involved at some level. The most important point of any epilepsy education is to help the child to feel secure and comfortable about the parent's seizures.

IMPACT ON FAMILY ROLES AND RELATIONSHIPS

Children in grade school, as well as teenagers, also face the burden of dealing with their peers who may have observed the parent's seizures. Negative peer or community reaction to seizures may cause the child or teenager to withdraw and thus become socially isolated. For example, they may withdraw from the parent, saying that they don't want to go shopping or be seen with them in case they were to have a seizure in public, or they may withdraw from friends and avoid asking them to come to their home for fear that the parent's seizure might be observed. These issues may be difficult to discuss, and the health professional can initiate the conversation by periodically asking the patient during visits how the children are doing. Do they seem to have friends? Do they go out together as a family?

Talking with other children who have coped with seizures in a parent may be helpful. Support groups for children are often available through EFA's affiliates or through hospital-based epilepsy programs. In addition, children and teenagers may feel less embarrassed and may cope more effectively with a parent's seizures if they learn more about it on their own, e.g., by doing a school report on epilepsy or seizures. Another option is to have the parent or other concerned and informed adult, such as the nurse, health educator, or social worker, give a presentation to the class or school on epilepsy. Local affiliates of the EFA may offer programs that are designed to increase awareness about seizures for children and teachers in the school setting. Age-appropriate educational materials designed for children about seizures, including hand-outs, films, and videos, are also readily available for these presentations (see Appendix D, EFA Resources).

Exchanges of roles or responsibilities between parents and children may occur, particularly if one of the parents has poorly controlled seizures. This parent may become dependent on a child for assistance, inadvertently giving the child inappropriate parental control and responsibility. This may take the form of the child monitoring the parent's medication compliance, charting seizures, or taking on household responsibilities, such as cooking, cleaning, and even budgeting, at a level that is inappropriate for the child's age. Initially, these behaviors may be welcomed by one or both parents. However, ultimately they may undermine the parent–child relationship as well as the spousal relationship. When this occurs, the child may shift dependence, reliance, and respect for the parent with epilepsy to the other parent or to someone else, such as grandparents, neighbors, or other significant adults (Greif and Matarazzo, 1982; Lechtenberg, 1984).

Alternatively, children may attempt to protect a parent with epilepsy from emotional situations that they feel are stressful and/or might exacerbate the seizures. Deceptive behavior by children or undue stress on them to conceal their own problems may occur. Although being cared for can be reassuring and helpful, it can also foster dependence and undermine self-confidence and self-esteem for both the child and the parent. However, if protective behavior is discontinued, the parent may fear that the child or spouse is giving up on or abandoning him. Referral to a family counselor is recommended, to assist the family in coping with the epilepsy and to establish appropriate roles and responsibilities for each family member.

Changes in roles and responsibilities may also occur between partners. Often the partner or spouse feels neglected because the parent with epilepsy is focused on parenting responsibilities and maintaining her/his own health. If both parents are working, roles and responsibilities may become even more complex. Balancing the multiple demands of family and work is not easy at best, and can be even more difficult for a parent with uncontrolled seizures. Time management and reevaluation of individual and family priorities is mandatory for both parents. Additional concerns may arise during attempts to choose appropriate daycare. In addition to the parents' usual concerns, they must consider the possibility that one parent may not be able to drive and pick up the children. Alternatives may include choosing a daycare center close to home, where friends or family members can assist in transporting the children, or considering alternatives such as in-home care. After selecting the daycare arrangement, the parents should talk with the providers about the parent's epilepsy and its impact on the child. The EFA has some excellent information for babysitters and daycare providers to assist them in being supportive of the child.

Changing roles and responsibilities in a family can be difficult. Encouraging family members to talk about their concerns may help to identify hidden issues. Often, family members feel overwhelmed by the burdens of juggling family life, work, and health problems, and feel that they need a break. A social worker, recreational therapist, nurse, or other professional can help to identify respite care options or even leisure or recreational activities that the family can pursue together.

FIRST AID FOR THE PARENT

Parents are often the best source for teaching their children appropriate first aid for their particular seizure type. They should be encouraged to use the term "seizure" rather than "sick" with children of all ages. This ensures that if someone must be notified of a seizure, it is not confused with illness. It also helps young children to understand that they are not susceptible to seizures when they are sick. Preprogrammed telephones, paging systems, or emergency access systems can be used so that children who are unable to dial a phone number can reach appropriate help if it is necessary, e.g., a neighbor, working parent, or relative. Speaker phones may be helpful so that the child can stay with the parent but also use the phone to call for help.

Parents often worry about how involved a child should be in taking care of them during a seizure. It is important for children of all ages to know what to do and to feel involved at a level appropriate to their age and development, but they should not feel burdened with too much responsibility (Shafer, 1993). Basic first aid for any child to know includes:

Remaining calm and remembering that the parent will be okay
Staying with the parent and preventing her from further injury, if possible, until an adult arrives
Knowing how to call for help by dialing the local rescue squad or by calling a responsible sibling or adult

Writing a list of very simple steps for a child to remember and posting it in a readily accessible area is helpful. Families should have "seizure drills" periodically to ensure that all family members know appropriate first aid, have a chance to ask questions, and reevaluate their responsibilities. Specific first aid measures are outlined in Chap. 16.

PARENTAL COPING AND HEALTH MANAGEMENT

All parents, regardless of whether or not they are coping with a chronic disorder or disability, need time for themselves. This includes time away from children and time dedicated specifically to the relationship with the spouse or partner. Parents with epilepsy also need to pay particular attention to lifestyle and stress management issues that may affect their seizures and the impact of the seizures on their parenting abilities and family life. Self-management strategies such as obtaining adequate rest, nutrition, recreation, and exercise, minimizing or avoiding triggers of seizures, and maintaining stable medication regimen are a few examples. These factors may enhance the ability of the parent to cope more effectively with the demands of parenting and may also assist in seizure control (Fletcher, 1985). Ultimately, these strategies may enhance feelings of self-esteem and self-worth. Health care professionals can reinforce these self-care needs and provide self-management education to parents with epilepsy.

The family support network should be evaluated and additional resources identified to balance the demands of parenting and other psychosocial consequences of epilepsy. Encouraging a parent to network with parents without epilepsy may provide reassurance that not all symptoms or problems are related to the seizures, and offers a chance to talk about common parenting concerns. For other families, involvement in a parent support network for epilepsy can be helpful to discuss concerns of parental disciplining, seizure control, impact of epilepsy on family life, driving restrictions, and children's reactions to seizures. Often, the informal discussion with one who has "been through it" is more helpful than anything else. Telephone networks to parents in similar situations can be helpful in areas where physical distance prohibits frequent meetings. The EFA has established a parent and family support network that can be easily replicated in communities. A resource manual and guide are available through the EFA or one of its affiliates. See Chap. 22 for additional information about family supports.

REFERENCES

Fletcher S. *The challenge of epilepsy.* Santa Rosa, CA: Aura Publishing, 1985.

Greif E, Matarazzo RG. *Behavioral approaches to rehabilitation: coping with change.* New York: Springer Publishing, 1982.

Hauser WA, Hesdorffer DC. *Facts about epilepsy.* New York: Demos, 1990.

Lechtenberg R. *Epilepsy and the family.* Cambridge: Harvard University Press, 1984.

Lechtenberg R, Ackner. Psychologic adaptation of children to epilepsy in a parent. *Epilepsia* 1984;25:40–5.

Middleton AH, Attwell AA, Walsh GO. *Epilepsy: a handbook for patients, parents, families, teachers, health and social workers.* Boston: Little, Brown, 1981.

Santilli N. Supporting breastfeeding in women with epilepsy. *Clin Nurs Pract Epilepsy* 1993;4:11.

Shafer PO. When a parent has epilepsy. *Clin Nurs Pract Epilepsy* 1993;4:7–10.

ADDITIONAL READING

Annegers JF, Hauser WA, Anderson VE, Kirkland LT. The risks of seizure control disorders among relatives of patients with childhood onset of epilepsy. *Neurology* 1982;32:174–9.

Children and seizures: information for babysitters (brochure). Landover, MD: Epilepsy Foundation of America; 1994.

Eisenberg MG, Sutkin Lafaye C, Jansen MA, eds. *Chronic illness and disability through the life span: effects on self and family,* Vol. 4. New York: Springer Publishing, 1984.

Epilepsy and having children (brochure). Stevens Point, WI: Midstate Epilepsy Association, Inc., 1984.

Epilepsy and parenting (brochure). Lorain, OH: Epilepsy Foundation of NE Ohio, 1985.

Epilepsy in pregnancy (2-page hand-out). Landover, MD: Professional Advisory Board of the Epilepsy Foundation of America, 1986.

Parenting and you: a guide for parents with seizure disorders. Landover, MD: Epilepsy Foundation of America, 1994.

Epilepsy—sex, marriage, and pregnancy (3 cassette tapes). Presentations by Andermann E, Ramsay RE, Stalland N. EFA Conference, 1985.

Fiol M, Leppik IE, Gates J. Epilepsy and oral contraceptives: a therapeutic dilemma. *Minnesota Med* 1983;66:551–2.

Goldin GJ, Margolin RJ. The psychological aspects of epilepsy. In: Wright GN, ed. *Epilepsy rehabilitation.* Boston: Little, Brown, 1975:66–80.

Guerrant J, Anderson WW, Fischer A, et al. *Personality in epilepsy.* Springfield, IL: Charles C Thomas, 1962.

Kuhnz W, Koch S, Jakob S, et al. Ethosuximide in epileptic women during pregnancy and lactation period: Placental transfer, serum concentrations in nursed infants, and clinical status. *Br J Clin Pharmacol* 1984;18:671–7.

Livingston S. Psychosocial aspects of epilepsy. *J Clin Child Psychol* 1977;6:6–10.

McCormick KB. Pregnancy and epilepsy: nursing implications. *J Neurosci Nurs* 1987;19:66–76.

Schneider JW, Conrad P. *Having epilepsy: the experience and control of illness.* Philadelphia: Temple University Press, 1983.

Seizure recognition and first aid: information for teachers and providers of day care to young children (brochure/poster). Landover, MD: Epilepsy Foundation of America, 1989.

Schumacher NC. *Epilepsy: a personal approach.* Cambridge, MA: Schenkman Publishing, 1985.

Yerby MS, Leppik I. Epilepsy and the outcomes of pregnancy. *J Epilepsy* 1990;3:193–9.

Yerby MS, McCormick KB. *Pregnancy and epilepsy: an information pamphlet for women with epilepsy who are planning a family.* Minneapolis: Minnesota Comprehensive Epilepsy Program, 1987.

Managing Seizure Disorders: A Handbook for Health Care Professionals, edited by N. Santilli, Lippincott-Raven Publishers, Philadelphia, 1996.
© 1996 Epilepsy Foundation of America.

18

Impact of Epilepsy on Employability

Dianne Chasen Lipsey

Employment is a primary life goal for most people. It is both a reward and indicator of independence. Many adults with epilepsy are working today in a full range of occupational fields. The Epilepsy Foundation of America (EFA) estimates that almost 80% of all people with epilepsy can work competitively. Most people with epilepsy will never have a seizure at work. Even so, people with epilepsy are often perceived by employers and job placement specialists as "difficult to employ." They often do have difficulty obtaining jobs suitable to their skills and interests.

The impact of epilepsy on a person's employability is highly individualized. However, there are general factors associated with epilepsy that may have the effect of limiting an individual's ability to gain and maintain employment— "employability." These include seizure activity, the presence of seizure-related conditions or other disabilities, seizure control medications and their side effects, social skill level, level of education, work skills and work history, and perceived limitations.

Although these factors may influence the types of jobs, duties, and environments in which a person with epilepsy can work, few would preclude a person from work altogether. The only clear factor that would automatically eliminate a person with epilepsy from a particular job is a lack of qualifications to do that job. The Americans with Disabilities Act (ADA), signed into law in July of 1990, prohibits discrimination in employment on the basis of epilepsy when a person with epilepsy is qualified, with or without a "reasonable accommodation," to perform the essential functions of the job in question.

This chapter reviews factors influencing employability, describes the employment alternatives for people with epilepsy, describes employer responsibilities under the ADA, reviews how health care professionals may interface with the work setting and people with epilepsy, and lists referral sources.

FACTORS INFLUENCING EMPLOYABILITY

Seizure Activity

It is estimated that 60% of people with epilepsy can be considered seizure-free. Approximately another 25% of people with epilepsy can work competitively but can be expected to have seizures during the course of their working years. Employment options may be different for those who have no seizures than for those who do.

For people who have been seizure-free for a significant period of time, there are few jobs from which they are absolutely barred on the basis of their history of seizures. However, the Federal Department of Transportation bars anyone with a history of seizures from obtaining a federal commercial driver's license. The Federal Aviation Administration (FAA) also bars anyone with a history of seizures from obtaining a commercial pilot's license. Beyond these "blanket restrictions," whether a person needs to be seizure-free for any particular period of time to be qualified to perform a job depends on the specific job. For many jobs, the fact that a person has a seizure will not prohibit them from doing their work.

For employment purposes, factors in addition to the length of time a person has not had a seizure may also be considered. For example, whether a person has an "aura" might be important if the person works around heavy machinery and might be injured if a seizure occurred suddenly and without warning. Likewise, an individual whose seizure activity is controlled only with heavy doses of antiepileptic drugs (AEDs) that impair memory, cognition, or coordination may have a problem doing a particular job if no special accommodations are available.

There is a growing body of knowledge about seizures, seizure recurrence, and overall prognosis. All of these factors should be considered when discussing employment potential for any given job.

People who are not seizure-free can be evaluated in terms of employability according to the characteristics of the seizures, among other factors.

A person whose seizures are characterized by impaired consciousness, loss of body tone, convulsions, and/or periods of disorientation may require certain environmental considerations in job placement. If such seizures are sufficiently likely to occur on the job and if a reliable warning preceding seizure onset is not assured, that person may be excluded from jobs involving exposure to toxic chemicals or hot surfaces, operation of heavy machinery, moving parts, or motor vehicles, or other environmental settings in which loss of consciousness could cause injury to the person or others.

A person whose seizures do not involve impaired consciousness is not necessarily be limited in the work environment. Employment decisions would, however, consider the exact type of functional loss that does occur during and after the seizure. For example, an individual who has simple partial seizures and who may lose function only in one arm but maintains full consciousness may be limited in certain climbing or lifting functions but be able to work in a wide range of jobs, even in potentially dangerous environments.

Some of the factors influencing employment decisions for people who are not seizure-free include specific characteristics of the seizures, frequency, and predictability of seizure occurrences.

Predictability can be one of the key factors. It includes likelihood of a seizure to occur during a particular time of day, the presence of a "warning" or "aura" before the onset of a seizure, and known precipitants of seizures, such as flashing or flickering lights, fatigue, dark/light patterns, or irregular schedules of eating or sleeping. If seizures occur with a predictable pattern, work environments, schedules, and circumstances can be adjusted to minimize the likelihood of a seizure occurring on the job.

Seizure-Related Conditions

Many people with seizures have no complications beyond maintaining seizure control. For those who do, these conditions can be more debilitating than the seizures themselves. They may include underlying neurologic factors, AED side effects, psychosocial adjustment issues, academic underachievement, the presence of another disability, or a combination of these factors. Cognitive and memory deficits, significant side effects of AEDs that may impair response rate and/or manual dexterity, fatigue, and drowsiness may also occur. The cognitive losses may result in difficulties with comprehension and specific skill deficits, such as math and reasoning. Memory deficits can make learning of complex tasks difficult and can have implications for work behavior as well. AEDs can impair cognitive functioning, which is characterized, in part, by slowed motor responses.

Fatigue and drowsiness can interfere with work productivity and accuracy. They are most often associated with AED levels and/or nocturnal seizures. If the seizures and AED levels are stable, the level of energy and alertness may be factors in the types of jobs and environments in which a person can work. If the fatigue and/or drowsiness seems unusual or changes, the AED levels may have to be reevaluated before the level of functioning can be determined.

One of the major concerns with related conditions is that they may not be understood by the individual, the service provider, or the employer. For example, a person who is seizure-free and who makes a good appearance during a job interview may encounter problems on the job because of undiagnosed deficits or misunderstood behavior, such as sleeping on the job. To the extent that these conditions can be understood before a person enters a job, they can be incorporated into the job placement and accommodation decisions. Neuropsychological test batteries have been developed specifically for people with epilepsy and can provide information directly relevant to job selection and job search.

Epilepsy may be associated with other types of disabilities. It often occurs in association with mental retardation or cerebral palsy or their combination, but it is not caused by these conditions (Hauser and Hesdorffer, 1990). Traumatic brain injury is often identified as a cause of epilepsy but does not account for a very large number of cases. The presence of epilepsy with these conditions complicates assessment of the individual and in many cases is not sufficiently dealt with when the other disability is considered and treated as "primary." The result has often been that people with other disabilities and active seizures do not or cannot participate in programs designed for people with those disabilities or, if they do, their success rate may be lower. There is a need to understand fully the interrelationship of the seizure condition with the other disabilities so that a successful service intervention can be planned.

Seizure Control Maintenance Regimens

Seizure control regimens can require individuals to take medication at specific intervals, to eat meals or snacks regularly, or to get regular amounts of rest. Some people should avoid environments with temperature extremes and highly stressful situations.

Attention to daily regimens can be important to maintain stable seizure activity and to reduce complications. Most often these workday regimens can be accommodated by an employer with little effort. They may require assigning the person to a regular shift rather than a swing shift and permitting more frequent but possibly briefer breaks. For people sensitive to stress, careful job placement with supportive supervision is important.

Social Skills and Work Habits

The EFA has operated a national employment assistance program, Training Applicants for Placement Success (TAPS), since 1976 (see Appendix D, EFA Resources). For many individuals served by TAPS, lack of appropriate social skills and work habits is a greater barrier to employment than their seizure activity, associated conditions, or daily regimens. The circumstances surrounding a seizure condition can directly affect an individual's ability to gain, maintain, and succeed in a job. These circumstances include, among others, age of onset and the degree to which it interrupts age-appropriate activities, and the response of family members to the individual during diagnosis and treatment.

Appropriate social skills and work habits result from vocational development, which begins very early in life and is an ongoing process. For young children this includes the first assignments of responsibilities by parents, learning to work and play with siblings and friends, learning to negotiate conflict, and gaining confidence in the ability to control the environment. As children age, development includes gaining greater personal autonomy and independence. For adolescents this often means driving and taking a first job. When these developmental phases are interrupted or perhaps are encountered with uncertainty, certain skills appropriate to interpersonal interactions on the job will not have been learned. Many young people who miss the opportunities for those first jobs may not have gained simple work habits that would be expected of more mature job applicants.

The consequences of a person's poor social skills and work habits will appear in personal conduct at work, productivity, reliability, and in the process of presenting to an employer for a job or promotion.

Families play an important role in encouraging children and adolescents with epilepsy to participate in their own care and in age-appropriate activities. They must overcome their own fears so that they can encourage their children to participate in activities that will promote their development and independence.

Adults and adolescents who exhibit poor social development and work habits can benefit from participation in job readiness programs that help people to gain the necessary skills to participate fully on the job. These include introductions to the world of work, trial work experiences, supported employment, and work enclaves. These programs help individuals to develop basic skills with which they can move into increasingly competitive environments.

Educational Level, Work Skills, and Work History

These are factors that influence the employability of everyone in the labor force. Among the successful clients of the EFA's TAPS National Project (during the period 1980–1994), most have had a high school education or an equivalency and many have had some previous work history. A person with good data processing skills, for example, can find a job with far less concern about seizure type than someone with no skills.

Depending on the age of onset, the quality and consistency of education can be affected. People with early-onset epilepsy may fall behind in school because of frequent interruptions required for treatment. This can be discouraging for a young person, who may stop trying or may be too fragmented to be effective, resulting in an inadequate educational experience.

Perceived Limitations

Employers, like members of the general public, may maintain views of epilepsy that are inaccurate. Because of these misconceptions, they may limit the types of jobs for which they would be willing to hire a person with epilepsy, may exclude people with epilepsy from participation in programs and opportunities offered by the company, or may deny employment altogether to people with epilepsy. Although the ADA prohibits these practices, an employer may be inclined towards them, believing that a person with epilepsy would harm him or herself or others, upset other employees or customers, and miss more work.

Interestingly, people with epilepsy themselves can reinforce these misconceptions because of their own misconceptions about their condition. Many TAPS participants, even those who have been seizure-free for several years, are fearful of having a seizure on the job. Without the help of a supportive employment service such as TAPS, they may allow those fears to limit their expectations and may represent their epilepsy to an employer as more of a problem than it really is. Once on the job, employees with epilepsy may be fearful of losing the job and may be hesitant to present legitimate concerns or needs for accommodations to employers.

Perceived limitations can often be overcome by effective training, availability of resources, and experience. TAPS, EFA affiliates, and other service providers can help to change these perceptions by providing information, in-service training programs, interview techniques, assistance with the placement decision, and supports for the employee on the job when needed. These supports give employers information, tools, and supports needed to change their attitudes and enable them to employ someone with epilepsy, even in a job previously believed to be inappropriate. Such programs also help people with epilepsy to develop appropriate expectations for their contributions to the work force, to develop an approach to discussing their epilepsy with their employer, when appropriate, and to learn how to represent themselves on the job.

CONTINUUM OF EMPLOYMENT OPTIONS

The overwhelming majority of people with epilepsy can work independently and in competitive employment. Many, however, benefit from greater levels of support in their work setting or from more support as they prepare to enter competitive employment. The continuum of employment options described here includes competitive employment, supported employment, work enclaves, sheltered employment, home employment, and self-selected unemployment. Each employment option can be an end in itself or a bridge for people moving toward more competitive work. This continuum reflects levels of independent functioning and work site integration.

Competitive Employment

Competitive employment covers jobs in the private or public sector for which a person with a disability can be expected to compete with persons who do not have disabilities. It is the goal for most people. Competitive employment is carried out in regular places of work, appropriately integrated within the functions of the employer, and usually requires some degree of independent functioning. Even though these jobs are in competitive settings, some are influenced by government incentives. A job in the federal government, for example, is in a "competitive" environment, even when an employee with a disability may have been hired for a job that offers preferential access to people with disabilities.

Programs such as the TAPS program, which target competitive employment as the goal, offer people with epilepsy supports that will help them to represent themselves in their job search and to compete for jobs appropriate to their skills and interests.

Supported Employment

Supported employment is considered to be the employment alternative of choice for people who may not be ready to work independently and may not ever be expected to. Employment occurs in competitive, integrated settings, but the nature of supported employment is characterized by a close collaboration between participating public and private sector employers and employment specialists knowledgeable about epilepsy and employment. "Job coaches" are employed by the program to establish opportunities with employers and to provide on-the-job supports. The supports usually include coaching employees with disabilities in performance of specific tasks or in handling work adjustment issues. Although the degree of on-site involvement varies, job coaches usually have considerable presence at the work site. In some cases they may be obligated to perform employee tasks in the employee's absence.

For some employees, the benefit of supported employment is the extension of their support system into the place of work. This can help them to gain skills and confidence in a competitive work environment while maintaining rehabilitation and training supports previously available only in sheltered, segregated settings. The advantage of supported employment over more sheltered employment is that it offers people an opportunity to work in a community-integrated setting. The goal for most people in supported employment is to be able to sustain themselves in their jobs independently.

Work Enclaves

Another type of supported employment is the work enclave. Enclaves offer the benefit of group support for employees who may not be able to work independently in the community and in more integrated settings. In work enclaves, a job coach and employer arrange for units of work to be assigned to a work group of employees with disabilities. They are intended to be small, including only four to six workers in any single enclave and integrating other employees without disabilities when possible. The tasks completed in enclaves are usually those that require little or no previous training or skills.

Sheltered Employment

Sheltered employment programs are often housed in rehabilitation facilities for people who, for a period of time or indefinitely, are perceived to need intensive intervention and support to learn skills to function independently. These are characteristically segregated environments for people with disabilities. They usually offer participants skill-building activities and a wage. Wages are earned by workers who complete tasks, often piecework, for which the facility has developed contracts with business. Pay is dispensed by the facility. The goal for most sheltered work programs is to help individuals to progress toward more independent settings.

Home Employment

Many people with severe and/or unpredictable seizures cannot or do not wish to work outside of their homes. Some people have been successful offering services such as telemarketing, subcontract service, and market research from their homes. People who elect to work from their homes often prefer to work in this setting so that transportation will not be a problem.

Self-Selected Unemployment

Some people have such severe seizures and related conditions that employment may not be an appropriate life goal for them. Many programs that serve people with epilepsy or other conditions consider their goal to be to help such people achieve the maximal independence appropriate to their needs and abilities. That goal can still be pursued in other areas of life, such as recreation or continuing education, for people who cannot or choose not to work.

EMPLOYERS' RESPONSIBILITIES UNDER THE ADA

In an effort to provide a person with epilepsy with the best possible support, service providers must understand and apply information regarding the range of issues and challenges associated with epilepsy. An employer, however, may not apply that information to the relationship with a person with epilepsy. Employers have less reason to understand all aspects of a person's medical or personal circumstances and are usually prohibited from seeking that information unless it is related to the performance of a job.

The ADA and regulations issued by the Equal Employment Opportunities Commission and the Department of Justice set forth requirements for employers with regard to their employment policies and practices as they affect the hiring of people with disabilities. Employers with 15 or more employees must comply with ADA regulations.

The ADA prohibits employers from discriminating against qualified individuals with disabilities because of such disabilities. These prohibitions apply to job application procedures, to hiring, advancement, or discharge of employees, to compensation, to job training, and to other terms, conditions and privileges of employment. A qualified person with a disability is an individual with a disability who "meets the legitimate skill, experience, education or other requirements of an employment position that he or she seeks or holds and who can perform the essential functions of the job, with or without a reasonable accommodation." (U.S. Department of Justice, 1991).

An employer is not required under the ADA to give preference to qualified applicants who have disabilities, but is required to provide a reasonable accommodation to allow a qualified person with a disability to perform the essential functions of the job, if the employer knows about the disability and the need for an accommodation and if the accommodation will not represent an "undue hardship."

In general, an employer will have no way of knowing about the presence of epilepsy or the need for an accommodation unless the individual discloses such information. This places responsibility on people with epilepsy to know when and how to present their condition to a potential or current employer. If an individual is able to perform the essential functions of the job in question, without the provision of a reasonable accommodation, there may be no reason to make the condition known and there is no obligation to do so.

Most accommodations for qualified people with epilepsy can be relatively easily and inexpensively achieved. Examples of reasonable accommodations for people with epilepsy include offering a person a day shift rather than a swing shift job to accommodate the need to maintain regular schedules for meals and rest, installing automatic cut-off switches on all power tools that an individual with seizures might use, painting over walls or covering floors with dark/light patterns when appropriate, or positioning an employee who has "warnings" before a seizure near an employee lounge equipped with a cot.

The ADA specifies requirements regarding appropriate use of pre-employment medical examinations and allows "employers to establish qualification standards that will exclude individuals who pose a direct threat to the health and safety of others, if that risk cannot be lowered to an acceptable level by the provision of a reasonable accommodation." Although a concern for safety has been the basis for employment discrimination in the past, the ADA requires "employers to make individualized judgments based on reliable medical evidence rather than on generalizations, ignorance, fear, patronizing attitudes, or stereotypes."

HEALTH CARE PROFESSIONALS INTERFACE WITH THE EMPLOYMENT PROCESS

Health care professionals are most likely to encounter the employment aspects of epilepsy in one of the following circumstances: as part of a pre-employment medical examination, when symptoms appear on the job that suggest the onset or change of seizures, or when a seizure on the job results in an injury. Two factors important for nurses and other health care professionals responding to such circumstances include the information they receive about the condition and the information they provide.

Information Received

During a pre-employment medical examination a nurse has the entire range of information about the individual's condition that would normally be available in a routine examination. Once the person is employed, the nurse may feel it necessary to obtain additional information regarding a seizure condition. Such information may include a detailed description of the seizure itself, signs and symptoms that may occur before the seizure, and behaviors normally expected after the seizure. The nurse and employer should discuss what first aid measures are most helpful, such as speaking quietly and in a reassuring manner, letting the person sleep for 20 min after the seizure, or giving the individual a tissue to wipe away the drool. Many people with epilepsy have preferences about responses to their seizures that lessen the severity and recovery time if followed by supportive people.

Information that a health care professional encounters when an individual is referred because of an accident or unusual behavior is less direct. If a person is referred for an evaluation after a convulsive seizure, the health care worker may be able to identify the seizure but also need to question observers about environmental causes or factors relative to recurrence.

If an individual is referred after an unrecognized seizure, the health care professional may have to infer certain conclusions on the basis of descriptions of behaviors observed by others. Such behaviors might include: not following instructions; forgetting information; having unusually large numbers of accidents or making unusually large numbers of mistakes; lack of attentiveness; drowsiness and irritability; unusually high frequencies of absences or tardiness; requests for more or longer breaks; or unusual behaviors such as running through the work place, getting up from work and roaming around the room, disrobing in public, or having sudden emotional outbursts. These behaviors could be symptoms of complex partial seizure activity, previously undiagnosed cognitive or memory deficits, inappropriate AED or nocturnal seizures.

Information Provided by the Health Care Professional

The ADA sets forth regulations for how and when an employer may conduct pre-employment medical examinations. When the pre-employment examination is appropriate, the information must be maintained as confidential medical records. Because the law allows sharing with managers or supervisors and first aid and safety personnel information for appropriate use, the health care professional may be able to provide information that will help such personnel to interpret the information relative to the functions of the job and to understand ways in which such limitations can be accommodated.

At times, medical professionals are asked by employers to make broad statements about an individual's ability to work or about the general state of health. Health care professionals should make an effort to state all medical information in functional terms. This provides the employer with sufficient information to make decisions about the individual's ability to perform the essential functions of the job or the appropriateness of providing a reasonable accommodation.

When questions cannot be answered in functional terms alone but may, in fact, raise questions about risk for seizures and about safety, the medical professional can provide factual information about the specific seizure type and encourage the employer to consult policies on hiring for jobs in which safety is a factor.

Health care professionals can also play an important role in helping educate employers and managers about how to identify seizures, factors likely to affect employee functioning, work site conditions that may contribute to seizure onset, job accommodations, and basic first aid for seizures. Their perspective could also contribute to an employer's policy development regarding people with seizures.

REFERRING EMPLOYEES FOR SERVICES

Neurologic Assessment

If conditions suggest that a person is experiencing first-time seizure activity, "breakthrough" or recurring seizures, increased seizure activity, or AED side effects, the most important referral is for a neurologic assessment or reassessment. All health care professionals should encourage the person to seek medical attention. If the person has no primary care provider or cannot consult with one, the professional can offer the names of some according to the policies of the employer.

Neuropsychological Assessment

A person with epilepsy who is experiencing problems on the job with attention, understanding or remembering instructions, or who consistently misses appointments with the nurse's or doctor's office, may benefit from a neuropsychological assessment. Neuropsychologists (psychologists with knowledge of neurologic deficits) can offer test batteries designed to assess difficulties sometimes encountered by people with epilepsy. These include memory difficulties, perceptual–motor difficulties, and problems with processing visual and/or spatial relationships.

Employee Assistance Programs

Many companies, especially those likely to have a nurse on site, have an Employee Assistance Program (EAP). The EAP can help the employee to identify options and needs and to negotiate with the employer concerning employment status.

EFA Resources and Services

Detailed information about the EFA's resources and services available to individuals with epilepsy is provided in Appendix D, EFA Resources.

Vocational Rehabilitation Agencies

These agencies are the most widely available programs for people with vocationally disabling conditions, including epilepsy. They are available throughout all states and, for eligible people, can provide the same range of services identified above. In addition, they can help to pay for medical evaluations, vocational assessment, treatment, retraining, transportation, and further education.

Protection and Advocacy Programs

When individuals feel that they have been discriminated against in an employment decision, protection and advocacy programs can help them to determine if they have legitimate complaints and can then help them to pursue appropriate remedies. For more information about legal protections, see Chap. 21.

EMPLOYMENT ISSUES

Unemployment may be twice as common among people with epilepsy compared with the general population

Many people with epilepsy are employed in positions less demanding than would be expected on the basis of their education and job skill levels; this pattern of "underemployment" may be due to fewer employment opportunities for people with epilepsy

The rates of absenteeism and accidents are no higher among persons with epilepsy than in the work force in general, and work performance does not differ; a small subgroup of employed people with epilepsy may have an increased risk for accidents at work

Job loss among employed individuals with epilepsy may be related to factors other than their seizures

Educational and rehabilitation interventions and job placement assistance programs appear to increase the likelihood that a person with epilepsy will find employment

Stigma, prejudice, and discrimination are all barriers to the employment of people with epilepsy

REFERENCES

Hauser WA, Hesdorffer D. *Facts about epilepsy.* New York: Demos Publications, 1990.
US Department of Justice, Civil Rights Division, Office on the Americans with Disabilities Act. *The Americans with Disabilities Act, questions and answers.* Washington, DC: 1991:2, 6.

Managing Seizure Disorders: A Handbook for Health Care Professionals, edited by N. Santilli, Lippincott-Raven Publishers, Philadelphia, 1996. © 1996 Epilepsy Foundation of America.

19

Adjustment Issues in Persons with Epilepsy

Joan Kessner Austin, Patricia Osborne Shafer, Mariah Snyder, and Bruce Hermann

This section briefly reviews adjustment issues for persons with epilepsy. It is particularly important for the health care professional to be aware of the behavioral correlates of adjustment problems, because these problems can pose major psychosocial complications for some individuals. Health care professionals, with their extended contact and familiarity with the patient and the extended family, are in an excellent position to screen the individual and family for these difficulties and to refer them for appropriate treatment.

The conceptual approach presented here may be helpful in understanding the major forces believed to contribute to the development of psychopathology in epilepsy, because it is a way or organizing the published literature for the reader who is not familiar with the epilepsy/psychopathology field. In addition, models can be of some clinical value for dealing with patients. The major behavioral problems associated with the epilepsies and the major risk factors associated with each behavioral problem are also reviewed. These problems are part of *interictal* (between seizure) behavior which is not explicitly associated with ictal (seizure) activity.

AN APPROACH TO UNDERSTANDING PSYCHOPATHOLOGY IN EPILEPSY

Considerable controversy has existed concerning many aspects of the relationship between epilepsy and psychopathology (Devinsky and Theodore, 1991). Much of this debate has centered on the role of specific variables, so-called risk variables, that may predispose individuals with epilepsy to a variety of behavioral and emotional problems. One well-known example of this controversy concerns the relationship between complex partial seizures and psychopathology. However, there are similar controversies about the importance of several other potential risk factors for psychopathology in people with epilepsy.

A model of psychopathology in epilepsy that would simultaneously consider

TABLE 1. *Factors that may influence cognitive functioning, behavior, and psychosocial adjustment in epilepsy*

Biologic	Psychosocial	Medication	Demographic
Age	Family/social	Number of	Education
Sex	support	medications	Ethnic and cultural
Types of epilepsy	Locus of control	Medication type	background
Etiology	Stigma	AED levels	Socioeconomic
Duration of epilepsy	Discrimination	Compliance	background
Seizure frequency	Social exclusion		
Number of episodes	Negative life events		
of status			
epilepticus			
Age at onset			
Related			
neuropsychological			
deficits			
Temperament			
Concurrent chronic			
medical problem			

Adapted from Herman et al., 1989.

many potential etiological factors has been developed (Hermann and Whitmann, 1986). Building on the work and writings of previous investigators, the developers suggest that four general forces represent potential etiologies of psychopathology in epilepsy. These broad forces include biologic, psychosocial, medication, and demographic factors. Many, if not all, of the specific variables of known or suspected etiological importance can be subsumed under one of these four guiding hypotheses (Table 1).

Table 1 presents these four groups of variables and several of the specific factors that may be subsumed under each. This table is not meant to be exhaustive; rather, it is meant to be illustrative. The major purpose of presenting this model is so that the reader will remember that the individual with epilepsy is subjected to a wide variety of influences that have the potential of adversely affecting mental health. Conceptualizing the potential risk factor in terms of four particularly significant forces may help in the understanding of the causes of behavioral disorders in those persons with whom the professional interacts.

This chapter highlights the global area of stress and reviews specific developmental issues. Finally, it offers some intervention strategies.

STRESS AND EPILEPSY

Response to stress is an often cited precipitant of seizures in people with epilepsy. Although a definitive relationship has not been clearly established, the association of high levels of stress with occurrence of seizures is accepted by many persons. Several hypotheses have been put forth for explaining the impact of high levels of stress on the occurrence of seizures. Areas in the temporal lobes, a common site of seizure origin, have low seizure thresholds and are closely aligned with emotions. Hyperventilation, which often occurs during high levels of stress, may alter the blood pH. Increased epinephrine secretion occurs in high levels of stress. Finally, hypoglycemia may be caused by increased metabolism during the stress response. Like many other chronic conditions, factors associated with epilepsy have the potential to create high levels of stress that may have a profound impact on the person's ability to function. Professionals can help to identify these factors and develop a plan of care that can reduce the stress response and promote psychological well-being.

STRESSORS IN EPILEPSY

Many interrelated factors may contribute to adjustment problems in persons with epilepsy. Simonds (1979) identified helpless feelings associated with lack of control over when a seizure will occur, feelings of alienation because of family and societal misconceptions about seizures, overprotection from family and friends, seizure type, and effects of some antiepileptic drugs (AEDs) as factors that can affect the mental health of persons with epilepsy.

Helplessness arising from lack of control over when seizures will occur is a prominent stressor for persons with epilepsy (Bagley, 1972; Snyder, 1986; Gehlert, 1994). Although lack of control over the condition is not unique to persons with epilepsy, the nature of the fear can be devastating. Bagley noted that human beings want to be in control, and the uncertainty regarding behavior during a seizure and when seizures will occur leads to feelings of helplessness. Fears about seizures and their consequences are common (Mittan, 1986; Goldstein et al., 1990) and are found even among persons who have comparatively good seizure control. Suggested treatment programs for such concerns have been reported (Helgeson et al., 1990).

Lack of understanding by others and the associated stigma of having epilepsy is another stressor experienced (Dell, 1986). Many persons with epilepsy still hide the existence of the condition from others because in the past they have experienced rejection when they shared the nature of their condition with others (Schneider and Conrad, 1983). Fear of being rejected may interfere with establishment of social networks or seeking employment. The public education programs sponsored by the Epilepsy Foundation of America (EFA) and its affiliates are beginning to have an impact on the public's understanding of epilepsy, but much work remains to be done. Although there is disagreement about the degree of stigma associated with epilepsy (Bagley, 1972; Ryan et al., 1980; Tan, 1986; Scambler and Hopkins, 1990), professionals should consider it in their evaluation of persons with epilepsy. Parents, family, friends, and teachers may be overprotective of individuals with epilepsy, thus preventing them from developing friends and a normal social life. Concern for the person prompts oversolicitous actions on the part of others. Although overprotectiveness is more prominent for younger persons, the long-term effects of this are seen in adults who have not acquired the social skills necessary for healthy interactions with others.

Other possible stressors for persons with epilepsy include having to take AEDs, difficulty in getting a driver's license or insurance, problems in obtaining and maintaining employment, and concern about offspring having epilepsy.

DEVELOPMENTAL TASKS AND EPILEPSY

Infancy

For optimal emotional development, babies need a safe, nurturing environment in which they are fed, touched, cuddled, talked to, and played with. Babies also need a stable adult in the environment for attachment and bonding to take place. A safe environment and attachment to an adult help children to cope with stress in later life (Lipsett, 1983).

Sometimes parents are unable to provide a safe, nurturing environment for a child with a chronic disorder, such as epilepsy (McCullum, 1973). Parents may be so burdened by their own inability to cope with the epilepsy that they are unable to respond to the child's needs. Some parents may be embarrassed that their children have epilepsy and feel guilty because they are not as proud of their children as they believe they should be. These parents do not derive as much satisfaction from interactions with their babies as parents who are not burdened with embarrassment and guilt. Therefore, epilepsy can indirectly have some adverse effect on a young infant by affecting the quality of parenting skills secondary to guilt, stigma, and other psychosocial consequences of epilepsy.

Early Childhood

Developmental tasks for children between 1 and 5 years of age include having daily routines, mastering toilet training and self-care activities, learning to communicate with others, and becoming socialized (Billingham, 1982). In emotional development, Erikson proposes that these children are involved in two nuclear conflicts: autonomy vs. shame and doubt and initiative vs. guilt (Freiberg, 1983). Children need an environment in which they can become increasingly independent and capable of providing their own bodily care. In addition, an atmosphere is needed in which children can develop autonomy and initiative.

Accomplishment of these developmental tasks can be hindered by epilepsy. Parents may be concerned about the possible occurrence of a seizure and may not allow the child to develop needed independence. Parents may over-restrict children's activities to the point that they experience shame, doubt, and guilt. Overindulgence and overprotection deprive children of achieving the needed tasks of autonomy and initiative. Consequently, they are deprived of feeling competent, a basis for later self-esteem (McCullum, 1973).

Middle Childhood

Once children reach school age they spend more time outside the family, with peers at school and in the neighborhood. They seek to become more independent from the parents and to become more attached to peers. Belonging to peer groups is very important in their emotional development. It is important for children to feel valued by their peers and to be a member of the group. Erikson proposes that school-aged children are involved in the nuclear conflict of industry vs. inferiority (Billingham, 1982). In the development of industry, success at school is very important. Achievement at school can enable children to derive a sense of pride in accomplishment and to win recognition from others. Experiences that make them feel inadequate or inferior can negatively affect emotional development and lead to feelings of inferiority (Freiberg, 1983).

When children reach school age, they have also developed cognitively to the point at which they can conceptualize illness more accurately (Billingham, 1982). During this period, children with a chronic physical condition, such as epilepsy, realize that they have a condition that most other children do not have. Feeling different, however, can interfere with their development of self-esteem and industry. Research has found that children with epilepsy have lower self-concepts than children with other chronic physical conditions (Matthews et al., 1982; Austin, 1988; Austin et al., 1994).

School-aged children with epilepsy have to cope with seizures and taking AEDs that may negatively impact memory and behavior (Stores, 1979) in addition to accomplishment of regular developmental tasks. Austin et al. (1994) found that children with epilepsy whose IQs were in the normal range experienced higher rates of academic retention. By the sixth grade, a greater number of the children with epilepsy had repeated a grade than children with asthma or their peers in the community. This could not be attributed to absenteeism. Therefore, although they were academically achieving, it took them more time to do it. In addition to academic concerns, parents of school-aged children with epilepsy are faced with fostering independence even though they may be worried that a seizure could subject the child to possible physical harm or rejection from peers. Even if the parents are comfortable with independent activities, school personnel, after-school care providers, and other activity directors may not feel as comfortable and may therefore impose undue restrictions.

ADOLESCENCE

Adolescence is a period of great change during which a person develops self-esteem, a sense of identity, capacity for intimacy, and capacity for independence from the family (McAnarney, 1985). An adolescent with epilepsy is confronted with adjusting to a chronic condition that can make accomplishment of normal developmental tasks more difficult.

The emotional reactions of adolescents in regard to their seizures do not have any set timetable for occurrence. They can develop at any point and usually recur frequently as these young people continually face new adjustments. Anger, fear, guilt, embarrassment, insecurity, and impaired self-esteem and self-image are just a few commonly reported emotional reactions. Seizures signify a loss of control over body, mind, and behavior. Individuals may either be unaware of what happens to them during a seizure or may be unable to stop a seizure if they are aware of it. Feelings may include a loss of control over life as they face restrictions or limitations, discrimination, overprotectiveness, or overpermissiveness from others. Adolescents may be unable to drive, may have difficulty making or keeping friends, experience difficulty at school due to learning problems or frequent absences, and may begin to experience vocational problems. As a result, they may feel that epilepsy is controlling their lives.

Early onset of seizures, especially uncontrolled seizures, may lead to cognitive or behavioral difficulties. There may be several reasons for these difficulties, such as the effects of underlying brain dysfunction, "silent" seizures interfering with cognitive processes such as memory or attention, and/or AED side effects. Cognitive and behavioral dysfunction may cause problems with learning (poor or underachievement) or psychosocial readjustment. For example, a student who has difficulty paying attention, completing assignments, or who acts impulsively may be labeled a "behavioral problem."

Adolescents with epilepsy may be at greater risk for depression and suicidal ideation than their peers (Austin et al., 1994). It is important for adolescents and their families to understand and be aware that these problems can occur. Potential or actual problems can then be more easily identified so that appropriate interventions can be started early. Individual and family expectations may also be more realistic, which will help in planning educational and vocational goals for the adolescent.

ADULTS

Developmental tasks of adulthood can include intimacy, marriage, economic independence, and parenting. The adjustment problems confronted by adults with epilepsy can interfere with the successful accomplishment of their developmental tasks. Some of the more frequently discussed adjustment problems associated with the epilepsies in adults are depression, aggression, sexual dysfunction, and personality change. An estimate of the magnitude of the risk involved is presented for each of these problems, as well as the specific factors that appear to predispose the individual with epilepsy to that particular problem.

Depression

Depression appears to be among the most common of the behavioral problems associated with epilepsy, although its exact prevalence in epilepsy is unknown (Robertson and Trimble, 1983; Altschuler, 1991). Several studies have reported high rates of depression, as well as anxiety, and examples of these studies are presented below.

In an investigation of patients with epilepsy admitted to a psychiatric hospital, Betts (1974) found depression to be the most common psychiatric diagnosis. Similarly, in a sample of 93 patients with complex partial seizures, Dalby (1971) found that depression was the most common diagnosis among those with significant psychopathology. Currie et al. (1971) found depression and anxiety to be the most frequent psychological complaints among 666 patients with complex partial seizures. Similar findings have been reported by others (Trimble and Perez, 1980).

On the basis of these findings, one might suspect that rates of suicide are elevated in epilepsy. Matthews and Barabas (1981) examined the mortality studies of epilepsy in which statistics pertaining to suicide were available. Although there were many methodologic problems with the previous studies, these investigators concluded that elevated rates of suicide appeared to be associated with epilepsy relative to the general population. Further data supporting the increased risk for suicide in epilepsy can be found in Hauser and Hesdorffer (1990) and in Barraclough (1987). Specific causative factors associated with suicide in epilepsy have been reported (Mendez et al., 1989).

Several research groups have tried to identify risk factors for depression. In general, a wide variety of biologic variables (such as seizure type, age at onset, side and site of seizure focus, seizure frequency, presence of an intracranial lesion) have been found to have some relationships with depression in epilepsy (Robertson and Trimble, 1983; Robertson et al., 1987; Altschuler, 1991; Devinsky and Vasquez, 1993; Victoroff et al., 1994). Psychosocial variables appear to be potentially powerful predictors of depression, but only a modest amount of investigation has occurred in this area (Hermann and Whitman 1984; Roth et al., 1994). Nevertheless, it appears that the stigma and discrimination associated with epilepsy, the loss of social support, increased life stressors, financial loss, and other social factors to which people with epilepsy are exposed represent significant risk factors for depression. Finally, the potential contribution of AEDs to depression cannot be overlooked. For example, barbiturate AEDs are now known to predispose to depression, particularly in susceptible individuals (Brendt et al., 1987), and alteration of the AED type can help to alleviate the depressive symptoms (Brendt et al., 1990). Helpful reviews of the more general effects of AEDs on cognition and mood are provided by Devinsky (1995), Dodrill (1991), and Meador and Loring (1991).

In summary, depression appears to be a significant interictal behavioral complication of the epilepsies, but understanding of the causes of interictal depression is still incomplete. The data that do exist suggest that seizure-related factors and biologic factors are involved, as are psychosocial variables and AED considerations. Because depression appears to be among the most common interictal behavioral complications, it is particularly important for health care professionals to be aware of the major symptoms of depression and to screen patients for their occurrence. Otherwise, this disorder may go unnoticed.

Aggression

Aggression has been a particularly controversial topic in the epilepsy behavioral literature (Fenwick, 1992). Two issues are really involved. The first concerns whether it is possible for an individual, during the course of a seizure, to commit a coordinated, goal-directed act of violence or aggression against others. This so-called "ictal violence" has been the subject of significant study, and it appears that such behavior occurs extremely rarely, if at all, during the course of a seizure (Escueta et al., 1981; Treiman, 1991). The larger and more controversial topic concerns whether individuals with epilepsy, particularly those with complex partial seizures, are more likely to manifest irritable, hostile, aggressive, or violent behavior between seizures. Among individuals with epilepsy, some risk factors for aggressive behavior have been identified. In general, a higher risk for aggressive behavior is associated with the following variables: younger chronological age, male gender, onset of seizures before the age of 10, history of a disrupted home environment, more generally disordered behavior, lower socioeconomic status, and more signs of organic cerebral disease manifested in the neurologic exam (Hermann and Whitman, 1984). Clearly, the determinants of aggressive behavior in epilepsy are multifactorial in nature (Herzberg and Fenwick, 1988).

Some mentally retarded individuals experience a concurrent problem of episodic dyscontrol syndrome (or rage attacks), which may be confused with aggressive behavior. As mentioned in Chap. 8, this is a separate problem.

In summary, although there has been a high degree of interest regarding the possible relationship between aggressive behavior and epilepsy in general and complex seizures in particular, the weight of the evidence has not shown a particularly strong relationship. Rather, a wide variety of specific risk factors are known to be associated with increased chances for aggressive behavior, and it is interesting to note that many of these risk factors are associated with aggressive behavior in the general population. Aggression and irritable behaviors are most likely to be seen in the postictal state, when the person is confused, and can be minimized by a calm atmosphere and a nonintrusive style of interaction.

Sexual Dysfunction

More research investigation into the area of sexual dysfunction in persons with epilepsy is occurring. Whereas past research focused primarily on issues for males, current attention is being focused on both sexes. A complete discussion of this issue for females can be found in Chap. 10. In addition, where appropriate, issues for both genders are discussed. Therefore, this section focuses on past research and is limited more to issues relevant to males.

There are relatively few investigations of sexual dysfunction in persons with epilepsy. Nevertheless, past data suggest that sexual dysfunction is not uncommon in epilepsy, particularly among persons with complex partial seizures. The most prominent dysfunction is so-called "hyposexuality" (Blumer, 1970). This hyposexuality has been called "global" because, in addition to a significant decrease in the incidence of sexual outlets, there is sometimes an accompanying and profound lack of libido. Therefore, sexual change pertains to both sexual function and sexual interest. There has been less investigation of this problem among women. However, the disorder seems to be particularly significant among men with epilepsy (Prichard, 1980), particularly those with complex partial seizures. Four investigations have compared individuals with complex partial seizures to those with other seizure types, and these studies have found a higher incidence of sexual dysfunction in complex partial seizures. Specifically, there were more complaints of impotence, a higher incidence of sexual hypoactivity, and more hyposexuality in patients with complex partial seizures (Guerrant et al., 1962; Kolarsky et al., 1967; Shukla et al., 1979). In addition to the association with seizure type, other risk factors are known. For example, there is a known relationship between sexual function and the person's psychiatric status in general, and level of depression in particular.

In addition to the role played by the type of seizure, there has also been some investigation into the importance of AEDs. Some evidence now suggests that AEDs may play a role in this disorder. Several studies in England (Toone et al., 1980, 1982, 1983) have identified alterations in the level of sex hormones, the most important of which is a decrease in levels of free testosterone, which underlies the disorder in sexual function. However, this is one of many physiologic factors that might contribute to sexual dysfunction, and if this is suspected to be the case, then monitoring in a certified sleep laboratory can help to untangle the causes of sexual dysfunction.

Finally, the social factors associated with epilepsy cannot be discounted. Taylor (1969) has discussed the limitations in opportunity and choice of sexual relationships, history of special care, low earning potential, and the inhibiting effects of these factors on adequate social functioning and sexual functioning.

In summary, there appears to be a significant rate of sexual dysfunction, particularly among males with epilepsy and with complex partial seizures in particular. This information is usually not volunteered by the individual, even though it is a significant source of worry and concern. It is suggested that some specific inquiry be devoted to this topic, either by the nurse or by the physician, so that further diagnostic procedures that may be of value in treating the problem can be pursued.

Interictal Personality and Behavioral Changes

The concept of a global "epileptic personality" has generally fallen into disfavor for lack of support from well-controlled investigations, but controversy regarding the hypothesis that persons with a particular seizure type (complex partial seizures of temporal lobe origin) are prone to show a syndrome of changes in personality and behavior continues (Bear and Fedia, 1977). This proposal has generated a remarkable amount of interest and debate. Some investigators see this topic as a way of investigating the biologic bases of personality, whereas others view the syndrome as a reincarnation of the pejorative "epileptic personality," and/or an unreliable pattern of findings (Mungas, 1982; Rodin et al., 1984; Benson, 1991). Suffice it to say that this notion remains quite controversial, with some investigators suggesting that the constellation of personality traits described has nothing to do with epilepsy or complex partial seizures in particular but is more closely associated with psychopathology of any type and is therefore seen among psychiatric patients as well as other special groups.

In terms of practical considerations, the presence of a certain personality type should not be used to diagnose the presence of a neurologic condition in general, or a particular seizure type in particular, until further research is conducted and the controversies settled.

Some major interictal behavioral correlates of the epilepsies and some of the risk factors associated with these behavioral problems have been identified. From a clinical perspective, it is important to be alert to the possibility of an associated emotional problem in patients with epilepsy. In trying to gain some understanding of the potential underlying causes of these difficulties, it may be helpful to keep in mind the major forces involved (biologic, psychosocial, medication, demographic) so that appropriate treatment/remediation procedures can be instituted.

ASSESSMENT AND INTERVENTIONS

Infants and Children

It is important to assess the level of adaptation of children with epilepsy on a regular basis. The assessment for infants should focus on the parent–infant interactions to determine how conducive the infant's environment is to the development of attachment and trust. Assessment in early childhood should focus on how conducive the environment is for the child to become independent in self-care activities and to have opportunities for becoming autonomous and developing initiative. Assessment of the school-aged child should include information on self-esteem, peer relationships, hobbies, coping patterns, academic achievement, and perceptions about epilepsy. For example, assessment should determine whether children are sharing with their peers the fact that they have a seizure condition and whether they are experiencing teasing or rejection by their peers. Parents should be assessed for parenting behaviors to determine if they are conducive to the development of self-esteem, competence, and peer relationships.

Interventions should be both parent-focused and child-focused to facilitate optimal development of children with epilepsy (Lewis et al., 1990). One goal of interventions with parents is to provide them with accurate information about epilepsy. Another goal is to make them aware of normal psychosocial development in children and their role in making the environment conducive to the accomplishment of these tasks. Final goals are for parents to recognize that children with epilepsy are at risk for poor self-esteem and to teach the parents strategies for enhancement of self-esteem. The goals for interventions with children are that they be given information when they are able to understand, be supported in their attempts to cope with a chronic physical disorder, and be supported in their attempts to meet age-appropriate developmental tasks.

Although most interventions with parents are educational in nature, professionals often need to intervene with parents who are not creating environments conducive to children's emotional development (Lewis et al., 1991). Some parents are unable to deal with their own feelings (e.g., depression, inadequacy, or guilt) and are consequently unable to help their children. Often education alone is not enough, and parents must be referred to mental health counseling by a psychiatric nurse, social worker, or psychologist. Although support groups do not offer therapy, they can be helpful to parents who are coping with epilepsy. Parents can also be taught to enhance their children's self-esteem using strategies suggested by McKay (1987), such as focusing on positive qualities, being an active listener, accepting the child's negative feelings, and involving the child in solving problems.

Children need both educational interventions and opportunities to talk about feelings. Professionals not only should tell children about epilepsy, but also should help them to develop strategies for telling their peers about seizures. Many times we focus all of our efforts on parents and expect them to translate the information to their child. Equal time should be devoted to the child, preferably with the parent present. This provides role modeling and the opportunity to receive information in a more simplistic format. For example, a professional can review with the child the videos and materials from the EFA that are specifically designed for young children. Together, the professional and the child can then decide what the child will tell his friends about epilepsy. Sometimes it helps for the child to practice before talking with friends.

Children who cope well are aware of their feelings about epilepsy and are able to communicate them. They are able to express how much they care for others and they feel that they are worthy of others' love and care. These children also feel competent that they can deal with problems that arise (Brenner, 1984). If assessment of children reveals poor coping strategies, it is imperative to work with both children and parents to help the children learn more adaptive coping strategies. For example, children can be encouraged to explore and communicate their feelings. They should be able to identify when they are mad, sad, glad, or scared and should be able to express these feelings appropriately. Children experience many of the same concerns that adults do. According to Austin (1994), they are afraid of dying, brain damage, "blood shots," and returning to the location where the first seizure occurred. Feelings of poor self-esteem should be explored and challenged. Often it is helpful to have children focus on what they can do well and on their positive qualities. Children can be taught to identify and deal with stressful situations in an adaptive manner. Sometimes the professional can model adaptive coping strategies for children. Children who are experiencing depression and serious behavioral problems should be referred for mental health counseling. Likewise, academic support should be provided to those who are struggling academically. Frequently, very simple accommodations can have a significant positive impact.

Adolescents and Adults

The first step in helping adolescents and adults with epilepsy is to assess feelings of loss of control and plan teaching and counseling accordingly. The individual must feel able to control epilepsy, not only the frequency of seizures, but also the effects of seizures on daily life and safety.

Evaluation of support systems helps to assess the extent of resources available to help teenagers with epilepsy cope with the demands of daily life. This type of evaluation should include family, friends, and classmates, teachers, and other school personnel. The ability of these support people to help teenagers maintain a safe environment without excessive limitations and to make necessary modifications in their daily life without discrimination is the key to their success. Often, the reactions of other people, either the overprotection or overpermissiveness, can be detrimental to children's development and functioning. For example, overprotectiveness may lead to rebellion and withdrawal from support systems or rejection of advice from others. It may also lead to chronic anxiety and insecurity that can hinder children's ability to become more independent and responsible for safety and activities of daily living. Overpermissiveness may lead to conflicts with authority figures, difficulty with limit-setting or restrictions, or more insecurity. The actions of other people toward those with epilepsy are important to determine for better understanding the basis of their reactions.

Stress management can be especially helpful for adolescents and adults. The first step is to conduct an individualized assessment of each patient to identify possible stressors. One cannot assume that all stressors are experienced in a similar manner by all persons. Snyder (1986) has developed a stressor inventory to determine stressors in persons with epilepsy and the degree to which these stressors interfere with functioning. Use of such an assessment guide may help adolescents and adults to identify areas that they are unable to handle adequately and that produce high levels of stress. In addition, the findings provide direction to the health care team in planning possible interventions.

The Washington Psychsocial Seizure Inventory (Dodrill et al., 1980) is another instrument that has been used in assessing adjustment of persons with epilepsy to determine problems that are interfering with well-being. The 132 items elicit information about family background, emotional adjustment, interpersonal adjustment, vocational adjustment, financial status, adjustment to seizures, medicine, and medical management, and overall psychosocial functioning. A downward extension for adolescents is now available (Batzel et al., 1991).

In addition to assessing possible stressors, the professional should determine coping mechanisms, including social support and access to health care, that the patient uses in dealing with stressors. Basic characteristics, such as cognitive ability, should be ascertained. It is important to share this assessment with other health and community professionals so that a comprehensive plan of care can be developed.

Classes that provide information on various aspects of a healthy lifestyle have proven to be useful. Not only persons with epilepsy but also family and friends can benefit from attending such classes. Topics for classes include information about sleep and rest, sexuality, nutrition, exercise, acquisition of skills for social interaction, use of community resources, and stress management skills. These classes are available at some local community mental health centers, EFA local affiliates, and health facilities specializing in treatment of epilepsy.

A number of stress management techniques have been described in the literature. Progressive relaxation, meditation, imagery, biofeedback, and autogenic therapy are some of the more commonly used techniques. Smith (1985) emphasized the need for working with the patient to determine which technique(s) the patient finds most appealing and then to proceed with intensive teaching of the technique. Several of these techniques have been used to reduce seizure frequency in persons with epilepsy. Although little attention has been given to the impact of stress management techniques on improving the overall well-being of persons with epilepsy, there is considerable documentation of the effectiveness of these interventions in other patient populations.

Progressive muscle relaxation involves alternate tensing and relaxing of muscle groups throughout the body. Bernstein and Borkovec (1973) developed a widely used procedure that teaches the tensing and relaxing of 16 muscle groups. Daily practice is needed to gain mastery of the technique. When stressful events are anticipated, the person can then institute the technique and avoid high levels of stress.

A number of meditative techniques exist: Benson's relaxation response (1975) is one of the best known of these techniques. In the relaxation response, patients sit quietly, close their eyes, relax all muscles, become aware of their breathing, and then employ a mental device that is synchronized with their breathing pattern. This is done for a 10–20-min period on a daily basis. A highly relaxed state is achieved.

A third stress management technique that can be readily implemented is imagery. In guided imagery, the teacher provides the patient with a description of a scene that elicits mental representations of visual, auditory, olfactory, gustatory, and tactile/proprioceptive qualities of the scene. Concentrating on the restful images helps to prevent stressful thoughts from entering consciousness and also helps to dispel stress.

SUMMARY

Counseling, behavioral therapy techniques, and changes in AEDs medications are used in treating these problems. Health care professionals also can refer clients to agencies that offer these services (see Chap. 22).

A relatively recent development in epilepsy research has been an interest in developing tools to formally assess quality of life. Clinicians and researchers have been concerned about the effects of epilepsy on important areas of function (cognition, behavior) for a very long time, but they had not used the models and tools that had been developed in related fields, particularly the health services research field, to study the effects of illness on functional status. However, new tools for both adults and children with epilepsy have been developed (Smith et al., 1991; Vickrey et al., 1992; Baker et al., 1993; Jacoby et al., 1993; Austin et al., 1994; Devinsky et al., 1995). These measures can serve as useful screening inventories and should enable health care professionals to screen patients for problems in an efficient manner.

REFERENCES

Altshuler L. Depression and epilepsy. In: Devinsky O, Theodore W., eds. *Epilepsy and behavior.* New York: Wiley Liss, 1991;47–65.

Austin JK. Childhood epilepsy: child adaptation and family resources. *J. Child Adolesc Psychiatr Ment Health Nurs* 1988;1:18–24.

Austin JK, Smith MD, Risinger MW, McNelis AM. Childhood epilepsy and asthma: comparison of quality of life. *Epilepsia* 1994;35:608–15.

Bagley C. Social prejudice and the adjustment of persons with epilepsy. *Epilepsia* 1972;13:33–45.

Baker G, Smith DF, Dewey M, Jacoby A, Chadwick DW. The initial development of a health-related quality of life model as an outcome measure in epilepsy. *Epilepsy Res* 1993;16:65–81.

Barraclough BM. The suicide rate of epilepsy. *Acta Psychiatr Scand* 1987;76:339–45.

Batzel LW, Dodrill CB, Dubinsky BL, et al. An objective method for the assessment of psychosocial problems in adolescents with epilepsy. *Epilepsia* 1991;32:202–11.

Bear D, Fedia P. Quantitative analysis of interictal behavior in temporal lobe epilepsy. *Arch Neurol* 1977;454–67.

Benson D. The Geschwind Syndrome. In: Smith DB, Treiman D, Trimble MR, eds. *Neurobehavioral problems in epilepsy.* New York: Raven Press, 1991:411–21.

Benson H. *The relaxation response.* New York: Avon, 1975.

Bernstein D, Borkovec, T. *Progressive relaxation training.* Champaign, IL: Research Press, 1973.

Betts TA. A follow-up study of a cohort of patients with eilepsy admitted to psychiatric care in an English city. In: Harris P, Maudsley C, eds. *Epilepsy: proceedings of the Hans Berger Centenary Symposium.* Edinburgh: Churchill Livingstone, 1974:326–38.

Billingham KA. *Developmental psychology for health care professions.* Boulder, CO: Westview Press, 1982.

Blumer D. Hyposexual episodes in temporal lobe epilepsy. *Am J Psychiatry* 1970;126:1099–106.

Brendt DA, Crumrine PK, Varma RR, et al. Phenobarbital treatment and major depressive disorder in children with epilepsy. *Pediatrics* 1987;80:909–17.

Brendt DA, Crumrine PK, Varma R, et al. Phenobarbital treatment and major depressive disorder in children with epilepsy: a naturalistic follow-up. *Pediatrics* 1990;85:1086–91.

Brenner A. *Helping children cope with stress.* Lexington, MA: Lexington Books, 1984.

Currie S, Heathfield, KW, Henson RA, Scott DF. Clinical course and prognosis of temporal lobe epilepsy: a survey of 666 patients. *Brain* 1970;94:173–90.

Dalby MA. Antiepileptic and psychotropic effects of carbamazepine (Tegretol) in the treatment of psychomotor epilepsy. *Epilepsia* 1971;12:325–34.

Dell J. Social dimensions of epilepsy: Stigma and response. In: Whitman S, Hermann BP, eds. *Psychopathology in epilepsy: psychosocial factors.* New York: Oxford University Press, 1986.

Devinsky O. Cognitive and behavioral effects of antiepileptic drugs. *Epilepsia* 1995;36(suppl 2):S46–65.

Devinsky O. Clinical uses of the quality-of-life in epilepsy inventory. *Epilepsia* 1993;34(suppl 4): S39–44.

Devinsky O, Theodore W, eds. *Epilepsy and behavior.* New York: Wiley-Liss, 1991.

Devinsky O, Vasquez B. Behavioral changes associated with epilepsy. *Neurol Clin* 1993;11:127–49.

Devinsky O, Vickrey B, Cramer J, et al. The development of the quality of life in epilepsy (QOLIE) inventory. *Epilepsia* 1995 (in press).

Dodrill CB. Behavioral effects of antiepileptic drugs. In: Smith DB, Treiman DM, Trimble MR, eds. *Neurobehavioral problems in epilepsy.* New York: Raven Press, 1991:213–24.

Dodrill CB, Batzel LW, Queisse HR, Temkin NR. An objective method for the assessment of psychological and social problems among epileptics *Epilepsia* 1980;21:123–35.

Escueta A, Mattson R, King L, et al. The nature of aggression during epileptic seizures. *N Engl J Med* 1981;305:711–6.

Fenwick P. Aggression and epilepsy. In: Devinsky O, Theodore W (eds). Epilepsy and behavior. New York: Wiley-Liss, 85–96.

Freiberg KL. *Human development: a life span approach,* 2nd ed. Monterey, CA: Wadsworth Health Sciences Division, 1983.

Gehlert S. Perceptions of control in adults with epilepsy. *Epilepsia* 1994;35:81–8.

Goldstein J, Seidenberg M, Peterson R. Fear of seizures and behavioral functioning in adults with epilepsy. *J Epilepsy* 1990;3:101–6.

Guerrant J, Anderson WW, Fischer A, et al. *Personality in epilepsy.* Springfield, IL: Charles C Thomas, 1962.

Hauser WA, Hesdorffer DC. *Epilepsy: frequency, causes, and consequences.* New York: Demos Publications, 1990.

Helgeson DC, Mittan R, Tan S, Chayasirisobhon S. Sepulveda epilepsy education: the efficacy of a psychoeducational treatment program in treating medical and psychosocial aspects of epilepsy. *Epilepsia* 1990;31:75–82.

Hermann BP, Whitman S. Behavioral and personality correlates of epilepsy: a review, methodological critique, and conceptual model. *Psychol Bull* 1984;95:451–97.

Hermann BP, Whitman S. Psychopathology in epilepsy: a multi-etiological model. In: Hermann BP, Whitman S, eds. *Psychopathology in epilepsy: social dimensions.* New York: Oxford University Press, 1986:5–37.

Hermann BP, Whitman S. Psychosocial predictors of interictal depression. *J Epilepsy* 1989;2:231–37.

Hermann B, Whitman S, Dell J. Correlates of behavior problems and social competence in children with epilepsy aged 6–11. In: Hermann B, Seidenberg M, eds. *Childhood epilepsies: neuropsychological, psychosocial and intervention aspects.* New York: John Wiley & Sons, 1989:143–57.

Herzberg JL, Fenwick PBC. The etiology of aggression in temporal lobe epilepsy. *Br J Psychiatry* 1988;153:50–5.

Jacoby A, Baker G, Smith D, Dewey M, Chadwick D. Measuring the impact of epilepsy: The development of a new scale. *Epilepsy Res* 1993;16:83–8.

Kolarsky A, Freund K, Machek J, Polak O. Male sexual deviation: association with early temporal lobe damage. *Arch Gen Psychiatry* 1967;17:735–43.

Lewis M, Salas I, de la Sota A, Chiofalo N, Leake B. Randomized trial of a program to enhance the competencies of children with epilepsy. *Epilepsia* 1990;31:101–9.

Lewis M, Hatton CL, Salas I, Leake B, Chiofalo N. Impact of the children's epilepsy program on parents. *Epilepsia* 1991;32:365–74.

Lipsett LP. Stress in infancy: toward understanding the origins of coping behavior. In: Garmezy W, Rutter M, eds. *Stress, coping and development in children.* New York: McGraw-Hill, 1983:161–80.

Matthews WS, Barabas G. Suicide and epilepsy: a review of the literature. *Psychosomatics* 1981;22: 515–24.

Matthews WS, Barabas G, Ferrari M. Emotional concomitants of childhood epilepsy. *Epilepsia* 1982;23:671–81.

McAnarney EF. Social maturation: A challenge for handicapped and chronically ill adolescents. *J Adolesc Health C* 1985;6:90–101.

McCullum AT. *The chronically ill child.* New Haven, CT: Yale University Press, 1973.

McKay J. Building self-esteem in children. In: McKay M, Fanning P. *Self esteem.* Oakland, CA: New Harbinger Publications, 1987:225–57.

Meador KJ, Loring D. Cognitive effects of antiepileptic drugs. In: Devinsky O, Theodore W, eds. *Epilepsy and behavior.* New York: Wiley-Liss. 1991:151–70.

Mendez M, Lanska D, Marion-Espaillat R, Burnstine T. Causative factors for suicide attempts by overdose in epileptics. *Arch Neurol* 1989;46:1065–68.

Mittan R. Fear of seizures. In: Whitman S, Hermann BP, eds. *Psychopathology in epilepsy: social factors.* Oxford University Press, 1986.

Mungas D. Interictal behavior abnormality in temporal lobe epilepsy: a specific syndrome, a nonspecific psychopathology. *Arch Gen Psychiatry* 1982;39:108–11.

Pritchard PB. Hyposexuality: a complication of complex partial epilepsy. *Trans Am Neurol Assoc* 1980;105:193–5.

Robertson M, Trimble MR. Depressive illness in patients with epilepsy: a review. *Epilepsia* 1983;24(suppl 2):S109–16.

Robertson M, Trimble MR, Townsend HRA. Phenomenology of depression epilepsy. *Epilepsia* 1987;28:364–72.

Rodin E, Schmaltz S. Twitty G. The Bear-Fedio personality inventory and temporal lobe epilepsy. *Neurology* 1984;34:591–96.

Roth DL, Goode KT, Williams VL, Faught E. Physical exercise, stressful life experience, and depression in adults with epilepsy. *Epilepsia* 1994;35:1248–55.

Ryan R, Kempner K, Emlen AC. The stigma of epilepsy as a self-concept. *Epilepsia* 1980;21:433–44.

Scambler G, Hopkins A. Generating a model of stigma in epilepsy: The role of qualitative analysis. *Soc Sci Med* 1990;30:1187–94.

Schneider J, Conrad P. *Having epilepsy.* Philadelphia: Temple University Press, 1983.

Saunders M, Rawson MR. Sexuality in male epileptics. *J Neurol Sci* 1970;10:577–83.

Shukla GD, Srivastava ON, Katiyas BC. Sexual disturbances in temporal lobe epilepsy: a controlled study. *Br J Psychiatry* 1979;134:288–92.

Simonds SK. What does high level wellness mean when you have epilepsy? 1979;3:144–50.

Smith JC. *Relaxation dynamics.* Champaign, IL: Research Press, 1985.

Smith DF, Baker GA, Dewey M, Jacoby A, Chadwick DW. Seizure frequency, patient-perceived seizure severity and the psychosocial consequences of intractable epilepsy. *Epilepsy Res* 1991;9:231–41.

Snyder M. Stressor inventory for persons with epilepsy. *J Neurosci Nurs* 1986;18:71–3.

Stores G. School children with epilepsy at risk for learning and behavior problems. *Dev Med Child Neurol.* 1979;30:502–508.

Tan S. Psychosocial functioning of adult epileptic and MS patients and adult normal controls on the WPSI. *J Clin Psychol* 1986;42:528–34.

Taylor DC. Sexual behavior and temporal lobe epilepsy. *Arch Neurol* 1969;21:510–6.

Toone BK, Wheeler M, Fenwick PBC. Sex hormone changes in male epileptics. *Clin Endocrinol* 1980;12:391–5.

Toone BK, Wheeler M, Fenwick PBC. Effects of anticonvulsant drugs on male sex hormones and sexual arousal. In: Sandler M, ed. *Psychopharmacology of anticonvulsants.* Oxford: Oxford University Press, 1982:136–42.

Toone BK, Wheeler M, Nanjee M, Fenwick PBC, Grant R. Sex hormones, sexual drive and plasma anticonvulsant levels in male epileptics. *J Neurol Neurosurg Psychiatry* 1983;46:824–5.

Treiman DM. Psychobiology of ictal aggression. In Smith DB, Treiman DM, Trimble MR, eds. *Neurobehavioral problems in epilepsy.* Raven Press: New York, 1991:341–56.

Trimble MR, Reynolds EH. Anticonvulsants and mental symptoms: a review. *Psychol Med* 1976;6:169–78.

Trimble MR, Perez MM. Quantification of psychopathology in adult patients with epilepsy. In: Kulig BM, Meinardi H, Stores G, eds. *Epilepsy and behavior '79.* Lisse: Swets and Zeitlinger, 1980:118–26.

Trimble MR, Thompson PT, Corbett JA. Anticonvulsant drugs, cognitive function and behavior. In: Sandler M, ed. *Psychopharmacology of anticonvulsants.* Oxford: Oxford University Press, 1982:106–21.

Vickrey BG, Hays RD, Graber J, Rausch R, Engel J, Brook RH. A health related quality of life instrument for patients evaluated for epilepsy surgery. *Med Care* 1992;30:299–319.

Victoroff J, Benson F, Grafton ST, Engel J, Mazziotta JC. Depression in complex partial seizures: Electroencephalography and cerebral metabolic correlates. *Arch Neurol* 1994;51:155–63.

ADDITIONAL READING

Brandt J, Seidman LJ, Kohl D. Personality characteristics of epileptic patients: a controlled study of generalized and temporal lobe cases. *J Clin Exp Neuropsychol* 1985;7:25–38.

Garmezy N, Rutter M, eds. *Stress, coping, and development in children.* New York: McGraw-Hill, 1983.

Hermann BP, Dikeman S, Schwartz MS, Karnes WE. Interictal psychopathology in patients with ictal fear: a quantitative investigation. *Neurology* 1982;32:7–11.

Perini G, Mendius R. Depression and anxiety in complex partial seizures. *J Nerv Ment Dis* 1984;172: 287–90.

Scambler G. Sociological aspects of epilepsy. In: Hopkins A, ed. *Epilepsy.* New York: Demos Publications, 1987:497–510.

Snyder M. Stress in persons with epilepsy. Unpublished paper, 1988.

Wright LM, Leahey M. *Families and chronic illness.* Springhouse, PA: Springhouse Corporation, 1987.

Managing Seizure Disorders: A Handbook for Health Care Professionals, edited by N. Santilli, Lippincott-Raven Publishers, Philadelphia, 1996.

20

Cultural Issues and Epilepsy

Patricia Dean

Caring for individuals with epilepsy and their families includes strategic support of the patient's and family's efforts to live with this disorder. Health care professionals do this by providing an explanation of what epilepsy is, why people have seizures, and what they must do to control them. We also attempt to help them incorporate this altered health status into their lifestyle. If these interventions are to be successful, an understanding of these patient's viewpoint is necessary. Because culture is the way that people perceive, behave in, and evaluate their world, intervention strategies must be culturally driven. Cultural sensitivity and appreciation are essential parts of providing holistic patient care in the present increasingly multiracial society. Health care providers must be sensitive to the unique cultural surroundings from which their clients emerge so that health problems can be adequately assessed and realistic interventions planned (Harwood, 1981). Increasing numbers of anthropologic studies involving various ethnic groups in the United States show that cultural identification and values are retained for generations and that these play a significant role in behavior under conditions of health or illness. Ethnic and cultural values influence people in their perception of health, reactions to illness, levels of information, trust in treatment sources, and attitudes towards health care services (Long et al., 1988). Demographic studies show that the United States is rapidly becoming a multicultural, pluralistic society. Health care professionals must recognize the value and importance of culturally appropriate care so that they can be effective health care providers. Intervention strategies planned for a Cuban–American with epilepsy must be different from those planned for an African–American. It is time to learn differing perspectives about culture.

DEFINITION OF CULTURE

To provide culturally sensitive care, an understanding of culture is necessary. Webster (1984) defines culture as the totality of socially transmitted behavior patterns, arts, beliefs, institutions, and all other products of human work and thought typical of a population or community at a given time. Other definitions of culture are offered in the nursing literature by a cadre of nurse theorists and researchers who are attempting to develop knowledge in this area. Leininger (1978) states that culture comprises the learned, shared, and transmitted values, beliefs, norms, and lifeway practices of a particular group, which guides thinking, decisions, and actions in patterned ways. Boyle and Andrews (1989) believe that culture represents a unique way of perceiving, behaving in, and evaluating the external environment, and therefore provides a blueprint for determining values, beliefs, and practices. Spector (1991) suggests that culture is a metacommunication system based on nonphysical traits, such as values, beliefs, attitudes, customs, language, and behaviors, which are shared by a group and passed down through generations. All of these definitions suggest that cultures are specific and distinctive. Culture defines who a person is and determines how that person will respond in a given situation. It consists of all the aspects of life that influence individual attitudes and behaviors. It is a universal phenomenon, and no one escapes the effects of cultural background (Charonko, 1992). The assumptions of one culture are not necessarily shared by another, a point that must be appreciated when the health care professional is dealing with patients from different cultural backgrounds.

CULTURAL ASSESSMENTS AND EPILEPSY

The professional must be prepared to provide culturally appropriate care for each patient, regardless of the person's cultural background. This requires some understanding of the patient's culture. Many aspects of a culture are important to understand, but it is not possible to learn the infinite details of every culture. It is, however, important to assume that such variations occur and to learn how they might affect health practices (Kleinman et al., 1978). Cultural background must include assessment of patients because it can give meaning to behaviors and attitudes that might otherwise be judged negatively. No cultural heritage can wholly explain how a given individual will think and act, but it can help health care professionals to anticipate and to understand how and why people make certain decisions (Groce and Zola, 1993).

Obviously, the first step to understanding a person's beliefs is being able to exchange information, and language and communication are therefore the first components of an assessment. Next, because health and illness are defined, perceived, and treated within a cultural context, it is imperative to develop an understanding of the range of epilepsy-specific beliefs, values, and practices within cultural milieu of a given patient (Long et al., 1988).

LANGUAGE AND COMMUNICATION

Language is a repository of culture and comprises a good deal of the individual's self-identity (Smart and Smart, 1992). Speaking the language of the country from which a person has emigrated suggests an affiliation with that cultural group and its belief systems. Although the ideal scenario is for the health care professional to speak the language of the individual, when this is not possible a translator is imperative. However, communications are altered when a translator is used. No two languages are identical, and it is never possible to provide an exact translation from one language to another. Translators have the power to quantify as well as qualify the information between the patient and practitioner. Therefore, it is important to clarify and review the information and situation with the interpreter (Halton, 1992).

Even without understanding of a person's spoken language, the health care provider can attempt to understand some of the nonverbal communication techniques. In dealing with patients from another culture, interactions should be conducted in a nonthreatening, unhurried manner, and should observe acceptable social and cultural amenities (Giger and Davidhizar, 1995). For example, eye contact and touching have some unique cultural implications in various groups. In dealing with Hispanic patients, even when a translator is present, good eye contact should be maintained, because the various Hispanic cultures tend to be very tactile in their expression. Some Hispanics may subscribe to the concept of *mal ojo* (evil eye), the belief that a stronger person can look at a weaker person and cause ill health or injury. This belief is particularly applied to children. When examining or admiring a child, the professional should maintain hands-on contact to dispel this fear (da Silva, 1984). Many Haitians also view eye contact as respectful and express themselves with touch. In contrast, many persons of Asian descent, as well as some Native Americans, consider avoidance of eye contact a sign of respect. The health care provider should recognize this, limit eye contact, and also understand that the patient may be attentive and interested even though eye contact is being avoided (Kozier et al., 1993). Respecting and recognizing these and other behaviors as characteristics of cultural background places the health care provider at an advantage in relationships with patients and families.

CULTURE, HEALTH BELIEFS, AND HEALTH PRACTICES

Although many studies, articles, chapters, and texts have addressed culturally perceived causes for illness, these are not necessarily specific to epilepsy. However, most ethnic health beliefs have common themes: natural forces, supernatural forces, and the imbalance between forces. There are many similarities among cultures regarding prevention and treatment of illness. For example, most cultures use a variety of home remedies, which are almost always benign. These folk remedies are usually compatible with a medical regimen and can be used to reinforce the treatment plan. Many ethnic communities possess folk healers who have the ability to "cure" maladies. In the Mexican–American community it is the *curandero*; in the Puerto Rican community it is the *espirituista*. Native Americans can consult a variety of healers. Some offer nonsacred treatments, whereas others perform services or effect cures through spiritual means. Some Asians subscribe to a belief in herbalists or practitioners knowledgeable in treatments practiced in Asia. In the Haitian culture, belief in the powers of supernatural spirits is prevalent. Many illnesses are viewed as caused by others wishing harm or evil. There are often "priests" within the community that can help them to reverse these curses. These healers are very powerful persons in their community. They speak the language of the family, combine ritual with prayer, and exhibit a sincere interest in the family and the problem. Although sometimes the belief in the folk practitioner might delay medical treatment, these practitioners usually suggest medical care if their treatment is not successful (Whaley and Wong, 1991).

Wearing of amulets, medals, and other religious relics believed by the culture to protect the individual or to promote healing is also common. The value of these practices to the patient must be recognized. People do not abandon their traditional beliefs just because they have been offered an explanation of the physiologic basis of epilepsy. Even if the explanation is readily accepted, this does not mean that the former belief will disappear. It is often more practical to find ways to incorporate these beliefs and practices into the treatment plan rather than wasting energy and time in trying to dispel them.

CULTURALLY PERCEIVED CAUSES OF EPILEPSY

Many people have beliefs and behaviors surrounding health and illness that are part of their culture. Even within general American society, beliefs and practices such as "feed a cold," "starve a fever," "disasters come in three," and "knock on wood" are still exercised, often unconsciously. It is not surprising, therefore, that a medical condition as mysterious as epilepsy can appear to have acquired multiple explanations regarding cause and treatment (Long et al., 1993). It is important to determine if there is a culturally perceived cause for the epilepsy or related disabilities because such a perception tends to color all other aspects of the family's and the community's attitudes toward the affected individual (Groce and Zola, 1993).

In some cultures, seizures are believed result from possession by an evil spirit or to represent a supernatural punishment for breach of taboo. Levy et al. (1987), in their book about seizures among the Navajo indians, report that the Navajo believe that sibling incest produces the signs of the major epileptic seizure. This Navajo disease, called "moth madness," creates a role for the patient that is entirely disvalued. This situation prompted them to study the attitudes of the families of Navajo children with epilepsy. They suspected that the families would withdraw emotional support and thus create emotional disturbances soon after the onset of the disorder. They hypothesized that community disapproval would intensify these problems during adolescence and adulthood, making adjustment to life very difficult. A study group of 46 Navajos and 42 Pueblos was identified.

The Pueblos were chosen as a comparison group because they do not believe that seizures are caused by incest or by any specific etiology. Inclusion criteria included having an active seizure disorder and onset of epilepsy before the age of 20. Exclusion criteria included convulsions that were a direct result of a preexisting emotional trauma (i.e., excessive drinking leading to head trauma) and mental retardation. Navajos were found to have social and emotional problems more often ($p<0.05$) than Pueblos.

These authors (Levy et al., 1987) also examined the attitudes of parents of young children from both groups. There were overprotective parents in both groups, but the overprotective Navajo parents tended to keep the child isolated. The characteristic attitude of the Navajo parents was withdrawal. Preschool-aged Navajo children tended to be brought to the hospital for treatment of seizures less often than Pueblo children. School-aged children were most often monitored and given medication by school nurses and counselors who maintained contact with the hospital. They reported that Pueblo parents tried to treat the child as normally as possible. Parents talked to the child's siblings and the neighbors' children so that they would act calmly when witnessing a seizure and would not tease the child. These children developed normally until they were old enough to realize that having seizures made them different from other children, which usually occurred in junior high school, at which time problems began to surface. The outward placidity of the Pueblo parents masked a tendency to deny the serious and chronic nature of the problem. Although children were brought to the hospital when seizures occurred, parents were resistant to the fact that it was a chronic condition and that the child would have to cope alone at some time in the future. By not discussing the epilepsy and answering questions, the parents did not help the child to develop any coping mechanisms. These authors found that after the age of 14 years Pueblo adolescents with epilepsy experienced emotional problems with the same frequency as Navajo teenagers, but not with the same degree of severity. Neither group was well maintained on medications, and seizures tended to recur frequently as a result (Levy et al., 1987). This work by Levy and colleagues confirms the importance of cultural assessment. Whereas one might have had the tendency to lump Native Americans into one group, it emphasizes the distinctiveness of cultures. It points out that individual intervention strategies must be formulated for persons of different cultural backgrounds. Moreover, it demonstrates the impact of a person's cultural beliefs on how health care is accessed and how standard treatment plans are followed.

THE TRANSCULTURAL DEMONSTRATION PROJECT

In recognition of the need to develop a better understanding of epilepsy among ethnic and cultural groups and to find more effective ways of reaching these groups and making services more accessible, the board of directors of the Epilepsy Foundation of America (EFA) called for an initiative that culminated in the launching of the Transcultural Demonstration Project in 1986. It targeted Afro–Americans, Cubans, and Haitians in Dade County, Florida, an ethnically and culturally diverse area. The first phase of the project consisted of an ethnographic field study among these communities, designed to elicit answers to the following questions:

How do individuals and families in these ethnic groups recognize epilepsy, and what do they consider to be its nature and treatment?

Who are the key figures that influence individual and family health care practices?

What are some of the special needs of the individuals with epilepsy and their families in the community?

What are some of the unique strengths and resources of these groups, and how can they be utilized to address the needs of people with epilepsy?

The Epilepsy Rapid Assessment Procedure (ERAP) was a tool developed to examine epilepsy-specific beliefs, attitudes, and behaviors in ethnic communities. Eighty-one individuals in 43 Cuban, Afro–American, and Haitian households participated in this study, which addressed general health beliefs, epilepsy-specific beliefs, access to, perceptions, and utilization of existing biomedical and traditional epilepsy-specific health services, and family interaction and psychosocial concerns related to epilepsy. Sample households included those from the general population, households in which a family member with epilepsy was currently using the general health care system, households whose family member with epilepsy was not currently using the health care system, and households in which a family member with epilepsy was using the Cuban–American clinical health care system.

Many of the results of the study emphasize the similarities of cultures rather than the differences. Most people in all three groups recognized tonic–clonic seizures as a form of epilepsy, a medical condition that could be controlled by medication. Likewise, spirit possession was listed as a label for these symptoms. Absence and complex partial seizures were usually not recognized as seizures. Cubans and Afro–Americans labeled absence seizures as daydreaming, distraction, or normal childhood behavior. Haitian informants often viewed absence seizures as symptoms caused by nutritional deficiencies, malnutrition, or exhaustion, and Cuban participants often interpreted symptoms of complex partial seizures as nervous conditions or reactions to stress. Afro–American informants viewed them as symptoms of nervous breakdowns, mental problems, stress, or substance abuse. The Haitians believed that these symptoms were related to mental problems or insanity. The informants cited both physical and nonphysical causes, whereas health professionals in general recognized only the physical causes of epilepsy. Perceived physical causes of seizures tended to be related to the brain, illness, substance abuse, and hot and cold belief systems. In addition, Haitians believed that deficiencies of proteins and vitamins were factors. The Cubans believed the causes to be emotional, spiritual, and occasionally the result of mental influence. Afro–Americans tended to believe in emotional and stress-related causes. Haitian informants' beliefs regarding the causes of seizures included spiritual, emotional, and mental components.

The beliefs in nonphysical causes of seizure symptoms among Cubans, Afro–Americans, and Haitians have important implications for treatment. Often, when seizure symptoms are believed to be caused by emotional, mental, or spiritual problems, individuals seek treatment from practitioners in these areas. Mental health professionals, herbalists, and spiritualists were sought out when seizure symptoms were viewed as physical but were believed to be caused by an underlying emotional or spiritual problem.

In each ethnic group there were specific names for symptoms other than seizures: "spells," "fits," "crisis," or *ataques*. Haitians used the Creole term *mal cadie* to refer to epilepsy. The term *crise* was used to refer to the individual's seizure. Epilepsy appeared to be a greater stigma in the Haitian community than in the Afro–American or the Cuban community. The perceived role of supernatural forces as a cause of epilepsy has a strong impact on the manner in which those with the condition were viewed in the community. In general, epilepsy was a "hidden condition" in the Miami Haitian community. Individuals with seizure disorders were often isolated and feared by those aware of their condition. Individuals with epilepsy in these communities reported that they were faced with considerable limitations because of the public's perception of their condition.

SUMMARY

The studies cited in this chapter about the epilepsy-related beliefs of the Navajo and Pueblo indians, and by some members of the Dade County community, are small ethnographic studies and do not reflect definitively the beliefs of all members of those cultures. They do suggest the need to explore cultural beliefs and behaviors as they apply to epilepsy. Providers of health care to people with epilepsy encounter people of many different racial and ethnic backgrounds. Some have become so acculturated to the majority culture that their health beliefs and practices are consistent with those of the health care system. However, there are those whose traditional practices and beliefs are still an integral part of their daily lives (Whaley and Wong, 1991). Providers must be sensitive to the uniqueness of these patients. They must include cultural background as part of their assessment and must try to adapt ethnic practices to fit into the plan of care rather than to attempt to change long-standing beliefs.

"The benefits of adding transcultural awareness to the provision of services for epilepsy go beyond improving access to services and treatment for populations which are chronically underserved. As the richness of each cultural perspective unfolds through the exploration and sensitive patient and family interviewing by health professionals, so does the fascination with the belief systems, as the bridges to better services are built" (Long et al., 1993).

REFERENCES

Boyle J, Andrews M. *Transcultural concepts in nursing care.* Glenview, IL: Scott, Foresman, 1989.

Charonko C. Cultural influences in "noncompliant" behaviors and decision making. *Holist Nursi Pract* 1992;6:73–8.

da Silva G. Awareness of Hispanic cultural issues in the health care setting. *Child Health Care* 1984;1: 4–10.

Giger J, Davidhizar R. *Transcultural nursing assessment and intervention,* 2nd ed. St. Louis, MO: Mosby, 1995.

Groce N, Zola I. Multiculturalism, chronic illness and disability. *Pediatrics* 1993;91:1048–55.

Halton D. Information transmission in bilingual, bicultural contexts. *J Commun Health Nurs* 1992;9: 53–9.

Harwood A. *Guidelines for culturally appropriate health care: ethnicity and medical care.* Cambridge, MA: Harvard University Press, 1981.

Kleinman A, Eisenberg L, Good B. Culture, illness and care: clinical lessons from anthropological and cross-cultural research. *Ann Intern Med* 1978;88:251–8.

Kozier B, Erb G, Blaise K, Johnson S, Smith-Temple J. *Techniques in clinical nursing,* 2nd ed. Menlo Park, CA: Addison-Wesley, 1993.

Leininger M. *Transcultural nursing: concepts, theories, and practices.* New York: John Wiley & Sons, 1978.

Levy J, Neutra R, Parker D. *Hand trembling, frenzy witchcraft and moth madness: a study of Navajo epilepsy.* Tuscon, AZ: University of Arizona Press, 1987.

Long A, Scrimshaw S, Hernandez N. Epilepsy in the transcultural community: Cubans, American blacks, and Haitians in Dade County, FL, 1993 [*unpublished*].

Long A, Scrimshaw S, Hurtado E. *Epilepsy Rapid Assessment Procedures (ERAP): rapid assessment procedures for the evaluation of epilepsy specific beliefs, attitudes and behaviors.* Landover, MD: Epilepsy Foundation of America, 1988.

Smart J, Smart D. Cultural issues in the rehabilitation of Hispanics. *J Rehab* 1992;April, May, June: 29–37.

Spector R. *Cultural Diversity in health and illness,* 3rd ed. Norwalk, CT: Appleton and Lange, 1991.

Webster's II New Riverside University Dictionary. Boston: Riverside Publishing, 1988.

Whaley L, Wong D. *Nursing care of infants and children.* 4th ed. St. Louis, MO: CW Mosby, 1991.

Managing Seizure Disorders: A Handbook for Health Care Professionals, edited by N. Santilli, Lippincott-Raven Publishers, Philadelphia, 1996.
© 1996 Epilepsy Foundation of America.

21

Legal Advocacy

David F. Chavkin

The nurse, along with other health care professionals, serves as a central player in identifying, diagnosing, and managing an individual's epilepsy. Each of these professionals can make a significant contribution in protecting the legal rights of that individual.

Health care professionals working with and in communities are in direct contact, often on a day-to-day basis, with the individual with epilepsy. They are directly familiar with the individuals and with their degree of seizure control, the type(s) of seizures, whether the person experiences an "aura" (warning), the person's reliability in taking prescribed antiepileptic drugs (AEDs), any side effects of such AEDs, and the functioning of the individual in home and work settings. Many of these aspects become critical in defining the legal rights and responsibilities of the person with epilepsy.

CONFLICTING TENSIONS

There are two related legal factors that might be described as conflicting tensions. These factors run throughout any discussion of the legal rights and responsibilities of an individual with epilepsy.

The first of these factors focuses on the rights of the individual with epilepsy. Although phrased somewhat differently, depending on the specific factual context and law being applied, the basic right is to be free from discrimination on the basis of disability. The goal, as defined by the Epilepsy Foundation of America (EFA), is to have an individualized determination of the individual based on that individual's strengths and weaknesses and not based on stereotypes or stigmas that bear little relation to reality. This is also the central theme of the Americans With Disabilities Act (ADA) of 1990.

The second of these factors focuses on the responsibilities of the person with epilepsy. The basic goal is to hold the individual accountable for volitional acts. In many ways, this is simply the mirror image of the antidiscrimination goal described above.

Any discussion of the legal rights and responsibilities of persons with epilepsy must necessarily focus on the first of these factors. The history of society's treatment of persons with epilepsy is largely a history of discriminatory treatment, due either to hostile or to protective motivations. However, with regard to the discussion of such issues as epilepsy as a defense for criminal conduct, some discussion of this second factor is also necessary.

THE ADVOCACY ROLE

Just as health care providers play a variety of roles in the context of medical care, they will play several roles in the context of legal advocacy. These roles will frequently include the following.

Identification

An individual or family will often discuss problems without labeling these problems as legal. A father may express concern over the appropriateness of an educational program for his son with epilepsy; a mother with epilepsy may discuss a pending custody battle with an ex-husband in which her fitness as a parent has been questioned; a worker with epilepsy may describe discrimination that she is experiencing on the job.

In each of these situations, the health care professional may be the person who will have to identify the potential legal aspects of each of these fact patterns. Identification of legal issues will therefore be a critical aspect of care.

Basic Advice

Although health care professionals will not be providing legal advice, basic information and advice will necessarily be provided. For example, a parent who is working through a special education problem should be advised to maintain copies of all correspondence with the school board and to send letters by certified mail. Similarly, a worker who is dealing with a job-related problem might be advised to review these job duties with a neurologist and to consider having the neurologist contact the employer to lessen the likelihood of discrimination.

In this way, the health care professional is not providing legal advice but is performing two critical duties: first, helping to ensure that a record will be preserved for legal review and second, identifying possible avenues for recourse and resolution short of formal legal intervention.

Legal Referral

The third basic role of the health care provider is to refer individuals and families to appropriate legal resources. Nurses and social workers already maintain or have access to inventories of community resources. By including legal resources within the framework of this referral role, they can help to link the individual or family with needed legal assistance.

Emotional Support

Sometimes the most important role that the professional can play is simply to support the client or patient. Legal disputes can take a significant toll on the individual or family. Level-headed persistence is often the key to achieving legal rights. The role of the professional in supporting, calming, redirecting, and encouraging should therefore not be underestimated.

IDENTIFYING THE CLIENT

One problem that frequently arises for lawyers and that will arise as well for health care professionals is keeping the identity of the client clearly in mind. Often a professional will be contacted by a parent, relative, or friend on behalf of a person with epilepsy. This well-meaning individual may have the best interests of the person with epilepsy at heart but may want to pursue a course of conduct that is not consistent with the wishes of the individual being "helped."

In such situations the professional must balance the desire to be responsive to the contacting person against the ethical obligation to the client or patient. As with other ethical dilemmas, no clear lines can be drawn. However, it is the wishes of the person with epilepsy that must ultimately be respected.

LEGAL ADVOCACY ISSUES

The following discussion of legal issues is by no means exhaustive in identifying the potential areas of legal concern or in discussing the specific subject areas. Rather, the discussion is designed to give a sense of the kinds of factual patterns that may involve legal rights. The goal should be to get a sense that if the treatment of a person with epilepsy does not seem fair, there may be a legal remedy to redress that grievance.

Adoption

Epilepsy may arise as an issue in adoption in one of two ways. First, a person's fitness as an adoptive parent may be questioned because of having epilepsy. Second, adoptive parents may try to annul the adoption of a child who develops epilepsy.

The main concern in adoption is the best interests of the child. The ability of the prospective parent or parents to care for and provide a suitable home for the child are necessarily relevant. In almost all states, the epilepsy of a prospective parent or parents would be considered along with all other factors in evaluating parenting ability.

For the vast majority of persons with epilepsy, the existence of epilepsy should not affect their ability to adopt. However, legal advocacy may be necessary to overcome an agency's resistance to adoption.

Only one state considers the development of a disability by a child as a legitimate basis for annulment of an adoption. Children with epilepsy should not be singled out as a class in adoption matters. Laws that promote unnecessary and unfair labeling of persons with disabilities may produce a life of segregation and resultant stigma.

To encourage adoption for "hard-to-place" children, special federal and state adoption assistance programs are available. Children with severe, disabling epilepsy may qualify under this program for special assistance. Legal advocacy may be appropriate to ensure that a child qualifies for this assistance to increase the likelihood of adoption. Provision of special assistance may also provide the incentive necessary to persuade a well-intentioned family to maintain an adopted child.

Child Custody

As in adoption, the best interests of the child or children are the main concern in a custody award. The disability of a parent is usually considered in deciding what custody arrangement is in the best interests of the child or children.

More and more courts have recognized that a parent's disability does not necessarily interfere with the fitness of that parent. Court decisions have therefore held that a parent's disability is simply one of the factors to be considered in making an award. This type of individualized evaluation is particularly important for parents with epilepsy, because it is rare that a parent's epilepsy will warrant denial of custody.

The issue of a child's epilepsy may also arise in a custody dispute. As with a parent's epilepsy, a child's epilepsy is a relevant factor but should not be the sole factor in determining what custody arrangement is best suited to the child's needs.

In both of these situations, legal advocacy is usually necessary to provide representation in the custody proceeding. Because knowledge of epilepsy is not ordinarily imparted in law school, health care professionals may have a special role in educating the attorneys and court about the effect of a person's epilepsy on the relevant issues. Pertinent information on the effect of a person's epilepsy on such issues is found in Chaps. 14 and 17.

Criminal Justice

Individuals with epilepsy may become entangled in the criminal justice system for the same reasons as persons without epilepsy. To the extent that epilepsy is not a factor in the specific conduct at issue, a person with epilepsy should be held to the same legal standard as anyone else. However, there are some special considerations that affect only individuals with epilepsy.

The first of these considerations relates to the misinterpretation of seizure-related conduct. During seizures or the period of confusion that may follow a seizure, people are sometimes mistaken for being under the influence of alcohol or illegal drugs. When this occurs, the person may be unjustifiably arrested for being drunk and disorderly, for creating a public disturbance, or for being under the influence of drugs. If the person wears or carries medical alert identification, this may be avoided. If seizures involving these behaviors are uncontrolled, it may be in the individual's best interest to discuss the situation with local authorities and the rescue squad to allow maximal independence. A number of educational materials have been developed just for this purpose. The video "Take Another Look," for police officers is just one. See Appendix D, EFA Resources, for a listing.

If these situations cannot be prevented, then legal advocacy will be necessary to defend the individual with epilepsy from criminal charges. This advocacy may require educating the defense attorney about epilepsy and providing materials necessary to educate the court and prosecuting attorney as well.

A different problem will arise if a person with epilepsy is incarcerated before trial or after being convicted of a criminal offense. The adequacy of medical care in correctional facilities has been a continuing topic of controversy. A nurse may provide service in one of these facilities or may have assisted an individual who now is incarcerated. In such cases, the nurse may have to assist the individual in seeking appropriate medical care while in custody, including provision of medication. Ultimately, legal advocacy may be necessary to enforce statutory or constitutional protections of appropriate health care.

Driver's Licensing

Especially for professionals working with teenagers, young adults, workers, and the elderly with new-onset seizures, driver's licensing is a commonly confronted legal issue. Most states require applicants for a driver's license with epilepsy to be seizure-free for a specified period of time and to submit a physician's evaluation of their ability to drive safely. Some states permit exceptions to the seizure-free period, e.g., for persons with strictly nocturnal seizures, for those who have a prolonged aura, or for those who had a seizure as a result of a physician-directed medication change but who are now expected to remain seizure-free. The EFA's model driver licensing law recommends that states generally use a 3-month seizure-free period, with exceptions if certain positive or negative factors exist. The model was developed in conjunction with the American Academy of Neurology and the American Epilepsy Society. Copies of the model law are available from EFA's Legal Advocacy Department.

Because of the importance of a driver's license in our society, the professional may need to assist a patient in securing a license or in maintaining one that is threatened with revocation. Ordinarily there is an opportunity for a hearing before a hearing officer or before a medical board. Although an attorney is usually needed to represent the individual, the health care professional can provide important information during the review proceeding.

It may be necessary to testify about the patient's compliance with a medication regimen. The health care professional may also be able to give an expert opinion about the likelihood that the patient will comply with license restrictions, and may therefore be of critical importance in increasing the mobility and opportunities of the individual with epilepsy.

Education

Educational issues may arise at almost any time in the life of the person with epilepsy. As children, persons with epilepsy may be prevented from engaging in certain school activities, or they may not receive an appropriate educational program because of unaddressed barriers related to the epilepsy. In higher education, students may be denied entrance into certain career training programs or may be denied requested accommodations.

Federal and state laws provide important protections from discrimination in education. The Individuals with Disabilities Education Act (IDEA) requires every state and local educational agency to provide every child with a disability with a free, appropriate public education. The ADA prohibits discrimination in public services and places of public accommodation. Section 504 of the Rehabilitation Act of 1973 prohibits discrimination on the basis of disability in educational programs by recipients of federal financial assistance. State antidiscrimination laws may also prohibit discrimination by public and private schools, colleges, and universities.

The role of the health care professional necessarily includes support for parents of children with epilepsy and encouragement not to accept an educational program that does not meet their children's needs. The professional may need to participate in interdisciplinary team meetings to plan a child's educational program. As in other areas, it may also be necessary to assist the parents or adult students in linking up with legal resources. For information on education resources, see Chap. 22.

Employment

People with epilepsy frequently experience great difficulty in obtaining and retaining employment. They are often denied jobs or not trained for work they could do well and safely because of an unreasoned fear of their seizures. Educating employers, co-workers, and the general public can help to break down these barriers and to increase the likelihood of full employment of persons with epilepsy. This has proven to be a long and difficult process. Until understanding and acceptance of people with epilepsy become more widespread, it is crucial for their employment rights and opportunities to be protected by effective, enforceable laws.

There are important federal and state laws that protect employees in many employment settings from discrimination on the basis of handicap. The ADA applies to employers with 15 or more employees. The ADA prohibits discrimination against qualified individuals with disabilities and requires employers to make reasonable accommodation. In addition, the Rehabilitation Act of 1973 protects employees of federal agencies, of private employers receiving significant government contracts, and of private employers receiving federal financial assistance. State laws frequently cover all but the smallest employers.

Legal protections vary from state to state. However, state laws commonly prohibit employers from refusing to hire, retain, or promote employees with disabilities who are able to safely and effectively perform the requirements of the job without accommodations or with reasonable accommodations. An accommodation is a modification in the job. An accommodation is reasonable if it is not too costly and if it does not require substantial modifications in job responsibilities.

A practice that often has the effect of screening out qualified applicants with epilepsy is the use of pre-employment inquiries. The ADA, the Rehabilitation Act, and many state laws prohibit such inquiries about an applicant's health or disability.

Professionals working with patients with epilepsy frequently identify fact patterns indicating possible employment discrimination. A long-standing employee with epilepsy who has consistently received high evaluations may be denied a promotion because of the perceived stress that the new position might create. Another employee may describe job safety restrictions that impede the performance of job duties and that are not required to accommodate the individual's epilepsy. Or, an employee may report being laid off or terminated after a seizure on the job.

These and similar actions by employers may be prohibited by state and federal antidiscrimination laws. However, enforcement actions usually depend on the filing of a timely complaint, either before the administrative agency with responsibility for enforcement or before an appropriate court. Because complaints usually must be filed within relatively short time limits (e.g., 180 days), it is important to encourage and, when necessary, assist the patient in pursuing these remedies. More information on epilepsy and employment is found in Chap. 18. For legal advice about specific job-related problems, individuals should consult with a local attorney.

Financial Assistance

The patient with epilepsy may need income support. This need may predominate over all other problems. Especially for those persons who are unemployed or underemployed, financial assistance may be necessary to meet basic requirements of food, shelter, and clothing. A social worker is usually in the best position to assist the individual with epilepsy in meeting these needs.

There are essentially two types of income assistance programs that should be kept in mind. The first of these types is the federally administered program. The second is the state or locally administered program.

The federal programs are usually administered by one of two agencies: the Social Security Administration or the Department of Veterans Affairs. The Social Security Administration administers the retirement, survivors, and disability social insurance programs for current and former workers and their families. The Social Security Administration also administers the welfare program of Supplemental Security Income (SSI) for aged, blind, and disabled low-income persons. The Department of Veterans Affairs provides financial assistance for veterans who are disabled by an injury or disease incurred in or aggravated by active service in the line of duty, whether during wartime or peacetime.

At the state or local level, financial assistance may be available through the Aid to Families with Dependent Children (AFDC) program for individuals with minor children. Financial assistance may also be available for low-income adults under general assistance or home relief programs.

Each of these programs has its own general eligibility criteria and may have specific provisions relating to people with epilepsy. Although the requirements are fairly complex and vary from program to program, one common thread runs through all of these programs. Eligibility is often the reward for persistence. Many qualified individuals are turned down initially and never pursue appeal rights. As a result, they do not receive the financial assistance they are qualified for and so desperately need.

The health care professional plays an essential role in encouraging the patient not to give up and to pursue appeal rights. The professional may be a necessary witness in any appeal proceeding to testify about the problems that the patient faces in performing activities of daily living or to testify about the extent to which the patient's epilepsy may interfere with employment, and may also be needed to ensure that the patient secures effective legal assistance.

Insurance

People with epilepsy have serious difficulties obtaining adequate insurance at reasonable rates. This problem applies particularly to health insurance and is due to the insurance industry's belief that people with epilepsy are likely to cost the companies money by submitting large or frequent claims. These difficulties have persisted for many years despite advances in medical treatment that enable the vast majority of people with epilepsy to achieve partial or complete seizure control.

Insurance is one of the areas that has been least touched by the disability rights movement. Although many states have laws that ban discrimination on the basis of disability in the issuance of insurance policies, few actions have been undertaken by state insurance commissions or by private parties. Because of the uncertain promise of legal actions in this area, families who have been denied insurance may want to consult with an independent insurance broker about their options. If they believe that an insurer has acted illegally, they may want to seek the advice of the state Insurance Commission or a local attorney.

The other alternative that may be available depends on state legislative initiatives on insurance. Many states have established assigned-risk auto insurance plans that include persons who have been unable to obtain insurance from the regular insurance market. Some states have also created shared-risk health insurance plans aimed at persons who have been unable to obtain standard health coverage. Many of the managed care programs available as part of employment benefits do not have preexisting waiting periods. Although insurance should be available without discrimination on the basis of disability or employment, until this goal is realized it is important to identify these types of special programs for use by affected families.

Medical Assistance

Just as persons with epilepsy may have a need for financial assistance to meet basic needs, such persons may also need government support for coverage of medical expenses. This need is compounded by the inadequate treatment provided by many private health insurance carriers.

There are two major governmental medical assistance programs: Medicare and Medicaid. These programs are frequently confused by individuals, and their eligibility and coverage requirements are seldom understood.

Medicare is a health insurance program provided by the federal government primarily to those persons eligible for Social Security benefits who are at least 65 years of age or who have received Social Security disability insurance benefits for at least 24 months. Part A of Medicare provides coverage, after payment of deductibles by the patient, for hospital services, skilled nursing services, and home health services. Part B of Medicare provides coverage, subject to co-insurance paid by the patient, for physician services, home health services, and durable medical equipment.

Medicaid is a welfare program administered by the states and provided with federal financial assistance primarily to families with children, to the aged, to the blind, and to the disabled. Eligibility requirements vary significantly from state to state, and coverage of services also varies widely. However, most states provide a range of inpatient and outpatient services, including physician services and prescription drugs, to low-income persons in the above groups.

Confusing eligibility requirements and frequently unresponsive bureaucratic systems combine to deny many eligible persons the coverage they deserve. As with financial assistance programs, level-headed persistence is the key to realizing the entitlement to services theoretically guaranteed by federal and state law.

Again, as with financial assistance programs, there is an important role for health care professionals in realizing this goal.

In focusing on the Medicare and Medicaid programs, the professional should not lose sight of the other programs that may be available to meet some or all of the costs of diagnosis and treatment of persons with epilepsy. For example, community health centers and migrant health centers are an important national resource for low-income persons with epilepsy. Maternal and child health programs may also be available to provide some needed services. Department of Veterans Affairs benefits may include outpatient medical and dental treatment, hospitalization, vocational rehabilitation, and educational training.

LEGAL RESOURCES

Throughout this discussion of legal advocacy there has been repeated reference to the need to link persons with epilepsy with legal resources. In addition to private attorneys, who can be identified by word of mouth or through local bar referral services, the following additional resources may be available in a local community.

Protection and Advocacy Systems

Every state has a protection and advocacy system funded in part by the federal government under the Developmental Disabilities Assistance and Bill of Rights Act. These systems have the responsibility for protecting the rights of persons with developmental disabilities, including epilepsy, and for advocating on their behalf. Many of these systems provide direct legal assistance; other systems have a comprehensive referral network.

Legal Services Programs

Every state and most local areas have a legal services (or legal aid) program funded in part under the federal Legal Services Corporation Act. These programs provide legal assistance in noncriminal matters to low-income persons.

Public Defender Programs

Every community has a public defender program designed to provide legal assistance in criminal matters to low-income persons. Some of these programs restrict representation to those persons faced with potential incarceration (rather than merely a fine) for a criminal offense. Public defender programs vary from staffed-office models to offices that contract with private attorneys.

Legal Services for the Elderly

Every state and most local areas have legal services programs funded in part under the Older Americans Act. For older persons with epilepsy (over 60 in many states), legal assistance in noncriminal matters will be available under eligibility requirements that are somewhat more generous than under the Legal Services Corporation Act. These programs for the elderly are sometimes established as separate offices in legal services programs.

Pro-Bono Projects

Many local bar associations have established pro-bono projects to provide free or reduced-cost legal services through private attorneys. These projects are usually targeted at persons who have too much income for free legal services but who cannot afford prevailing private attorney fees.

State Human Rights Commissions

Most states have an agency that enforces state antidiscrimination laws and may also be designated to handle complaints under the ADA.

Legal Advocacy Department of the Epilepsy Foundation of America

Although there is no substitute for capable local counsel, the Legal Advocacy Department of the EFA can be an important resource for attorneys handling legal claims for persons with epilepsy. The Legal Advocacy Department maintains information on the various federal and state laws and the court decisions interpreting these laws. The department's phone number is (301) 459-3700. Clients can receive general information on legal and psychosocial issues such as employment and driver's licensing by calling EFA's information and referral department at (800) EFA-1000.

CONCLUSION

By the end of this section the health professional will probably not be in a position to square-off with Perry Mason in a courtroom. However, the role of the professional is probably even more important.

Every day many persons with epilepsy are subjected to discrimination based on their epilepsy. Too many of these individuals have no idea of their legal rights and never pursue legal remedies. By working with individuals and families, if appropriate, the professional can help them to calmly review their factual situations, assess their options, secure legal assistance when needed, and provide expert input to the attorney and client. In performing these functions, the professional can help to realize the overall goal of a society that treats individuals on the basis of their actual strengths and weaknesses and not on the basis of stereotypes or stigma.

Managing Seizure Disorders: A Handbook for Health Care Professionals, edited by N. Santilli, Lippincott-Raven Publishers, Philadelphia, 1996. © 1996 Epilepsy Foundation of America.

22

Accessing Community Resources

Marie Ormsby

Whether patient, parent, spouse, or sibling, the person who is dealing with a seizure disorder may discover the need for services beyond good medical care. Epilepsy, like other chronic disorders, can have an impact on many aspects of daily life. The loss of driving privileges because of uncontrolled seizures may jeopardize employment and thus insurance coverage, ability to be self-supporting, or ability to obtain medical care. A child's seizures may lead to academic failure, labeling as a "behavior problem," and difficulties in getting along with classmates.

Often, it is possible to avoid escalating problems through timely intervention and the use of suitable community resources. Even in small communities, public programs are available to meet many basic needs. In addition to tax-supported programs, private agencies and organizations provide a wide range of services to individuals and families. The nurse, social worker, or any other health care provider can be in a pivotal position to suggest resources for families or individuals.

SERVICES AVAILABLE

Although many health care providers can and often do provide community referrals to patients or families, it is important to be aware that information and referral (I & R) services are uniquely prepared to assist in identifying resources. These I & R services have comprehensive community information and are skilled in assessing needs and available services. For people with epilepsy, the following services might be explored.

The Epilepsy Foundation of America (EFA): Local affiliates provide information on community services in addition to their own programs. If there is no local listing under "Epilepsy," call 1-800-EFA-1000, the national toll-free number of the EFA. The EFA can also be contacted via Internet (postmaster@efa.org).

A local I & R service. Check social service listings, or call the toll-free number listed above. Information and referral services maintain a current database of local community resources.

A local United Way: Many offer formal information and referral services. If there is none serving your community, call EFA's toll-free number or contact them through the Internet (postmaster@efa.org).

The Area Agency on Aging: These agencies serving the elderly population maintain information and referral capacity; many of the agencies they list serve all ages. Check city or county listings.

Infant, Youth, and Family Services and Parenting Centers

These service organizations provide a wide variety of information on daycare providers, recreational programs, support services, educational services, and in some instances a toy lending library. If available, they are listed in the Yellow Pages or can be located through local listings or by contacting I&R services.

Community Service Boards

These agencies serve individuals and families in need of mental health and mental retardation services. They often provide direct services through a variety of programs and supports. Likewise, staff will serve as case managers.

Of the resources noted above, the local EFA affiliate is most directly involved with the problems of epilepsy and may have the services and programs that will most benefit a patient. In areas where no affiliate exists, the other agencies suggested may be tapped for information.

THE SOCIAL SERVICE SPECTRUM

The categories of services that follow have been arranged as an outline to help identify possible sources of help for patients and family members. If there is no community I & R serving your area, the outline might be used to develop the professional's own file of community services.

Support Groups

There are several types of support groups that have been developed to meet varying needs. Among them are:

Self-help groups, run by and for those with a personal involvement in epilepsy.

General support groups, using a professional as a leader or as a resource person; many serve an educational purpose for members.

Parent groups, offering a place where parents can share experiences and feelings; they may be self-run or professionally led. Parent groups are often instrumental in working for better community services as well.

Counseling groups, professionally led, which may deal with a wide variety of goals and purposes, from job preparation to psychotherapy.

Social or recreational groups, whose purpose is primarily to provide a way for people to get out and meet others. Add the local recreation or parks department to the list of general resources given above. Many religious organizations also have such programs.

Counseling Resources

There are many levels of counseling, and it is important to be sensitive to individual needs in suggesting services to a patient. A word of caution: The professional should know the resources and should be sure that they have some understanding of epilepsy and its special consequences.

Hospital social service departments, which are geared to helping with the practical aspects, e.g., discharge planning, but can also help a patient to deal with the personal and family impact of a diagnosis of epilepsy.

Social workers, who can be found in many of the settings suggested below. They also may be found in private practice; check the social service listings in the telephone book. Again, know the resource; many have specialized practices.

Psychologists, also providing counseling and therapy in a variety of settings. In addition, the majority of psychological and educational testing is administered by psychologists. For patients with epilepsy, the services of a neuropsychologist may facilitate more effective treatment, education, and habilitation.

Psychiatrists, as physicians, may be a resource for patients with complex or overwhelming psychiatric problems. Patients should be encouraged to consult with their neurologist about the need for psychiatric help.

Mental health clinics are staffed by the disciplines described above; in addition, they may refer patients to vocational or other community services.

Family service agencies provide individual and family counseling; some have special programs, such as therapy groups, which may meet particular needs.

School counselors can serve as liaison between home, school, and medical resources. They can also assist an individual child with problems and can work with the parents when referral to special services is being considered.

Clergy may also be considered as a counseling resource; this can be explored with individual patients.

Education

Epilepsy can affect a child's education in several ways. Absence seizures may be perceived as inattentiveness or behavior problems, and concentration, memory, and alertness may be affected by seizures or medications. Under federal and state laws, schools must provide appropriate education and special services to any child whose disability is impeding the ability to benefit from regular classroom education. If a child with a seizure disorder is having difficulty in school, the parents should be encouraged to work with both the doctor and the school to help the child achieve his or her full potential. The following resources can be suggested to parents:

The National Information Center for Handicapped Children and Youth
PO Box 1492
Washington, DC 20013
(800)-695-0285
1-(202)-884-8200
This is a national information clearinghouse for parents of children with disabilities.

The local director of special education, or the state office of special education. For addresses of state offices, contact the center noted above, or call EFA's toll-free line.

Head Start programs, which enroll a percentage of 3- and 4-year-olds with medical problems or disabilities.

Preschool Handicap Programs enroll children 2–5 years of age who have special needs that could potentially interfere with cognitive development. These are typically sponsored by the school system but sometimes are a joint venture with a local nonprofit organization such as The ARC.

Early Intervention Programs are emerging in each state as the result of Part H of the Individuals with Disabilities Education Act (IDEA). The state defines which children will be eligible for the services. Their purpose is to provide service to children from birth to 2 years who are at risk for developing disabilities. The lead agencies responsible for the program vary from state to state.

College aid, to assist young people with epilepsy. There are few special resources, but an excellent digest of scholarship resources for students with disabilities is available from:
HEATH Resource Center (Higher Education Adult Training for People with Handicaps)
One Dupont Circle
Washington, DC 20036
1-(800)-544-3284

The following organization may also be of help:
Federal Student Aid Information Center
Washington, DC
1-(800)-433-3243

Employment

Employment may become a difficult problem for people who have a seizure disorder or who develop seizures as adults (see Chap. 18). Employers' perceptions are frequently more of a barrier than the seizures themselves. Through its network of employment programs, the EFA has shown that people with seizure disorders are capable and competent employees. For employment questions, contact:

Employment, Training and Youth Services
Epilepsy Foundation of America
4351 Garden City Drive
Landover, MD 20785
1-(301)-459-3700

Local or state EFA affiliate: Many have employment programs; if not, they may be able to offer materials or guidance.

The national office of EFA: EFA has developed materials and offers programs through its local affiliates to link employers and job seekers. If there is a question of discrimination, EFA's Legal Advocacy Department can provide information about these issues by phone at (301) 459-3700.

The Department of Vocational Rehabilitation: This is a federally funded program designed to assist job-seekers with disabilities. Check local or county listings, or call the EFA.

Legal Assistance

Although the rights of people with epilepsy have been greatly enhanced through legislative changes and initiatives, there are issues, such as driving, for which specific requirements and restrictions are in place. The EFA has a Legal Advocacy Department that maintains current information on state and federal laws affecting the rights of people with epilepsy with regard to employment, driving, and other legal issues. The Department does not represent individual clients but it does provide information and resources to attorneys whose clients have epilepsy-related legal problems. Clients can be referred to direct services, such as:

Protection and advocacy agencies, directed to provide services that protect the rights of those with developmental disabilities.

Legal rights services, available to low-income clients.

Lawyer referral services, often operated by local bar associations.

Disability rights centers, specializing in issues related to disability law. For more information on legal issues, see Chap. 21.

Financial Aid

Most financial aid programs in the United States have statutory requirements for eligibility. They are typically administered by state and local social service departments, health departments, and Social Security offices; the specific agency structure may vary from state to state. It helps to build a network of contacts at these agencies who can help to assess the most likely source of help for a patient. If available, use the local EFA affiliate or I & R service as a way to seek help for patients who are not eligible for public programs. Major financial aid categories and possible resources include:

Income support, with three major categories: Supplemental Security Income (SSI), Social Security Disability Insurance (SSDI) for ex-workers who meet eligibility requirements, and Aid to Families with Dependent Children (AFDC) for unemployed parents with minor children.

Medical care, where the major public categories are Medicare (for the elderly and eligible disabled), Medicaid (for eligible low-income persons) and Services to Children with Special Health Needs, which offers health service to eligible children through age 21. The services of this program vary; check with the local or state health department.

Hospital care, which can sometimes be obtained through the provisions of the Hill–Burton Act. This federally administered program requires hospitals that receive Hill–Burton funds to provide a certain amount of free care to patients. Talk with the patient financial services of the local hospital, or call 1-(800)-638-0742 [in Maryland, 1-(800)-492-0359] for information about services.

Medications, often available at lower cost through local or national EFA membership. Members of national EFA can use the mail-order service operated by the American Association of Retired Person Services, Inc. (AARP). Explore local affiliates as well; some have local programs; some may have suggestions for arranging emergency supplies. Physicians and other health professionals can contact the following organization regarding the availability of a medication free of charge:

Prescription Drug Indigent Program (sponsored by the Pharmaceutical Manufacturers Association) 1-(800)-762-4636.

Health Care

Patients with seizures that are difficult to control may benefit from a consultation or from going to a comprehensive, multidisciplinary center for evaluation. This should also be considered for those whose daily lives are seriously impaired by drug side effects. Consider the following sources of information:

EFA, 1-(800)-332-1000: A national database, continually updated and expanded, contains information on hospitals, clinics and individual neurologists who have indicated that they treat people with epilepsy. Staff will discuss the patient's needs and send three or more names, with service description provided by the physician or facility to EFA.

Local EFA affiliates can provide specific local information on health care resources.

Local medical referral services.

Epilepsy Education

Patients and families who are well-informed about epilepsy are likely to be more successful in dealing with compliance, control of seizures, and the psychosocial aspects of seizure disorders. Current professional information and materials are available from:

The EFA's National Epilepsy Library, 1-(800)-332-4050, through which health professionals can receive a sample packet of patient education materials. In addition, the NEL has an in-house database of journal articles and other publications about the medical and psychosocial aspects of epilepsy, as well as an extensive collection of monographs, reports, symposia proceedings, government documents, and other materials about the comprehensive management of epilepsy. The NEL provides individualized responses to requests and document delivery.

Local EFA affiliates, which may provide in-school programs to educate teachers, school nurses, other school personnel, and students about epilepsy. These programs may include information on first aid, self-help and parent support groups, family action service programs, recreational programs for children and adults, public outreach programs and community education, community residences, and counseling. To contact an EFA affiliate, look under "Epilepsy" in the local telephone directory or call EFA's toll-free number, 1-(800)-EFA-1000.

Recreation

Everyone needs to have fun, but this is sometimes restricted for people with seizure disorders. It is important to encourage normal activity; restrictions (if any) should be determined by the physician, not by arbitrary rules. Many children and adults with seizure disorders participate in regular sports and recreation programs. If special programs are appropriate, check with:

Local EFA affiliates, who may have or know of programs in camping, social outings, and recreational groups.

Parks and recreation departments, many of which offer adapted programs.

Easter Seal Societies: This national organization also operates camping programs for people with disabilities. Check for local or state listings.

Service clubs, lodges, and religious groups can be checked for special programs.

This overview is not all-inclusive but it offers a vehicle for health care professionals to search for community resources on epilepsy in their locale.

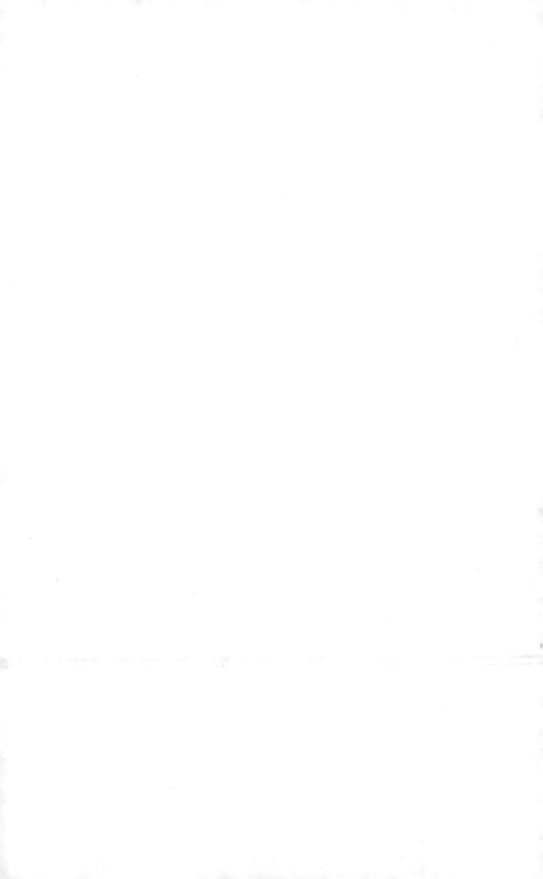

Managing Seizure Disorders: A Handbook for Health Care Professionals, edited by N. Santilli, Lippincott-Raven Publishers, Philadelphia, 1996.
© 1996 Epilepsy Foundation of America.

Appendix A

Psychosocial Nursing Diagnoses and Interventions in Epilepsy[1]

Judy Ozuna

This list of psychosocial nursing diagnoses is provided to assist in developing both short- and long-term health management plans. This list is designed as a reference. Plans of care must be individualized for each person.

I. Fear
   A. Next seizure
   B. Injury during seizure
   C. Prejudice/rejection
      1. History of epilepsy
      2. Societal values
   D. Death
   E. Brain damage
   F. Malformed or affected offspring
   G. Interventions
      1. Fear of the location of first seizure and where most seizures occur
         a. Support efforts to return or go to that location (e.g., school, bedroom)
         b. Explore positive reasons a seizure in that particular location is safe
         c. Make appropriate adjustments in environment when possible
      2. Fear of injury (from trauma, aspiration, drowning)
         a. Avoid precipitating factors
         b. Avoid dangerous activities
         c. Ensure compliance
         d. Practice appropriate first aid
      3. Fear of prejudice/rejection
         a. Assess personal, family, school, work, community attitudes
         b. Educate about epilepsy
         c. Counsel about attitudes

---

[1] Adapted from Santilli N, Dodson WE, Walton AV. *Students with seizures: a manual for school nurses.* Landover, MD: Epilepsy Foundation of America, 1991.

      4. Fear of death
        a. Assess source of fear
        b. Compare death rates for general population with those for people with epilepsy
        c. Reinforce healthy fear of injury during seizure
      5. Fear of brain damage
        a. Review present abilities
        b. Provide information re: seizures and effect on brain
        c. Introduce to others who have seizures (refer to self-help or parent group)
      6. Fear of affected offspring
        a. Recommend good pre-pregnancy counseling
        b. Refer to genetic counselor

II. Ineffective Coping/Denial
  A. No correlation to type/frequency of seizures
  B. Manifestations
    1. Poor compliance
    2. Continuing dangerous activities
    3. Concealing or lying about diagnosis
  C. Interventions
    1. Assess feelings
    2. Correct misconceptions
    3. Counsel
    4. Refer to school and/or community resources
    5. Introduce to others with seizures, refer to self-help groups

III. Social Isolation
  A. Due to feared or actual rejection, medication side effects, school or vocational activity restrictions
  B. Interventions
    1. Assess cognitive function, personality, routine, behavior
    2. Establish individual goals
      a. Specific number of interactions
      b. Participation in novel activity
      c. Participation in own care
    3. Encourage group discussions/support groups
    4. Practice role playing
    5. Encourage participation in extracurricular and community activities

IV. Altered Role Performance
  A. Conflict based on discrepancy between desired and actual role
  B. Related to academic performance, job for teens, independence, activity restriction (athlete role may change), competitive employment, parenting

C. Interventions
    1. Offer counseling for person, family
    2. Refer to vocational counselor, social services, recreational therapy community service agencies (EFA)
V. Noncompliance with medication regimen
  A. Most common cause of poor seizure control
  B. Related to aspects of chronic illness
    1. To take medication regardless of presence of symptoms
    2. Change in lifestyle
    3. Drug side effects
    4. Denial, rebellion
    5. Forgetfulness
  C. Interventions
    1. Encourage physical and laboratory assessment to determine possible deviations
    2. Rule out other causes of low blood levels
      a. Drug interaction
      b. Altered drug metabolism (liver or kidney disease, pregnancy)
      c. Dose in relation to age (children, teenagers, elderly)
      d. Generic/trade drug substitution
    3. Assess
      a. Drug level
      b. Degree of compliance
      c. Reasons for poor compliance
        1. Forgetfulness
        2. Confusion about prescription
        3. Reluctance to take pills in front of others
        4. Attitude toward condition
        5. Family problems
        6. Poor social support
        7. Poor patient–provider interaction
        8. Denial
        9. Cost of medication
    4. Use Health Belief Model as patient education guide
    5. Teach strategies to enhance memory
      a. Use written instructions
      b. Keep calendar of medication doses
      c. Use Medi-set, pill boxes, multiple alarm watches
      d. Associate medication taking with daily activities
    6. Teach about medications
      a. Drug action
      b. Pharmacokinetics
      c. Side effects

         d. Dosing schedule

         e. Simplify regimen

     7. Increase supervision

         a. Provide feedback about drug levels

         b. Discuss seizures, medication taking habits

         c. Improve patient–provider relationship

     8. Other

         a. Provide clear, concise instructions

         b. Encourage natural social support systems

         c. Help person and family feel competent to manage his/her treatment regimen

         d. Refer to medical assistance programs which can decrease Rx cost

VI. Knowledge Deficit

   A. Involving: disease, diagnosis, first aid, medication, follow-up, self-care, legal restrictions, school, community resources

   B. Interventions

     1. Provide verbal/written information

     2. Show or lend EFA's Family Video Library series

     3. Inform about seizure type, use correct term

     4. Remind not to call ambulance for single seizure

     5. Inform about drugs, side effects, warn about abrupt withdrawal

     6. Remind about follow-up

     7. Inform about driving laws

VII. Memory Deficit

   A. Related to seizures, medications

   B. Ranges from mild to severe

   C. Interventions

     1. Assess patient, interview family

     2. Rule out drug toxicity, adjust drugs

     3. Keep written reminders

     4. Use consistent daily routine

VIII. Sexual Dysfunction

   A. Related to fear of, or frequency of, seizures, underlying neuropathology and/or neuropsychology, medication

   B. Intervention

     1. Obtain history

     2. Assess patient needs, feelings, attitude, mood, cultural values

     3. Correct misconceptions

     4. Identify precipitating factors

     5. Distinguish between problems of desire and performance

     6. Refer to appropriate medical and support services

BIBLIOGRAPHY

Beniak JA, Beniak TE. Social isolation. In: Snyder M, ed. *Care of the neurological patient: a nursing perspective.* New York: John Wiley and Sons, 1983:260–90.

Caveness WF, Gallup GH. A survey of public attitudes toward epilepsy in 1979 with an indication of trends over the past thirty years. *Epilepsia* 1980;21:509–18.

Devinsky O, Penry JK. Quality of life in epilepsy: a clinician's view. *Epilepsia* 1993;34(suppl 4): S4–7.

Green L, Roter D. The literature on patient compliance and implications for cost-effective patient education programs in epilepsy. In: *Plan for nationwide Action on epilepsy,* Vol II, Part I, Sections I–VI. Washington, DC: Commission for the Control of Epilepsy and Its Consequences, DHEW, 1977.

DiIorio C, Faherty B, Manteufell B. The development and testing of an instrument to measure self-efficacy in individuals with epilepsy. *J Neurosci Nurs* 1992;24:9–13.

DiIorio C, Faherty B, Manteufell B. Learning needs of persons with epilepsy: a comparison of perceptions of persons with epilepsy, nurses, and physicians. *J Neurosci Nurs* 1993;25:22–9.

Hartshorn JC, Byers VL. Impact of epilepsy on quality of life. *J Neurosci Nurs* 1992;24:24–9.

Harshorn JC, Byers VL. Importance of health and family variables related to quality of life in individuals with uncontrolled seizures. *J Neurosci Nurs* 1994;26:288–97.

Haynes RB. Determinants of compliance: the disease and the mechanics of treatment. In: Haynes RB, Taylor DW, Sackett DL, et al., eds. *Compliance in health care* Baltimore: Johns Hopkins University Press, 1979:49–62.

Haynes RB. Strategies to improve compliance with referral, appointments, and prescribed medical regimens. In: Haynes RB, Taylor DW, Sackett DL, et al., eds. *Compliance in health care.* Baltimore: Johns Hopkins University Press, 1979:121–43.

Hogue CC. Nursing and compliance. In: Haynes RB, Taylor DW, Sackett DL, et al., eds. *Compliance in health care,* Baltimore: Johns Hopkins University Press, 1979:247–59.

Lannon SL. Epilepsy in the elderly. *J Neurosci Nurs* 1993;25:273–82.

Loiseau P, Strube E, Broustet D, et al. Learning impairment in epileptic patients. *Epilepsia* 1983;24: 183–92.

Marston MV. Compliance with medical regimens: a review of the literature. *Nurs Res* 1970;19:313–23.

Mungus D, Ehlers C, Walton N, et al. Verbal learning differences in epileptic patients with left and right temporal lobe foci. *Epilepsia* 1985;26:340–5.

Morrell MJ. Sexual dysfunction in epilepsy. *Epilepsia* 1991;32(suppl 6):S38–45.

Ozuna J. Intermittent loss of arousal. In: Bronstein K, Stewart-Amedei C, Kunkel J, et al., eds. *AANN's neuroscience nursing text,* 2nd edition. Philadelphia: W.B. Saunders (in press).

Ozuna J, Cammermeyer M. Learning needs of the epilepsy patient. In: VanMeter MJ, ed. *Neurologic care: a guide for patient education.* New York: Appleton-Century-Crofts, 1982:133–50.

Pellock JM. Standard approach to antiepileptic drug treatment in the United States. *Epilepsia* 1994;35(suppl 4):S11–18.

Sackett D. A compliance practicum for the busy practitioner, In: Haynes RB, Taylor DW, Sackett DL, et al., eds. *Compliance in health care.* Baltimore: Johns Hopkins University Press, 1979:286–94.

Sackett D. Why don't patients take their medicine? *Can Fam Physician* 1977;23:452–64.

Shope JT. The patient's perspective. In: Black RB, Hermann BP, Shope JT, eds. *Nursing management of epilepsy.* Rockville, MD: Aspen Systems Corporation, 1982:54–5.

Snyder M. Effect of relaxation on psychosocial functioning in persons with epilepsy. *J Neurosurg Nurs* 1983;15:250–4.

Appendix B
Plans of Care (for Inpatients)

Judy Ozuna

Care of Patient with Epilepsy (General)

Nursing diagnosis	Outcome criteria	Nursing interventions	
Potential for injury R/T seizures Defining characteristics: Previous history of falls with seizure activity Antiepileptic drugs (AED's) in toxic range	Patient is free of injury from seizures. Patient complies with unit safety policies. Patient/family verbalize appropriate safety measures prior to discharge.	Allow patient, if approved by RN, to participate in off-unit recreational activities 24 h after admission. Assess seizure frequency upon admission and initiate Safety Precautions. –Allow tub-bath or shower only with staff member or significant other in attendance; maintain voice contact. –Place bed in low position, side rails up at nap and bedtime. –Place call light within easy reach of patient.	–Lock wheels on bed. –Keep furniture and equipment out of patient's pathway. –Have staff or significant other accompany patient when off the unit. If prone to falls, continually assess need for protective head gear, face mask, wheel chair and/or elbow and knee pads.
Alteration in home maintenance management R/T seizures	Patient/family state components of discharge plans.	Provide patient with medic alert information and ID jewelry. Continually assess patient's discharge needs.	Review first aid and safety/precautions for seizures Emphasize need for regular medical follow-up

continued

Appendix B (Continued)

Nursing diagnosis	Outcome criteria	Nursing interventions
Knowledge deficit of epilepsy R/T lack of information	Patient/family verbalize understanding of basic anatomy, physiology and pathology associated with seizure type	Review with patient/family and document AED therapy –Name, dosage and time of AEDs –Most common side effects –Possibility of drug interactions –Risk of changing from trade name to generic AEDs Encourage maintenance of seizure calendar Review self-management guidelines –Avoidance of known seizure triggers –Moderation in alcohol consumption –Adequate rest and exercise –Appropriate management of stress –Avoidance of hazardous activities –Compliance with driving restrictions –Use of social and vocational resources
	Patient/family verbalize understanding of first aid and safety precautions for seizure type. Individualize teaching materials.	Assess patient/family's understanding of first aid and safety precautions for seizure type. Individualize teaching materials. Inform patient/family of available films and printed materials, contact: Epilepsy Foundation of America 1-800-EFA-1000
Knowledge deficit of AED therapy R/T lack of information	Patient/family verbalize accurate knowledge of AED therapy and potential adverse effects of medications.	Assess patient/family knowledge of AEDs Teach patient and family –Purpose of medication –Potential side effects –Importance of compliance with medication schedule and serum drug level monitoring –Risk of changing to generic from trade name medications Document patient/family level of understanding

Care of Patient with Absence Seizures

Nursing diagnosis	Outcome criteria	Nursing interventions
Sensory/perceptual alteration R/T absence seizures	Patient is free of injury from seizure. Patient/family verbalize/demonstrate first aid	Assess: –Frequency of seizures –History of injury R/T absence seizures If seizures occur: Document seizure: –Frequency –Duration –Level of consciousness

Nursing diagnosis	Outcome criteria	Nursing interventions	
	measures for absence seizures.	–Keep calm –Protect from injury –Continue to talk with patient and assess cognition –Assess seizure progression	–Body parts involved In postictal phase: –Provide emotional support –Inform patient of seizure –Allow resumption of routine activity –Continually assess clinical seizure activity

Care of Patient with Generalized Tonic-Clonic (GTC) and Tonic Seizures

Nursing diagnosis	Outcome criteria	Nursing interventions	
Potential for injury R/T GTC or tonic seizure	Patient is free of injury from seizure. Patient/family verbalize/demonstrate first aid measures for GTC or tonic seizures.	Assess: –Frequency of seizures –History of injury seizures –Need for protective head gear, face mask, wheel chair, and/or elbow and knee pads If seizure occurs: –Keep calm –Protect from injury –Do not put anything in mouth (unless airway is needed) –Remove harmful objects –Loosen tight clothing –Stay with patient until seizure ends –Do not offer food, drink, or medications –Allow patient to rest/sleep after seizure –Reassure, support patient when consciousness returns If seizure occurs when patient in wheel chair: –Support body by standing behind chair, slipping arms under patient's arms	–Support patient's chin in neutral position to facilitate breathing –Place patient in side-lying position in bed after seizure stops Document: –Precipitating factors, if known –Prodrome or aura, if any –Level of consciousness –Vital signs –Pupillary reaction –Motor response –Incontinence –Nature of body movements –Head and/or eye deviation –Skin color change –Distortion of facial features –Duration of ictal phase –Duration of unresponsiveness to verbal and/or physical stimuli

continued

Appendix B (*Continued*)

Care of Patient with Complex Partial Seizures

Nursing Diagnosis	Outcome criteria	Nursing interventions	
Sensory/perceptual alteration R/T complex partial seizures	Patient is free of injury from a seizure. Patient/family verbalize or demonstrate correct first aid measures for complex partial seizures.	Assess: –Frequency of complex seizures –History of injury related to complex partial seizures –Need for protective head gear, face mask, wheelchair, and/or elbow and knee pads If seizures occur: –Keep calm –Remove harmful objects from patient's path –Do not restrain the patient's movements (unless in danger) but follow them if they wander about –Stay with person during and after the seizure as he/she may be confused for a period of time –Do not offer any food, drink or medications –Let patient rest and/or sleep afterwards –Be reassuring and supportive after the confusional state is over Assess neurologic function during a seizure –Level of consciousness –Cognitive function –Vital signs –Pupillary reaction –Automatisms	Document seizure Prodrome or aura: –Note subjective symptoms before seizure began Active phase: –Describe automatisms –Note length of active phase Postictal phase: –Note duration of confusional state Recovery phase: –Note time of return to baseline neurologic state

266

Managing Seizure Disorders: A Handbook for Health Care Professionals, edited by N. Santilli, Lippincott-Raven Publishers, Philadelphia, 1996. © 1996 Epilepsy Foundation of America.

Appendix C

Seizure Recognition and First Aid

Seizure type	What it looks like	What it is not	What to do	What not to do
Generalized tonic–clonic (also called grand mal)	Sudden cry, fall, rigidity, followed by muscle jerks, shallow breathing or temporarily suspended breathing, bluish skin, possible loss of bladder or bowel control, usually lasts a couple of minutes. Normal breathing then starts again. There may be some confusion and/or fatigue, followed by return to full consciousness.	Heart attack Stroke	Look for medical identification. Protect from nearby hazards. Loosen ties or shirt collars. Protect head from injury. Turn on side to keep airway clear. Reassure when consciousness returns. If single seizure lasted less than 5 min, ask if hospital evaluation wanted. If multiple seizures, or if one seizure lasts longer than 5 min, call an ambulance. If person is pregnant, injured, or diabetic, call for aid at once.	Don't put any hard implement in the mouth. Don't try to hold tongue. It can't be swallowed. Don't try to give liquids during or just after seizure. Don't use artificial respiration unless breathing is absent after muscle jerks subside, or unless water has been inhaled. Don't restrain.
Absence (also called petit mal)	A blank stare, beginning and ending abruptly, lasting only a few seconds, most common in children. May be accompanied	Daydreaming Lack of attention Deliberate ignoring of adult instructions	No first aid necessary, but if this is the first observation of the seizure(s), medical evaluation should be recommended.	

continued

Appendix C (Continued)

Seizure type	What it looks like	What it is not	What to do	What not to do
	by rapid blinking, some chewing movements of the mouth. Child is unaware of what's going on during the seizure, but quickly returns to full awareness once it has stopped. May result in learning difficulties if not recognized and treated.			
Simple partial	Jerking may begin in one area of body, arm, leg, or face. Can't be stopped, but patient stays awake and aware. Jerking may proceed from one area of the body to another, and sometimes spreads to become a convulsive seizure.	Acting out, bizarre behavior	No first aid necessary unless seizure becomes convulsive, then first aid as above.	
	Partial sensory seizures may not be obvious to an onlooker. Patient experiences a distorted environment. May see or hear things that aren't there, may feel unexplained fear, sadness, anger, or joy. May have nausea, experience odd smells, and have a generally "funny" feeling in the stomach.	Hysteria Mental illness Psychosomatic illness Parapsychological or mystical experience	No immediate action needed other than reassurance and emotional support. Medical evaluation should be recommended.	
Complex partial (also called psychomotor or temporal lobe)	Usually starts with blank stare, followed by chewing, followed by random activity. Person appears unaware of	Drunkenness Intoxication on drugs Mental illness Disorderly conduct	Speak calmly and reassuringly to patient and others. Guide gently away from obvious hazards.	Don't grab hold unless sudden danger (such as a cliff edge or an approaching car) threatens.

Seizure type	Description	Differential	First aid
	surroundings, may seem dazed and mumble. Unresponsive. Actions clumsy, not directed. May pick at clothing, pick up objects, try to take clothes off. May run, appear afraid. May struggle or flail at restraint. Once pattern established, same set of actions usually occur with each seizure. Lasts a few minutes, but postseizure confusion can last substantially longer. No memory of what happened during seizure period.		Stay with person until completely aware of environment. Offer to help getting home. Don't try to restrain. Don't shout. Don't expect verbal instructions to be obeyed.
Atonic seizures (also called drop attacks)	A child or adult suddenly collapses and falls. After 10 seconds to a minute he recovers, regains consciousness, and can stand and walk again.	Clumsiness Normal childhood "stage" In a child, lack of good walking skills In an adult, drunkenness, acute illness	No first aid needed (unless he hurt himself as he fell), but the child should be given a thorough medical evaluation
Myoclonic seizures	Sudden brief, massive muscle jerks that may involve the whole body or parts of the body. May cause person to spill what they were holding or fall off a chair.	Clumsiness Poor coordination	No first aid needed, but should be given a thorough medical evaluation.

continued

Appendix C (*Continued*)

Seizure type	What it looks like	What it is not	What to do	What not to do
Infantile spasms	These are clusters of quick, sudden movements that start between 3 months and 2 years. If a child is sitting up, the head will fall forward, and the arms will flex forward. If lying down, the knees will be drawn up, with arms and head flexed forward as if the baby is reaching for support.	Normal movements of the baby Colic	No first aid, but doctors should be consulted.	

Managing Seizure Disorders: A Handbook for Health Care Professionals, edited by N. Santilli, Lippincott-Raven Publishers, Philadelphia, 1996.
© 1996 Epilepsy Foundation of America.

Appendix D

Epilepsy Foundation of America Resources and Materials

The Epilepsy Foundation of America (EFA) is the national organization that works for people affected by seizures through research, education, advocacy and service. EFA is governed by an all-volunteer board of directors and its programs are reviewed by a volunteer professional advisory board. The organization has its national office in Landover, Maryland, a suburb of Washington, D.C. It is represented in 125 communities nationwide by more than 75 local organization affiliated with EFA. To contact an EFA affiliate, look under "Epilepsy" in the local telephone directory or call EFA's toll-free information service (1-800-EFA-1000). EFA's Internet address is: postmaster@efa.org.

The following programs conducted by the Epilepsy Foundation of America may be of particular interest to health professionals:

NATIONAL PROGRAMS

The national office of EFA conducts national programs and produces program materials that can be used at the local level to provide local services. Major national programs include the following.

Research to develop better treatments, new drugs, and to find a cure.

Information and education to improve public understanding of epilepsy through mass media campaigns and educational materials.

Advocacy to fight discrimination and support independent living. Volunteers and staff monitor government actions affecting people with epilepsy and work to remove inequities and barriers affecting people with epilepsy.

Membership through which individuals receive a free subscription to EpilepsyUSA, the Foundation's national newspaper, as well as access to other benefits. Membership in EFA is open to all.

Employment programs to increase and enhance the employment of persons with epilepsy. The programs aid people with epilepsy to find and keep competitive work. They have helped thousands of people find jobs.

A *National Epilepsy Library* provides authoritative information to professionals and to the public. The Library maintains its own database of articles on the clinical and psychosocial aspects of epilepsy and has computer access to major collections of medical information.

Toll-free access to information about epilepsy for patients, parents, and the public (1-800-EFA-1000).

A *Parent and Family Network* to bring families together for mutual support.

LOCAL PROGRAMS

The state and local affiliates of EFA provide and obtain needed services to meet the needs of people with epilepsy in the community. Local programs may include the following.

Information and referral services to help families get the help they need.

School Alert programs to improve the school environment for the child with epilepsy.

Support groups for people with epilepsy or their parents in which they can share common experiences and solve individual problems through discussion and mutual support.

Camping programs for youngsters with epilepsy.

Community education especially during November (National Epilepsy Month).

Professional education through conferences for local physicians, nurses and other health care professionals.

Community residences for people with epilepsy who need additional help to live independently.

Counseling for people with epilepsy and their families.

Advocacy for those who are being discriminated against on the basis of epilepsy.

Job finding and employer education programs.

Respite care for children and adults with severe epilepsy.

SELECTED PRINTED AND AUDIOVISUAL MATERIALS

New materials from the EFA are being developed on an ongoing basis. A current catalog, titled Videos, Pamphlets, Posters & Books, of all available EFA materials may be obtained from the EFA Catalog Sales Department. Their toll-free phone number is 1-800-213-5821. EFA members receive a discount on selected items.

Books and Monographs

Children with Epilepsy: A Parent's Guide
This book familiarizes parents with therapy, coping skills and some of the special issues that arise when a child has severe seizures. (314-page softcover book)

Epilepsy: Frequency, Causes and Consequences

This definitive statistical study addresses the causes, incidence, prevalence, natural history, risk factors, and prognosis of epilepsy in specific populations and its impact on the individual and community. (378-page hardcover book)

Facts About Epilepsy

This pamphlet provides a synopsis of the book *Epilepsy: Frequency, Causes and Consequences.* (16-page softcover booklet)

Guide to Understanding and Living with Epilepsy

Easy-to-understand resource for people with epilepsy and their families. Covers a wide range of medical, social, and legal issues. (345-page softcover book)

How to Recognize and Classify Seizures and Epilepsy

Discusses the causes of seizures and epilepsy, the classification of epileptic seizures and epileptic syndromes, seizure types, electroencephalography, and treatment. A companion video of the same name is also available. (21-page monograph)

Living Well with Epilepsy

Encourages people with epilepsy to take charge of their lives and try new experiences to enrich existence. (166-page softcover book)

Seizure Recognition and Observation: A Guide for Allied Health Professionals

Aids allied health professionals in observing, recording, and reporting seizure behavior to the physician. A companion piece to the video and monograph titled *"How to Recognize and Classify Seizures and Epilepsy."* (12-page monograph)

Students With Seizures: A Manual for School Nurses

Designed for use by the school nurse with the purpose of creating a more accepting and understanding school environment for children with seizure disorders. (131-page manual)

The Americans With Disabilities Act: A Guide to Provisions Affecting Persons With Seizure Disorders

Focuses on the employment provisions of the ADA, and helps to explain essential terms in relation to epilepsy such as: reasonable accommodation, essential job functions, and who is eligible under this act. (46-page manual)

The Comprehensive Clinical Management of the Epilepsies

Focusing on the parallel and interdependent process of diagnosis, treatment, and followup, this monograph discusses the clinical aspects of epilepsy management, highlighting the importance of utilizing a complete team of epilepsy service providers. A companion video of the same name is also available. (32-page monograph)

The Legal Rights of Persons with Epilepsy

An in-depth overview of the many important issues which persons with epilepsy, their families and advocates may face. (124-page softcover book)

Parents, Family and Caregiver Resource Materials

Answers to Your Questions About Epilepsy (32-page booklet)

Because You Are My Friend (16-page pamphlet)

Brothers and Sisters: A Discussion Guide for Families of Children With Epilepsy (95-page guide)

Epilepsy and Learning Disabilities (Fold-out reprint)

Epilepsy, Part of Your Life (26-page pamphlet)

Epilepsy: You and Your Child (30-page pamphlet)

Epilepsy: You and Your Treatment (14-page pamphlet)

Epilepsy: Questions and Answers (18-page pamphlet)

Finding Out About Seizures: A Guide to Medical Tests (Fold-out pamphlet)

Issues and Answers: A Guide for Parents of Teens and Young Adults With Epilepsy (110-page guide)

Issues and Answers: Exploring Your Possibilities--A Guide for Teens and Young Adults with Epilepsy (110-page guide)

Issues and Answers: Guide for Parents of Children with Seizures, Birth to Age Six (105-page guide)

Issues and Answers: Guide for Parents of Children with Seizures, Ages Six to Twelve (102-page guide)

Me and My World Packet for Children (pamphlets)

Medical Aspects About Epilepsy (6-page reprint)

Medicines for Epilepsy (14-page pamphlet)

Parent and Family Network Resource Materials (3-ring binder)

Parenting and You: A Guide for Parents with Seizure Disorders (130-page guide)

Preventing Epilepsy (16-page pamphlet)

Recognizing the Hidden Signs of Childhood Seizures (fold-out pamphlet)

School Planning: A Guide for Parents of Children with Seizure Disorders (125-page guide)

Seizure Recognition and First Aid (Fold-out pamphlet and poster)

"Speaking Out" Series: Partners in Advocacy-Understanding the Process; Partners in Advocacy-Tools & Resources; Partners in Advocacy-Family Action Guide (set of 3 guides)

Spider-Man Battles the Myth Monster (16-page comic book)

Surgery for Epilepsy (12-page pamphlet)

Talking to Your Doctor About Seizure Disorders (fold-out pamphlet)

The Child With Epilepsy at Camp (14-page pamphlet)

Time Out for Families: Epilepsy and Respite Care (66-page guide)

What Everyone Should Know About Epilepsy (16-page booklet)

Videos

Comprehensive Clinical Management of the Epilepsies
Illustrations through narration and demonstration of the multidisciplinary approach to the treatment of the epilepsies. Several different seizure types and their attending psychosocial problems are presented with suggested comprehensive treatment approaches. A companion monograph of the same title is also available. (17-min VHS videocassette)

Epilepsy In Children: A Primary Care Perspective
Contains footage of actual seizures to illustrate diagnosis, how to recognize and differentiate between seizure types in children; and an initial approach to pediatricians and other medical personnel. (22-min VHS videocassette)

Epilepsy Is—Program I (Ages 5-12)
Epilepsy Is—Program II (Ages 12-adult)
Curriculum aid to help teachers explain epilepsy to students. Examines common seizure types through interviews with children and young adults with epilepsy. Reviews first aid for epilepsy and why the support of friends is important. (11-min videotape; 14-minute videotape)

Epilepsy: Quality of Life
Includes a panel discussion between experts, patients, and family members. (41-min VHS videocassette)

How to Recognize and Classify Seizures and Epilepsy
Contains actual footage depicting six seizure types. A companion monograph of the same title is also available. (25-min VHS videocassette)

Meeting the Challenge—Employment Issues and Epilepsy
This video answers the questions most often asked by employers and covers a multitude of employment issues. (9-min videocassette)

Seizure Disorders and the School I (Elementary School Personnel)
Seizure Disorders and the School II (Secondary School Personnel)
A tool for teaching teachers and other school personnel about epilepsy; the videotapes address fears and concerns school personnel may have about epilepsy, review how epilepsy may affect learning, and discuss how the teacher can make the school experience a positive one. (14-min VHS videocassettes)

Seizure First Aid

Combines footage of real seizures with reenactments to demonstrate proper first aid procedures. (10-min VHS videocassette)

Seizures in Later Life

This video addresses issues that older people face when they have epilepsy. (14-min VHS videocassette)

Understanding Complex Partial Seizures

Describes symptoms and experiences of simple and complex partial seizures. (12-min VHS videocassette)

Voices from the Workplace

Individuals with epilepsy describe personal and social challenges in the workplace. Ideal for employers, co-workers and the public. (14-min VHS videocassette)

And Life Goes On: Severe Seizures of Early Childhood

Three sets of parents discuss the feelings, the changes they have made in their home lives, and resources that can help families to cope when a child has a severe seizure disorder. (16-min videocassette)

A Question of Epilepsy

Individuals and families discuss how epilepsy has affected their lives; what they felt when they learned about epilepsy, how they learned to cope, what adjustments they have made. (25-min videocassette)

Epilepsy: The Child and the Family

Upbeat introductory video that answers common questions of parents and families. (Slides on tape with narration, 14-min videocassette, English or Spanish)

Family Video Library Series

Includes 12 videotapes which address a range of subjects to help patients, parents, and family members gain a better understanding and appreciation of the condition and the adjustments needed to achieve a satisfying lifestyle. All videotapes in the series are available in closed captioned formats.